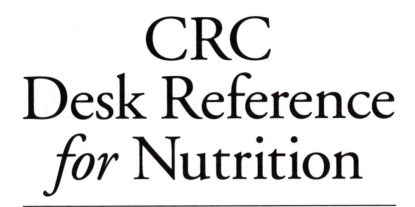

CRC
Desk Reference
for Nutrition

Third Edition

CRC
Desk Reference
for Nutrition

Third Edition

Carolyn D. Berdanier

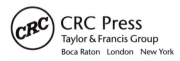
CRC Press
Taylor & Francis Group
Boca Raton   London   New York

CRC Press is an imprint of the
Taylor & Francis Group, an **informa** business

CRC Press
Taylor & Francis Group
6000 Broken Sound Parkway NW, Suite 300
Boca Raton, FL 33487-2742

© 2011 by Taylor & Francis Group, LLC
CRC Press is an imprint of Taylor & Francis Group, an Informa business

No claim to original U.S. Government works

Printed in the United States of America on acid-free paper
Version Date: 20110511

International Standard Book Number: 978-1-4398-4844-9 (Hardback)

Visit the Taylor & Francis Web site at
http://www.taylorandfrancis.com

and the CRC Press Web site at
http://www.crcpress.com

$ 99.\frac{95}{xx}

REF/613.203/BER/3rd Ed.

Contents

List of Figures

List of Tables

List of Longer Topics

Preface to the Third Edition

As in the previous editions of this *CRC Desk Reference for Nutrition*, terms of interest to the nutritionist are listed alphabetically. Included are medical terms, food science terms, metabolic terms, physiologic terms, drug terms, biotechnology terms, and nutrition terms. Since nutrition and foods are integrated sciences, not all of these terms will be useful to all readers. However, there should be a large number of terms useful to many readers. The third edition provides many more terms than were provided in the earlier editions. There have been some notable changes and inclusions that hopefully will make this edition more useful than the earlier ones. A web address has been included to give the reader access to the extensive tables of food composition maintained by USDA. In addition, a web address for dietary reference intakes (DRIs) has been included to again provide the most current recommendations for nutrient intakes. These recommendations are in a state of flux. As the information base expands with respect to nutrient use and need, the DRIs are changed to reflect this newer knowledge. The recommended dietary allowance (RDA) table found in the first edition has been omitted, as have the many tables of food composition.

Included in this edition are the many drugs that are used to manage nutrition-related conditions. Cardiovascular disease, diabetes, hypertension, obesity, and so forth are diseases that, while incurable, are manageable. Many medical conditions have a nutrient component to their development as well as a genetic component, and the major ones are described. Some of the rare genetic diseases relevant to nutrition and metabolism are also listed. Many drugs used in the management of chronic disease are of interest to the nutritionist, so these drugs are listed. Some may have an impact on the nutritional well being of the individual. Dietitians helping their clients with their food choices may wish to know what drugs their clients are taking. The drugs included in this book are listed as generic compounds along with their trade names. Not all drugs have been included. Omitted are the drugs used to manage mental illness, drugs used as anticancer medications, anti-AIDS drugs, and drugs used for Parkinson's, Alzheimer's, and other diseases. Of course, as new drugs are constantly entering the prescription world, this current list may not include them.

It is hoped that you, the reader, will find this book an essential addition to your library.

About the Author

Carolyn D. Berdanier, PhD, is a professor emerita of nutrition at the University of Georgia in Athens, Georgia. She earned her BS degree from the Pennsylvania State University and MS and PhD from Rutgers University. After a postdoctoral fellowship year with Dr. Paul Griminger at Rutgers, she served as a research nutritionist at the USDA Human Nutrition Institute in Beltsville, Maryland. At the same time, she also served as an assistant professor of nutrition at the University of Maryland. Following these appointments, she moved to the University of Nebraska, College of Medicine, and then in 1977, she joined the University of Georgia where she served as department head of foods and nutrition, for 11 years. She stepped down from this position to resume full-time research and teaching with a special interest in diabetes. Her research has been funded by a variety of funding agencies.

Dr. Berdanier has authored more than 150 research articles, contributed 40 chapters to multiauthored books, prepared 45 invited reviews for scientific journals, and edited, coauthored, or authored 17 books. She has served on the editorial boards of the *FASEB Journal,* the *Journal of Nutrition, Biochemistry Archives, Nutrition Research*, and the *International Journal of Diabetes Research.* She serves as an ad hoc reviewer for articles in her specialty for a wide variety of scientific journals.

Acknowledgments for the Third Edition

The author would like to express her appreciation to the contributors of the first edition, Anne Datillo, Wilhelmine P.H.G. Verboeket-van de Venne, and Toni Adkins White. Some of their contributions have been reused in this third edition. Appreciation is also extended to her husband, Reese, who put up with the many hours at the computer preparing this third edition. His patience and support are much appreciated. Lastly, this third edition would not have been possible without the encouragement and support of Randy Brehm, her gracious editor at Taylor & Francis.

How to Use This Book

Terms of importance to nutritionists, dietitians, and clinicians are listed alphabetically. Cross-referencing is used when more than one term is used for the same definition. Two appendices are in the back of the book. One contains general information about meal planning and food selection and the other provides a variety of metabolic maps. These maps are general in nature and lack the considerable detail found in detailed books on biochemistry. They are in the appendix to provide a general idea of the pathways involved in the important metabolic systems of interest to the nutritionist. Because the terms are listed in alphabetical order, there is no index.

A

ABCESS

A circumscribed collection of pus.

ABETALIPOPROTEINEMIA

One of the lipoprotein disorders. (See Lipoproteins.) The characteristic lack of apoB lipoprotein is due to a mutation in the gene for a microsomal triglyceride transfer protein that is essential for apoB lipoprotein translocation to the surface of the enterocyte and subsequent synthesis of the intestinal chylomicrons. This is a rare disorder inherited as an autosomal recessive trait. It is characterized by a complete lack of apoB-containing lipoproteins. It is associated with the clinical symptoms of lipid malabsorption, acanthocytes, retinitis pigmentosa, and myoneuropathy. In addition, clinical signs of fat-soluble vitamin deficiency may appear due to inadequate absorption of these vitamins.

ABNORMAL APPETITE (PICA)

Habitual consumption of items of no nutritional value. In some cases, the item in question will have a deleterious effect on the person's health. The habit is called pica, after the Latin word for magpie. Many different items are consumed; however, the most common are clay (geophagia), laundry starch (amylophagia), and ice (pagophagia). Pregnant women and children are the most frequently affected, and black women are three to four times more affected than white women of the same socioeconomic group.

ABSORPTION

Nutrients in the diet are absorbed by cells lining the gastrointestinal tract (enterocytes) by one of three mechanisms: (1) active transport, (2) facilitated diffusion, and (3) passive diffusion. The absorption of both micro- and macronutrients is described as separate entries.

Mechanisms for nutrient transport into the enterocyte:

1. Active transport: A process that moves essential nutrients against a concentration gradient and requires energy (usually from ATP) and a nutrient carrier. Many carriers are specific for specific nutrients. Many of the essential nutrients are actively transported. The exceptions are the minerals and the essential fatty acids. The minerals are absorbed by processes that involve either passive diffusion and/or carrier-mediated transport.
2. Passive diffusion: Movement of compounds across the cell membrane so as to equalize the concentration of these compounds on both sides of the membrane. This process applies to water, some electrolytes, small sugars, and small, nonessential amino acids. Essential fatty acids diffuse across the lipid portions of the membranes.
3. Facilitated diffusion: Movement of nutrients against a concentration gradient. It usually requires a carrier but may not require energy.

Amino Acid Absorption

Although single amino acids are liberated in the intestinal contents, there is insufficient power in the digestive enzymes to render all of the amino acids singly for absorption. Thus, the brush border of the absorptive cell absorbs not only the single amino acids but also di- and tripeptides. In the process of absorbing the peptides, the enterocytes hydrolyze them to their amino acid constituents. There is little evidence that peptides enter the blood stream. There are specific transport systems for each group of functionally similar amino acids. The carriers for the amino acids are listed in Table 1.

Most of the biologically important L-amino acids are transported by an active carrier system against a concentration gradient. This active transport involves the intracellular potassium ion and the extracellular sodium ion. As the amino acid is carried into the enterocyte, sodium also enters in exchange for potassium. This sodium must be returned (in exchange for potassium) to the extracellular medium, and this return uses the sodium-potassium ATP pump. In several instances, the carrier is a shared carrier. That is, the carrier will transport more than one amino acid. The mechanism whereby these carriers participate in amino acid absorption is similar to that described for glucose uptake.

Carbohydrate Absorption

Once the monosaccharides are released through the action of the carbohydrate-hydrolyzing enzymes, they are absorbed by one of several mechanisms. Glucose and galactose are absorbed by an energy-dependent, sodium-dependent, carrier-mediated active transport system. Because the transport is against a concentration gradient, energy is required to "push" the movement of glucose into the enterocyte. This transport is illustrated in Figure 1.

Glucose and galactose appear to compete for the same transport system. They also compete for a secondary transporter, a sodium-independent transporter (the mobile glucose transporter, GLUT 2), found in the basolateral surface of the enterocyte membrane. The two transporters differ in molecular weight. The sodium-dependent transporter has a molecular weight of 75 kDa while the sodium independent transporter weighs 57 kDa. The sodium-independent transporter is a member of a group of transporters called GLUT 1, 2, 3, or 4. Each of these transporters is specific to certain tissues. They are sometimes called mobile glucose transporters because when not in use they reside in the endoplasmic reticulum. Under the appropriate conditions, they move from the endoplasmic reticulum to plasma membrane, where they fuse with the plasma membrane, and bind glucose. Upon binding, the transporter and its associated glucose is released from the membrane. Through this mechanism, the glucose enters the absorptive cell.

TABLE 1
Carriers for Amino Acids

Carrier	Amino Acids Carried
1	Serine, threonine, alanine
2	Phenylalanine, tyrosine, methionine, valine, leucine, isoleucine
3	Proline, hydroxyproline
4	Taurine, β-alanine
5	Lysine, arginine, cysteine, cysteine
6	Aspartic and glutamic acids

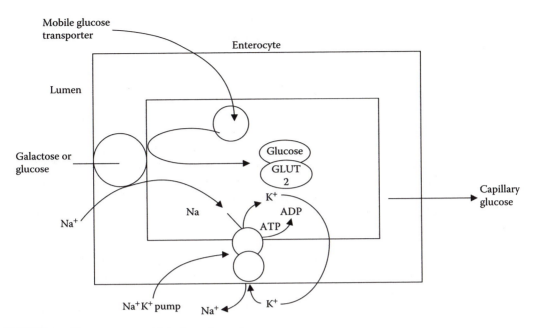

FIGURE 1 Glucose transport into the enterocyte.

Fructose is absorbed by facilitated diffusion. This process is independent of the sodium ion and is specific for fructose. In the enterocyte, much of the absorbed fructose is metabolized such that little fructose can be found in the portal blood even if the animal is given an intraluminal infusion of this sugar. On the other hand, an infusion of sucrose will sometimes result in measurable blood levels of fructose. This may be due to the location of sucrase (the enzyme that catalyzes the hydrolysis of sucrose to fructose and glucose) on the enterocyte. Rather than extending out into the lumen as do the other disaccharidases that are anchored to the enterocyte by a glycoprotein, sucrase is more intimately anchored. The sucrose molecule then is closely embraced by the enzyme, which in turn facilitates both the hydrolysis of sucrose and the subsequent transport of its constituent monosaccharides. Thus, both monosaccharides enter the enterocyte simultaneously. For the other monosaccharides present in the lumen, passive diffusion is the means for their entry into the enterocyte. Pentoses such as those found in plums or cherries, and other minor carbohydrates will find their way into the system only to be passed out of the body via the urine if the carbohydrate is not used.

CHOLESTEROL ABSORPTION

Only 30%–40% of the dietary cholesterol is absorbed; it is absorbed by diffusion with the other lipid components of the diet. Absorption requires the emulsification step with the bile acids as emulsifiers. Absorbed cholesterol passes into the lacteals and thence into the thoracic duct. The percent cholesterol absorbed depends on a number of factors including the fiber content of the diet, the gut passage time, and the total amount of cholesterol present for absorption. At higher intake levels less is absorbed, and vice versa at lower intake levels. Compared with fatty acids and the acylglycerides, the rate of cholesterol absorption is very slow. It is estimated that the half-life of cholesterol in the enterocyte is 12 hours. With high-fiber intakes, less cholesterol is absorbed because the fiber (cellulose and lignens) acts as an adsorbent, reducing cholesterol availability. These carbohydrates also shorten the residence time of the ingesta in the intestine. Thus, high-fiber diets reduce gut passage time, which in turn results in less time for cholesterol absorption. The mode of action of pectins and gums in lowering cholesterol absorption is different. These carbohydrates decrease transit time also, but rather than acting as adsorbents, they lower cholesterol absorption by creating a gel-like consistency of the chyme, rendering the cholesterol in the chyme less available for absorption.

GLYCERIDE (TRI-, DI-, AND MONOACYLGLYCERIDE) ABSORPTION

Before the glycerides can be absorbed they must be hydrolyzed to their component fatty acids and glycerol. The glycerol is absorbed into the portal blood stream while the fatty acids pass into the lacteals and thence into the thoracic duct. The hydrolysis begins in the mouth with the action of the lingual lipase. Although the action of lingual lipase is slow relative to lipases found in the duodenum, its action to release diacylglycerol and short-chain and medium-chain fatty acids serves another function: These fatty acids serve as surfactants. Surfactants spontaneously adsorb to the water-lipid interface, stabilizing emulsions as they form. Other dietary surfactants are the lecithins and the phospholipids. All together these surfactants plus the churning action of the stomach produce an emulsion, which is then expelled into the duodenum as chyme.

Once the chyme enters the duodenum, its entry stimulates the release of the gut hormones pancreozymin and cholecystokinin into the blood stream. Cholecystokinin stimulates the gall bladder to contract and release bile. Bile salts serve as emulsifying agents and serve to further disperse the lipid droplets at the lipid-aqueous interface, facilitating the hydrolysis of the glycerides by the pancreatic lipases. The bile salts impart a negative charge to the lipids, which in turn attracts the pancreatic enzyme, colipase.

Pancreozymin (secretin) stimulates the exocrine pancreas to release pancreatic juice, which contains three lipases (lipase, lipid esterase, and colipase). These lipases act at the water-lipid interface of the emulsion particles. One lipase acts on the fatty acids esterified at positions 1 and 3 of the glycerol backbone, leaving a fatty acid esterified at carbon 2. This 2-monoacylglyceride can isomerize, and the remaining fatty acid can move to either carbon 1 or 3. The pancreatic juice contains another less specific lipase (called a lipid esterase) that cleaves fatty acids from cholesterol esters, monoacylglycerides, or esters such as vitamin A ester. Its action requires the presence of the bile salts. The lipase that is specific for the ester linkage at carbons 1 and 3 of the triacylglycerols does not have a requirement for the bile salts and, in fact, is inhibited by them. The inhibition of pancreatic lipase by the bile salts is relieved by the third pancreatic enzyme, colipase. Colipase is a small protein that binds to both the water-lipid interface and to the lipase, thereby anchoring and activating it. The products of the lipase-catalyzed reaction, a reaction that favors the release of fatty acids having 10 or more carbons, are these fatty acids and monoacylglyceride. The products of the lipid esterase–catalyzed reaction are cholesterol, vitamins, fatty acids, and glycerol. Phospholipids present in food are attacked by phospholipases specific to each of the phospholipids. The pancreatic juice contains these lipases as prephospholipases that are activated by the enzyme trypsin.

As mentioned earlier in this definition, the release of bile from the gall bladder is essential to the digestion and absorption of dietary fat. Bile contains the bile acids, cholic acid and chenodeoxycholic acid. These are biological detergents or emulsifying agents. At physiological pH, these acids are present as anions, so they are frequently referred to as bile salts. They form aggregates with the fats at concentrations above 2–5 mM. These aggregates are called micelles. The micelles are much smaller in size than the emulsified lipid droplets. Micelle sizes vary depending on the ratio of lipids to bile acids but typically range from 40 to 600 Å. Micelles are structured such that the hydrophobic portions (triglycererols, cholesterol esters, etc.) are toward the center of the structure, whereas the hydrophilic portions (phospholipids, short-chain fatty acids, bile salts) surround this center. The micelles contain many different lipids. Mixed micelles have a disc-like shape in which the lipids form a bilayer and the bile acids occupy edge positions, rendering the edge of the disc hydrophilic. During the process of lipase and esterase digestion of the lipids in the chyme, the water-insoluble lipids are rendered miscible and transferred from the lipid emulsion of the chyme to the micelle. In turn, these micelles transfer the products of digestion (free fatty acids, glycerol, cholesterol, etc.) from the intestinal lumen to the surface of the epithelial cells where absorption takes place. The micellar fluid layer next to this cell surface is homogenous, yet the products of lipid digestion are presented to the cell surface, and these products are transported into the absorptive cell by passive diffusion. Thus, the degree to which dietary lipid is absorbed once digested depends largely on the amount of lipid to be absorbed relative to the amount of bile acid available to make the micelle. This, in turn, is dependent on the rate of bile acid synthesis by the liver and bile release by the gall bladder. Virtually all of the fatty acids, monoacylglycerides, and glycerol are passively absorbed by the enterocyte.

The fate of the absorbed fatty acids depends on chain length. Those fatty acids having 10 or fewer carbons are quickly passed into the portal blood stream without further modification. They are carried to the liver bound to albumin in concentrations varying between 0.1 and 2.0 µeq/mL. Those fatty acids remaining are bound to a fatty acid–binding protein and transported through the cytosol to the endoplasmic reticulum, whereupon they are converted to their CoA derivatives and re-esterified to glycerol or residual diacylglycerides or monoacylglycerides to re-form triacylglycerides. These re-formed triacylglycerides adhere to phospholipids and fat-transporting proteins that are members of the lipoprotein family of proteins. (See Lipoproteins.) This relatively large lipid-protein complex migrates to the Golgi complex in the basolateral basement membrane of the enterocyte. The lipid-rich vesicles fuse with the Golgi surface membrane, whereupon the lipid-protein complex is exocytosed or secreted into the intercellular space, which, in turn, drains into the lymphatic system. The lymphatic system contributes these lipids to the circulation as the thoracic duct enters the jugular vein prior to its entry into the heart.

AFTER GASTRIC RESECTION

When the stomach is fully or partially removed or bypassed, the individual loses storage capacity as well as the acidification of the ingested food. Gastric resection can also result in the loss of secretion of pepsin and vitamin B_{12} intrinsic factor. The loss of pepsin affects the digestibility of protein. Anemia due to the loss of the gastric intrinsic factor needed for the absorption of vitamin B_{12} can occur. With gastric resection, there is a loss of the churning/mixing function of this organ and this can result in a reduction of food digestibility. Patients who have undergone bypass surgery for weight loss (bariatric surgery) may have some of the same concerns with respect to protein digestion and vitamin B_{12} absorption.

AFTER INTESTINAL RESECTION

Depending on which section of the intestine is removed and how much of this section is lost, digestion and absorption can be reduced. If the resection involves the duodenum, a reduction in the absorption of glucose and amino acids as well as some of the minerals and vitamins may occur.

IN LACTOSE INTOLERANCE

Lactose must be hydrolyzed to glucose and galactose. These monosaccharides are then actively transported into the enterocyte. In the absence or graded loss of normal lactase activity, this hydrolysis does not occur fully and lactose can accumulate in the lumen of the intestine exerting an osmotic effect on the gut. Water diffuses into the lumen and increases the volume of the lumen contents. This, in turn, stimulates peristalsis and results in diarrhea. Some of the lactose is fermented by the gut flora and produces gas (flatulence) and discomfort. Some people experience these symptoms only when large amounts of lactose-containing foods are consumed; others are extremely sensitive to lactose presence and cannot tolerate any lactose in their diets.

IN GLUTEN-INDUCED ENTEROPATHY

Diarrhea, flatulence, and discomfort are the results of an inability to digest the grain protein, gluten. The undigested gluten remains in the intestinal tract, exerting an osmotic effect on the contents and surrounding tissues. Water is drawn into the tract, increasing the volume of the lumen contents. This stimulates peristalsis with the expulsion of watery stools. If undiagnosed and gluten is not removed from the diet, the absorptive cells are abraded from the lumen surface and the absorption of other nutrients is impaired.

MINERAL ABSORPTION

The essential minerals enter the absorptive cell by one of several mechanisms. Iron, copper, and zinc are absorbed via specific proteins that have an affinity for these minerals. The minerals are loosely bound and released to the body after absorption. These proteins can also serve as transport proteins for these minerals in the blood. Sodium and potassium enter (or are exchanged) by an ATPase specific for these ions. Chloride, iodide, and fluoride enter by way of an anion-cation exchange mechanism. Calcium uptake occurs via two mechanisms: (1) passive diffusion, and (2) via a vitamin D-dependent carrier (calbindinD_{9k}). Neither system is particularly efficient with between 20% and 50% of ingested calcium being absorbed. Absorption efficiency is related to the calcium content of the diet, the amount of phytate in the diet, the calcium status of the individual, and the presence of other diet ingredients that affect calcium availability and the acidity of the gut contents. Phosphorus is absorbed via an active, saturable, sodium-dependent mechanism that is facilitated by the vitamin D-dependent protein, calcitriol. Calcitriol also facilitates the absorption of calcium. Magnesium is absorbed by both passive and active transport. Neither system is very efficient. Absorption can vary between 30% and 70% of ingested mineral.

Many of the microminerals (iron, zinc, copper, selenium, iodine, fluorine, manganese, chromium, molybdenum, chromium, silicon, vanadium, nickel, and arsenic) are toxic if consumed in excess. The body absorbs these minerals very poorly so some protection against excess intake is provided by the gastrointestinal tract. Some of these minerals are absorbed via a carrier-mediated process. For iron, the protein is ferritin; for zinc, it is metallothionein. Copper absorption uses either albumin or transcuprein. Selenium is very efficiently absorbed from the gut on the very-low or low-density lipoproteins. Iodine and fluorine are absorbed via passive diffusion. The absorption of the other ultratrace minerals is not completely known.

VITAMIN ABSORPTION

Some of the vitamins are absorbed via active transport. The largest of the vitamins, vitamin B_{12}, requires a factor, called intrinsic factor produced in the stomach, for absorption. The fat-soluble vitamins are absorbed along with the fat component of the diet. Vitamin A requires a retinal-binding protein. Vitamin D requires a specific transport protein. Ascorbic acid is actively absorbed; the B vitamins are generally assumed to be passively absorbed.

ACANTHOCYTOSIS

A rare blood condition characterized by deformed red blood cells having irregular cell surfaces and pseudopod-like projections. These cells are very fragile.

ACARBOSE

A drug that inhibits α-glucosidase, an enzyme important to the digestion of starch. It can serve as an adjunct to metformin or insulin in the management of type 2 diabetes mellitus.

ACAT

Acetyl coenzyme A: cholesterol acyltransferase. An enzyme that catalyzes the formation of an ester linkage (–O–) between a fatty acid and cholesterol.

ACCEPTABLE DAILY INTAKE (ADI)

Estimation of the maximum allowable level of a food component or contaminant. These values serve as guides in health policy. For noncarcinogenic compounds, the ADI is derived from the no observed adverse effect level (NOAEL) determined in experimental animals. NOAEL is divided by safety factors (e.g., 10 for taking into account the extrapolation from animals to humans and 10 for taking into account a susceptible human subpopulation such as infants), resulting in an integral safety factor of 100. Factors considered in establishing the ADI are as follows:

- Biochemical studies, including absorption kinetics, distribution, excretion route, excretion rate, metabolic conversion, biological half-life, effect on enzymes, and other critical factors
- Toxicological studies, including carcinogenicity, mutagenicity, neurotoxicity, potentiation, and antagonism; and reproductive effects such as teratogenicity and acute and chronic toxic effects on either the progeny or mother, involving several species and multigenerational effects
- Epidemiological studies, including observations in occupational or accidental exposures
- Results of human volunteer studies

ACE INHIBITORS

Antihypertensive drugs. Compounds that inhibit the angiotensin-converting enzyme (ACE). This enzyme catalyzes the conversion of angiotensin I to angiotensin II. Angiotensin II stimulates water and sodium resorption and vasoconstriction. Through inhibition of this enzyme, both sodium and water are lost to a greater extent than without inhibition of the converting enzyme and blood pressure is reduced. Figure 2 illustrates the interacting roles of several hormones on water balance and blood pressure regulation. Drugs that act in this way are separate entries in this reference.

ACEBUTOLOL HYDROCHLORIDE

An antihypertensive drug that works as a beta blocker. This drug also has a use in regulating heart rhythm. Trade name: Sectral.

ACETALDEHYDE

An aldehyde formed from the oxidation of ethanol; it can be converted to acetate and thence to acetyl CoA.

ACETALDEHYDE DEHYDROGENASE

An enzyme that catalyzes the conversion of acetaldehyde to acetate.

ACETAMINOPHEN

An over the counter drug that reduces headache, fever, and inflammation. Trade names include Aspirin-Free Anacin, Tylenol, Apacet, and others.

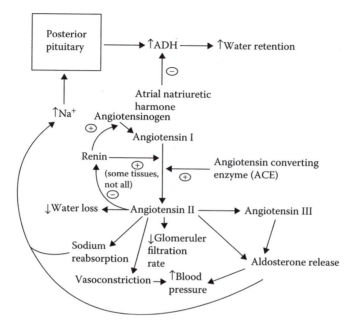

FIGURE 2   Hormones that affect water balance and blood pressure.

ACETOACETATE

A four-carbon compound found in large amounts in uncontrolled insulin-dependent diabetic patients. It is a normal end product of fatty acid oxidation and can be further metabolized and used as fuel by normal tissues. Its further metabolism yields carbon dioxide and water.

ACETONE

A three-carbon ketone found in normal tissues and blood. It can accumulate if the citric acid cycle is not working properly. Levels of acetone are high in the uncontrolled insulin-dependent diabetic patients and can be toxic.

ACETONEMIA

Higher than normal levels of acetone in the blood. Normal levels can be between 3 and 20 mg/mL. In the uncontrolled insulin-dependent diabetic individual, acetone levels can significantly exceed 20 mg/mL.

ACETONURIA

Higher than normal (1 mg/L/24 h) levels of acetone in the urine.

ACETYL CoA

A two-carbon metabolic intermediate that is the starting substrate for fatty acid synthesis. It is also the end product of fatty acid degradation (fatty acid oxidation). When joined to oxalacetate, acetyl CoA enters the citric acid cycle as citrate and the CoA portion of the molecule is removed for use in other reactions. (See Metabolic Maps, Appendix 2.)

ACETYLCHOLINE

A neurotransmitter released by a calcium-dependent process in response to the arrival of an action potential. Acetylcholine initiates changes in ion permeability that occur at the neuromuscular junction. Acetylcholine is hydrolyzed by acetylcholinesterase to choline, which is then reused.

ACETYLCHOLINESTERASE INHIBITORS

Natural toxins with alkaloids as active components. They have been detected in several edible fruits and vegetables such as potatoes, eggplant, and tomatoes. The most potent inhibitor is found in the potato. It is a glycoalkaloid, solanine. The solanine concentration in the potato varies with the degree of maturity at harvest, the rate of nitrogen fertilization, storage conditions, greening by exposure to light, and by variety. Commercial potatoes have a solanine content of 2–15 mg/100 g fresh weight. Greening of potatoes may increase the solanine content to 80–100 mg/100 g fresh weight. Most of the alkaloid is concentrated in the skin and potato sprouts. It is generally accepted that a solanine content of 20 mg/100 g fresh weight is the upper safe limit of consumption. Potatoes also can contain other glycoalkaloids (chaconine and tomatine) with properties similar to solanine. The symptoms seen in potato poisoning may be due to the combined effects of these alkaloids. Potato poisoning is a very rare event and would require the consumption of enormous quantities of potatoes.

ACHALASIA

Constriction or malfunction of muscles controlling peristalsis by the esophagus. Because the muscles do not readily relax in this condition and there is a loss in the synchrony of constriction and relaxation, ingested food does not readily pass into the stomach.

ACHLORHYDRIA

Absence of hydrochloric acid in the stomach either through gastric cell malfunction or through the surgical removal of the acid-producing cells in this organ. Iron absorption is impaired in this condition as is the conversion of pepsinogen to pepsin, a proteolytic enzyme important for protein digestion.

ACID-BASE BALANCE

Minute to minute regulation of the hydrogen ion concentration (pH) in the body; this is accomplished through the action of the bicarbonate buffering system, the phosphate buffering system, and the body proteins.

ACIDIC AMINO ACIDS

Amino acids having two carboxyl groups in their structures. These amino acids are aspartic and glutamic acids.

ACIDOSIS

When the blood pH falls below 7.4, acidosis develops. Metabolic acidosis refers to changes in the bicarbonate concentration in the blood; respiratory acidosis refers to changes in carbon dioxide pressure. Dehydration, uncontrolled insulin-dependent diabetes mellitus, low carbohydrate diets, cardiac failure, and pulmonary insufficiency can result in acidosis.

ACNE

Skin disease characterized by eruptions of infected sebaceous cells.

ACP (ACYL CARRIER PROTEIN)

A protein that has pantothenic acid as its prosthetic group. It is active in fatty acid synthesis as it carries the acyl groups that are bound to the CoA molecule in the multienzyme complex called fatty acid synthetase.

ACRODERMA ENTEROPATICA

A rare genetic disease characterized by an inability to absorb zinc.

ACROLEIN

An oxidation product of excessively heated fats and oils.

ACROMEGALY

A disease that results from excess growth hormone production and release from the anterior pituitary. It is characterized by coarsening of facial features through growth of the facial bones. Excess fatty acid mobilization and glucose intolerance are also observed. In the young, excess growth hormone production is characterized by gigantism. In the adult, it is termed acromegaly because the long bones are closed, making further growth impossible. In adults, treatment consists of removing the source of the excess growth hormone. Usually this is a tumor in the anterior pituitary.

ACTINOMYCIN D

An antibiotic containing D-amino acids.

ACTIVE SITE

A three-dimensional region of a catalyst, receptor, or carrier where the substrate binds prior to catalysis, binding, or transport.

ACTIVE TRANSPORT

See Absorption.

ACTIVITY INCREMENT

The energy needed to sustain body activities. The typical energy costs of a variety of activities are shown in Table 2.

ACTUARIAL DATA

Information used to create mortality tables and life expectancy numbers.

ACUTE RENAL FAILURE

Cessation of renal (kidney) function.

TABLE 2
Energy Cost of Activities Exclusive of Basal Metabolism and the Energy Cost of the Digestion of Food

Activity	kcal/kg/h	kJ/kg/hr
Bed making	3.0	12.6
Bicycling (century run)	7.6	31.9
Bicycling (moderate speed)	2.5	10.5
Boxing	11.4	47.9
Carpentry (heavy)	2.3	9.7
Cello playing	1.3	5.5
Cleaning windows	2.6	10.9
Crocheting	0.4	1.7
Dancing, moderately active	3.8	16
Dancing, rhumba	5.0	21
Dancing, waltz	3.0	12.6
Dishwashing	1.0	4.2
Dressing and undressing	0.7	2.9
Driving car	0.9	3.8
Eating	0.4	1.7
Exercise		
Very light	0.9	3.8
Light	1.4	5.6
Moderate	3.1	13
Severe	5.4	22.7
Very severe	7.6	31.9
Fencing	7.3	30.7
Football	6.8	28.6
Gardening, weeding	3.9	16.4
Golf	1.5	6.3
Horseback riding, walk	1.4	5.9
Horseback riding, trot	4.3	18.0
Horseback riding, gallop	6.7	28.0
Ironing (5-lb iron)	1.0	4.2
Knitting sweater	0.7	2.9
Laboratory work	2.1	8.8
Laundry, light	1.3	5.4
Lying still, awake	0.1	0.4
Office work, standing	0.6	2.5
Organ playing (1/3 handwork)	1.5	6.3
Painting furniture	1.5	6.3
Paring potatoes	0.6	2.5
Playing cards	0.5	2.1
Playing ping-pong	4.4	18.4
Piano playing (Mendelssohn's song without words)	0.8	3.3
Piano playing, mildly vigorous	1.4	5.9
Piano playing, strenuous	2.0	8.4
Reading aloud	0.4	1.7
Rowing	9.8	41.0
Rowing in race	16.0	66.9

(*Continued*)

TABLE 2 (*Continued*)
Energy Cost of Activities Exclusive of Basal Metabolism
and the Energy Cost of the Digestion of Food

Activity	kcal/kg/h	kJ/kg/hr
Running	7.0	29.3
Sawing wood	5.7	23.8
Sewing, hand	0.4	1.7
Sewing, foot-driven machine	0.6	2.5
Sewing, electric machine	0.4	1.7
Singing in loud voice	0.8	3.3
Sitting quietly	0.4	1.7
Skating	3.5	14.6
Skiing (moderate speed)	10.3	43.1
Standing at attention	0.6	2.5
Standing relaxed	0.5	2.1
Sweeping with broom	1.4	5.9
Sweeping with carpet sweeper	1.6	6.7
Vacuum cleaning	2.7	11.3
Swimming (2 mph)	7.9	33.1
Tailoring	0.9	3.8
Tennis	5.0	20.9
Typing, rapidly	1.0	4.2
Typing, electric typewriter	0.5	2.1
Violin playing	0.6	2.5
Walking (3 mph)	2.0	8.4
Walking rapidly (4 mph)	3.4	14.2
Walking, high speed (5.3 mph)	8.3	34.7
Washing floors	1.2	5.0
Writing	0.4	1.7

ACUTE TOXICITY

A potentially lethal condition caused by a very large intake of a substance that the body cannot metabolize or excrete.

ACUTE TUBULAR NECROSIS

Most common form of acute renal failure that results when an ischemic event or a nephrotoxin damages the renal tubules.

ACYLATION

The addition of an acyl group (carbon chain) to a substrate.

ACYLCARNITINE TRANSPORT SYSTEM

Essential for the oxidation of fatty acids in the mitochondria. The fatty acids are activated by conversion to their CoA thioesters. This activation requires ATP and the enzyme, acyl CoA synthase or thiokinase. There are several thiokinases, which differ with respect to their specificity for the different fatty acids. The activation step is dependent on the release of energy from ATP. Once the fatty acid is activated, it is bound to carnitine with the release of CoA. The acylcarnitine is then translocated through the mitochondrial membranes into the mitochondrial matrix via the carnitine–acylcarnitine translocase. As one molecule of acylcarnitine is passed into the matrix, one molecule of carnitine is translocated back to the cytosol and the acylcarnitine is converted back to acyl CoA. The acyl CoA can then enter the β-oxidation pathway. Without carnitine, the oxidation of fatty acids, especially the long-chain fatty acids, cannot proceed. Acyl CoA cannot traverse the membrane into the mitochondria and thus requires a translocase for its entry. The translocase requires carnitine.

AD LIBITUM

A Latin term meaning to eat freely or to have unrestricted access to food.

ADDISON'S DISEASE

A disease that is the result of insufficient production of the adrenal cortical hormones, notably, cortisol and aldosterone.

ADDITIVES

Substances added to food to enhance its flavor, texture, appearance, or keeping qualities. Terms used to describe these additives are listed in Table 3, and Table 4 gives a list of additives.

TABLE 3
Terms Used to Describe the Function of Food Additives

Terms

Anticaking agents, free flow agents
Antimicrobial agents
Antioxidants
Colors and coloring adjuncts
Curing and pickling agents
Dough strengtheners
Drying agents
Emulsifiers
Enzymes
Firming agents
Flavor enhancers
Flavor agents or adjuvants
Flour treating agents
Formulation aids
Fumigants
Humectants
Leavening agents
Lubricants and release agents
Nonnutritive sweeteners
Nutrient supplements
Nutritive sweeteners

(Continued)

TABLE 3 (*Continued*)
Terms Used to Describe the Function of Food Additives

Terms

Oxidizing and reducing agents

pH control agents

Processing aids

Propellents, aerating agents, gases

Sequestrants

Solvents, vehicles

Stabilizers and thickeners

Surface active agents

Surface finishing agents

Synergists

Texturizers

Note: These agents serve to improve the quality and shelf life of the products to which they are added during manufacture. The terms are self-explanatory. The agents on this list are Generally Recognized As Safe (GRAS) by the U.S. Food and Drug Agency (FDA).

TABLE 4
Common Additives and Their Functions in Food

Item	Function
Acetic acid	pH control; preservative
Adipic acid	pH control; sometimes a buffer and neutralizing agent as in confectionary manufacture
Ammonium alginate	Stabilizer and thickener; texturizer
Annatto	Color
Arabinogalactan	Stabilizer and thickener; texturizer
Ascorbic acid (vitamin C)	Nutrient; antioxidant; used to prevent rancidity
Aspartame	Nonnutritive sweetener especially in soft drinks
Azodicarbonamide	Flour bleaching agent; preservative
Benzoic acid	Preservative
Benzoyl peroxidide	Flour bleaching agent; may also be used in certain cheeses
Beta-apo-8′-carotenal	Color
BHA (butylated hydroxyanisole)	Antioxidant; preservative
BHT (butylated hydroxytoluene)	Antioxidant; preservative
Biotin	Nutrient
Calcium alginate	Stabilizer, thickener; texturizer
Calcium carbonate	Nutrient; mineral supplement
Calcium lactate	Preservative
Calcium phosphate	Leavening agent; sequestrant; nutrient
Calcium proprionate	Preservative
Calcium silicate	Anticaking agent
Canthaxanthin	Color
Caramel	Color
Carob bean gum	Stabilizer; thickener
Carrageenan	Emulsifier; stabilizer; thickener
Cellulose	Emulsifier; stabilizer; thickener
Citric acid	Preservative; antioxidant; pH control agent; sequestrant

TABLE 4 (*Continued*)
Common Additives and Their Functions in Food

Item	Function
Citrus red no. 2	Color
Cochineal	Color
Corn endosperm oil	Color
Cornstarch	Anticaking agent; drying agent; formulation aid; processing aid; surface finishing aid
Corn syrup	Flavoring agent; humectant; nutritive sweetner; preservative
Dextrose (glucose)	Flavoring agent; sweetner; humectant; preservative
Diglycerides	Emulsifiers
Dioctyl sodium sulfosuccinate	Emulsifier; processing aid; surfactant
Disodium guanylate	Flavor enhancer
Disodium inosinate	Flavor adjuvant
EDTA (ethylenediaminetetraacetic acid)	Antioxidant; sequestrant
FD & C colors (Blue # 1, Red # 40, Yellow # 5)	Color
Gelatin	Stabilizer and thickener; texturizer
Glycerine (glycerol)	Humectant
Grape skin extract	Color
Guar gum	Stabilizer, thickener, texturizer
Gum arabic	Stabilizer, thickener, texturizer
Gum ghatti	Stabilizer, thickener, texturizer
Hydrogen peroxide	Bleaching agent
Hydrolyzed plant protein	Flavor enhancer
Invert sugar	Humectant, nutritive sweetener
Iron	Nutrient
Iron ammonium citrate	Anticaking agent
Karraya gum	Stabilizer, thickener
Lactic acid	Preservative, pH control
Lecithin (phosphatidylcholine)	Emulsifier, surface active agent
Mannitol	Anticaking agent, nutritive sweetener; stabilizer, thickener, texturizer
Methylparaben	Preservative
Modified food starch	Drying agent, formulation aid, processing aid, finishing agent
Monoglycerides	Emulsifiers
MSG (monosodium glutamate)	Flavor enhancer
Papain	Texturizer, tenderizer
Paprika	Color, flavoring agent
Pectin	Stabilizer, thickener, texturizer
Phosphoric acid	pH control
Polyphosphates	Nutrient, flavor improvement, pH control
Polysorbates	Emulsifiers, surface active agents
Potassium alginate	Stabilizer, thickener, texturizer
Potassium bromide	Flour treatment
Potassium iodide	Nutrient
Potassium nitrite	Curing and pickling agent
Potassium sorbate	Preservative
Propionic acid	Preservative
Propyl gallate	Antioxidant, preservative
Propylene glycol	Emulsifier, humectant, stabilizer, thickener, texturizer
Propylparaben	Preservative
Saffron	Color, flavoring agent

(*Continued*)

TABLE 4 (*Continued*)
Common Additives and Their Functions in Food

Item	Function
Silicon dioxide	Anticaking agent
Sodium acetate	Preservative, pH control
Sodium alginate	Stabilizer, thickener, texturizer
Sodium aluminum sulfate	Leavening agent; pH control
Sodium benzoate	Preservative
Sodium bicarbonate	Leavening agent, pH control
Sodium chloride(salt)	Flavor enhancer, formulation aid, preservative
Sodium citrate	Curing and pickling agent, sequestrant, pH control
Sodium diacetate	Preservative, sequestrant
Sodium nitrate (Chile saltpeter)	Curing and pickling agent, preservative
Sodium nitrite	Curing and pickling agent, preservative
Sodium propionate	Preservative
Sorbic acid	Preservative
Sorbitan monostearate	Emulsifier, stabilizer, thickener
Sucrose	Nutritive sweetener, preservative
Tagetes (Aztec marigold)	Color
Tartaric acid	pH control
Titanium dioxide	Color
Tocopherols	Antioxidants, nutrient
Tragacanth gum	Stabilizer, thickener, texturizer
Turmeric	Color
Vanilla	Flavor
Vanillin	Flavor
Yellow prussiate	Anticaking agent

Source: Adapted from Ensminger et al. 1994. *Foods and Nutrition Encyclopedia.* 2nd ed., p. 13–18. Boca Raton FL: CRC Press. Many of the additives listed above are on the GRAS (Generally Regarded As Safe) list.

ADDITIVES: LEGAL DEFINITION

The U.S. Food and Drug Administration (FDA) defines food additives as follows:

> The intended use of which results or may reasonably be expected to result, directly or indirectly, either in their becoming a component of food or otherwise affecting the characteristics of food. A material used in the production of containers and packages is subject to the definition if it may reasonably be expected to become a component or to affect the characteristics, directly or indirectly, of the food packaged in the container. "Affecting the characteristics of food" does not include such physical effects as protecting contents of packages, preserving shape, and preventing moisture loss. If there is no migration of a packaging component from the package to the food, it does not become a component of the food and thus is not a food additive. A substance that does not become a component of food, but that is used, for example, in preparing an ingredient of the food to give a different flavor, texture, or other characteristic in the food, may be a food additive.

(Code of Federal Regulations, Title 21, Section 170.3; revised 4/1/78).

ADENINE

A purine base that is an essential component of the genetic material, DNA; when joined to ribose via a phosphate bond, adenine becomes adenylnucleotide or adenosine. It is also a component of the high-energy material, ATP (three phosphate groups), ADP (two phosphate groups), and AMP (one phosphate group).

ADENOSINE

See Adenine.

ADENYL CYCLASE

The enzyme responsible for the conversion of ATP to cyclic AMP, an important second messenger for hormones that stimulate catabolic processes.

ADENYLATE

See AMP (Adenosine Monophosphate).

ADH (ANTIDIURETIC HORMONE)

ADH, also called vasopressin, is synthesized by the supraoptic and paraventricular neurons of the posterior pituitary. The synthesis of ADH occurs in the ribosomes and proceeds via the formation of a macromolecular precursor or prohormone. This precursor or propressophysin has a molecular weight of about 20,000 Da. The prohormone contains several subunits, each of which has a biological function. One of these subunits, ADH, is preceded by a signal peptide. When the osmoreceptors located in the anterolateral hypothalamus perceive a change in the osmolarity of the blood (normal range: 275–290 mOsm/kg), this signal peptide is alerted and ADH is released. ADH binds to receptors in the glomerulus and renal convoluted tubules with the result that water is reabsorbed. The sensitivity of the system is affected by the physiological status of the individual. For example, the phase of the menstrual cycle in females affects the sensitivity to the action of ADH such that water balance (water retention) varies through the cycle.

The osmoregulatory mechanism is not equally sensitive to all plasma solutes. Sodium and its anions (which contribute roughly 95% of the osmotic pressure of the plasma) are the most potent solutes with respect to the stimulation of the osmoreceptors. Certain sugars such as sucrose and mannitol have been shown to stimulate these receptors in vitro, but these sugars do not normally appear in the plasma. Urea concentrations above 2 pg/mL stimulate ADH release, as does sustained hyperglycemia. Both uncontrolled diabetes and end stage renal disease are characterized by abnormal water balance. People with uncontrolled diabetes are polyuric (excess urine production) and very thirsty. In severe hyperglycemia, the solute load in the blood is increased. This triggers both thirst and ADH release. Both serve to dilute the excess solute load. The body then responds by increasing urine production and release. This excess urination gets rid of the excess solute and the excess consumed water. In principle, the same thing happens in the early phase of renal disease. In this instance, the solutes are not excreted because of the disease state of the kidney. ADH functions to retain water so as to dilute these solutes. In the end stage of this disease, the patients are thirsty and polyuric because their condition renders them less able to reabsorb water via the convoluted tubules. They may have the signals to release ADH, but the target tissue (the renal convoluted tubules) is not able to respond. Other stimuli for ADH release include emesis (vomiting), changes in blood volume or pressure, excessive sweating, hemorrhage, diarrhea, drugs that act as diuretics or that are antihypertensive agents, hyperinsulinemia, and other hormones related to water balance (i.e., angiotensin, renin, and aldosterone).

Infusion of epinephrine, acetylcholine, or other monoamines into the third ventricular cavity has been shown to elicit thirst and ADH release. These effects are due to their transmitter action at the various synapses in the ventricular cavity. In doing so, they act directly on the juxtaventricular receptors involved in the control of water balance (see Figure 2). Angiotensin II, norepinephrine, and prostaglandin E have all been found to elicit ADH release and thirst and, in addition, have been shown to activate the Na$^+$–K$^+$ ATPase in cerebral as well as other tissues. This activation relates Na$^+$ concentration to thirst (since Na$^+$ activates this ATPase), and this enzyme may be essential to receptor excitation. An inhibitor of transmembrane Na$^+$ transport, hydrochlorothiazide, markedly reduces drinking in sodium-loaded nephrectomized rats. Inhibition of drinking can also be shown with ouabain, an inhibitor of Na$^+$–K$^+$ ATPase, and with glycerol. Glycerol also suppresses the thirst induced by dehydration.

ADHESIONS

Fibrous bands of material that connect two surfaces that are normally separate.

ADIPOCYTES

Cells that store fat.

ADIPOSE TISSUE

Anatomical location of fat stores that can be raided in times of energy deficit. Adipose tissue also is an endocrine organ secreting a variety of bioactive factors including cytokines, inflammatory mediators, fatty acids, and adipokines such as leptin and adiponectin. Most of these act at both the local (autocrine/paracrine) and systemic (endocrine) levels. In addition to these efferent signals, adipose tissue also expresses various receptors (see Receptors) that allow it to respond to afferent signals from traditional hormone systems as well as from the central nervous system (CNS). Hormones such as insulin, glucagon, glucagon-like peptide (GLP-1), glucocorticoids, thyroid hormones, and catecholamines are active signals for adipose tissue.

ADIPSIA

Lack of thirst sensation.

ADIPSIN

Also known as complement factor D. It is a protein that is a member of the trypsin family of peptidases. It is a component of the alternative complement pathway best known for its role in the humoral suppression of inflammation by infectious agents. The protein is also a serine protease that is secreted by adipocytes into the bloodstream. It has a high level of expression in the fat pads and may play a role in the association of the inflammatory response associated with obesity.

ADOLESCENCE

The period of growth during which the transition between childhood and adulthood occurs.

ADP

Adenosine diphosphate; metabolite of ATP. Energy is released when ATP is split to ADP and inorganic phosphate (Pi).

ADRENAL GLAND

A bean- or pea-shaped gland attached to the superior surface of each kidney. It consists of an outer cortex and an inner portion, the medulla. The cortex releases cortisol, hydrocortisone, corticosterone (the glucocorticoids), aldosterone, and in some species, dehydroepiandrosterone (a steroid hormone intermediate). The medulla releases the catecholamines (epinephrine and norepinephrine) and the enkephalins. These hormones play a role in the fight or flight reaction or the sudden alarm response.

ADRENALCORTICAL HORMONES

Steroid hormones produced by the adrenal cortex.

ADRENOCORTICOTROPIN HORMONE (ACTH)

Hormone released by the anterior pituitary that stimulates the release of the adrenal cortical steroid hormones (cortisol, corticosteroid, hydrocortisone, dehydroepiandrosterone, and aldosterone). Its release, in turn, is stimulated by the corticotropin-releasing hormone (CRH) that is released by the hypothalamus.

ADSORB

To attract and retain substances on the surface. For example, dietary fiber can adsorb cholesterol and facilitate its excretion via the feces.

ADULT RESPIRATORY DISTRESS SYNDROME (ARDS)

Condition characterized by increased capillary permeability in the lung circulation resulting in noncardiogenic pulmonary edema.

ADVANCED CARDIAC LIFE SUPPORT (ACLS)

Advanced resuscitation techniques including airway management, arrhythmia detection, drug therapy, and defibrillation.

AEROBIC METABOLISM

Metabolic reactions that require oxygen.

AEROPHAGIA

The habit of swallowing air.

AFLATOXINS

Food contaminants produced by molds. The most important of these mold-produced contaminants are the aflatoxins, and these compounds can be toxic. They are produced by the molds *Aspergillus flavus* and *A. parasiticus*. They are derivatives of coumarin fused to either a cyclopentanone (B group) or a six-membered lactone (G group). Different types of aflatoxins include aflatoxin B_1, B_2 (dihydroderivative of B_1), G_1, G_2 (dihydroderivative of G_1), M_1 (metabolic product of B_1), and M_2 (metabolic product of B_2). In view of occurrence and toxicity, aflatoxin B_1 is the most important, followed by G_1, B_2, and G_2. Aflatoxins are heat stable and hard to transform to nontoxic products. They are produced in foods when the environmental conditions consist of relatively high humidity and temperatures. The toxicity of the aflatoxins involves hepatotoxicity. Factors affecting aflatoxin toxicity and carcinogenicity are as follows:

- Species (very susceptible: dog, duckling, guinea pig, neonatal rat, rabbit, turkey poult, rainbow trout; moderately susceptible: chicken, cow, ferret, hamster, mink, monkey, pheasant, pig, rat; very resistant: mouse, sheep)
- Gender (male animals more susceptible than female animals)

- Age (young animals more susceptible than mature animals)
- Nutritional status (animals fed diets deficient in protein, methionine, choline, or vitamin A more susceptible than animals fed sufficient diets)
- Other factors (cocarcinogenic compounds such as ethionine, cyclopenoid fatty acids, malvalic acid, sterculic acid; anticarcinogenic compounds such as urethane, diethylstilbestrol, phenobarbitol)

Foodstuffs most likely to become contaminated with aflatoxins are peanuts, tree nuts, cottonseed, corn, figs, and certain grasses. Human exposure can also occur through the consumption of milk or meat from contaminated animals. Prevention of aflatoxin contamination is achieved by discouraging fungal growth, particularly by adequate post harvest crop drying. Aflatoxin consumption has been associated with an inability to respond to oxytocin (dystocia), an inability to lactate, and certain forms of cancer.

AGAR

A food additive that is extracted from seaweed; it acts as a gelling agent. (See Table 4.)

AGARITINE

A member of a series of hydrazine derivatives occurring in mushrooms, including the common edible mushroom *Agaricus bisporus*.

AGE-ADJUSTED DEATH RATE

The number of deaths in a specific age group for a given calendar year divided by the population of that same age group and multiplied by 1000.

AGING

The processes involved from conception to death; an evolution of metabolic, endocrinological, and physiological change that occurs in the individual from inception through birth, childhood, adolescence, adulthood, and senescence. In the United States, the segment of the population over the age of 65 has grown rapidly.

AGONIST

A compound that enhances the activity of another compound in the body.

AGRANULOCYTOSIS

Considerable decrease in leukocytes resulting from depression of granulocytes formed in the bone marrow.

AIDS (ACQUIRED IMMUNE DEFICIENCY SYNDROME)

A disease that results when a specific virus (HIV) attacks elements of the immune system, rendering it unable to respond to incoming antigens or infective agents.

ALANINE

A nonessential amino acid. (See Table 5.) Alanine can be synthesized from pyruvate with an amino group donated by glutamate or aspartate.

ALANINE CYCLE

A cycle that plays an important role in maintaining blood glucose levels within the normal range (80–120 mg/dL, 4–6 mmol/L). The cycle uses alanine released by the muscle and deaminated by the liver to produce glucose via gluconeogenesis. This glucose is transported to the muscle where it is oxidized to pyruvate that in turn is converted back to alanine. The cycle is an important defense against hypoglycemia during starvation. The cycle is illustrated in Figure 3.

TABLE 5
Essential and Nonessential Amino Acids for Adult Mammals

Essential	Nonessential
Valine	Hydroxyproline
Leucine	Cysteine
Isoleucine	Glycine
Threonine	Alanine
Phenylalanine	Serine
Methionine	Proline
Tryptophan	Glutamic acid
Lysine	Aspartic acid
Histidine	Glutamine
[a]Arginine	Asparagine
[b]Taurine	Hydroxylysine
	Tyrosine

[a] Not essential for maintenance of most adult mammals.

[b] Felines require taurine, a metabolite of L-cysteine as a component of their diets.

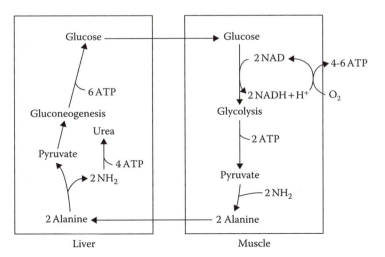

FIGURE 3   The alanine cycle.

ALAR

A plant growth regulator; chemical name: daminozide.

ALBINISM

A rare genetic disease characterized by the failure of the body to synthesize melanin (the pigment that gives skin its color). The disease is due to one or more mutations in the gene for tyrosine hydroxylase.

ALBUMIN

Small molecular weight protein found in blood and sometimes in urine. It is a single-chain globular protein consisting of 610 amino acids. It assists in the maintenance of the osmotic pressure of the intravascular spaces. It is also a major carrier for free fatty acids in the blood. Albumin found in the urine is considered an early warning sign of renal disease. Normally, it does not cross the renal cell membranes but is conserved by the glomerular cell.

ALBUMINURIA

Abnormal condition where albumin is found in the urine.

ALCAPTONURIA

A rare genetic disease in which homogentisic acid (a metabolite of phenylalanine and tyrosine) accumulates because of a mutation in the gene for homogentisic acid oxidase.

ALCOHOL

A hydrocarbon containing a hydroxyl group (–OH) attached to one of the carbons in the carbon chain. The most common alcohol in the diet is the two-carbon compound, ethanol, (CH_3CH_2OH). Excess addictive consumption is referred to as alcohol abuse or alcoholism. Ethanol is metabolized in the liver. The pathway for metabolism is shown in Figure 4.

ALCOHOL ABUSE AND CARDIOMYOPATHY

Although the precise cause of cardiomyopathy in alcoholism is unknown, alcohol abuse is the major cause of dilated cardiomyopathy, which leads to intractable congestive heart failure.

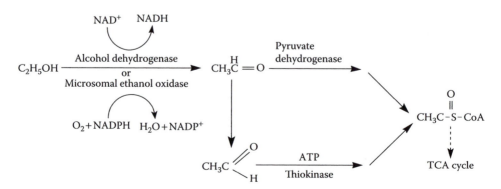

FIGURE 4   The metabolism of ethanol (alcohol) in the liver.

Alcohol Abuse and Diabetes Mellitus

Significant alcohol consumption (>2 ounces of alcohol/day) by people with diabetes has been associated with hypoglycemia. Alcohol decreases gluconeogenesis in the liver, and as a result, hypoglycemia can readily develop several hours after alcohol ingestion. If light to moderate quantities of alcohol (1–2 drinks) are consumed with a mixed meal, blood glucose is not adversely affected.

Alcohol Abuse and Gout

Hyperuricemia (excess uric acid in the blood) is positively correlated to alcohol intake in adult males. When significant quantities of alcohol are consumed, lactic acid accumulates that in turn inhibits the excretion of ureates. Ureate accumulation is a characteristic of gout. If the alcohol is consumed with a mixed meal there seems to be little effect on ureate accumulation.

Alcohol Abuse and Hyperlipidemia

Significant intakes of alcohol are associated with significant rises in serum triglycerides. Light alcohol intake, in contrast, appears to result in an increase in the levels of high-density lipoproteins.

Alcohol Abuse and Hypertension

Significant alcohol intake is positively associated with hypertension. Light intakes have little or no effect on blood pressure.

Alcohol Abuse and Hypomagnesmia

Alcoholism appears to increase the need for magnesium in the diet.

Alcohol Abuse and Hyponatremia

Alcoholism may be characterized by low blood levels of sodium.

Alcohol Abuse and Hypophophatemia

Alcoholism is characterized by low blood levels of phosphate. This impairs blood pH regulation.

Alcohol Abuse and Metabolic Acidosis

Metabolic pH falls when excessive alcohol intake occurs.

Alcohol Abuse and Niacin Deficiency

Niacin is part of the coenzyme NADH and NADPH. Both are needed for the metabolism of alcohol. Excess alcohol consumption drives up the need for this vitamin.

Alcohol Abuse and Septic Shock

Due to a decreased immune response, alcoholics are at high risk for developing the end result of a process initiated by sepsis known as septic shock.

Alcohol Abuse and Vitamin Need

The metabolism of alcohol drives up the need for thiamin, niacin, pantothenic acid, and pyridoxine.

ALCOHOL WITHDRAWAL

Abstinence of alcohol by an alcoholic individual is associated with neurologic symptoms, cardio-vascular symptoms, and fluid volume deficit.

ALCOHOLIC LIVER

Damage to the liver due to excessive ethanol (alcohol) consumption.

ALCOHOLISM

An addictive disease with strong genetic factors concerning the excessive consumption of ethanol.

ALDEHYDE

A carbon compound containing a $-C=O$ group.

$$-C=O$$
$$|$$
$$H$$

ALDOLASE DEFICIENCY

A mutation in the gene for aldolase that results in an accumulation of fructose 1,6-bisphosphate. Aldolase catalyzes the cleavage of fructose 1,6-bisphosphate to glyceraldehydes-3-phosphate and dihydroxyacetone phosphate. (See Glycolysis and Metabolic Maps, Appendix 2.)

ALDOSTERONE

A steroid hormone produced by the adrenal cortex that acts on the cells bordering the distal tubules of the kidney stimulating them to reabsorb sodium. When sodium is reabsorbed, water is retained. Thus, aldosterone plays an important role in sodium and water conservation (see Figure 2).

ALENDRONATE SODIUM

An anti-osteoporosis drug. Trade name: Fosamax.

ALIMENTARY CANAL

See Gastrointestinal Tract.

ALIMENTARY TOXIC ALEUKIS (ATA)

See Mycotoxins and Trichothecenes.

ALIPHATIC

A chain of carbon atoms with associated hydrogen and/or hydroxyl groups.

ALIPHATIC AMINO ACIDS

Amino acids that consist of a chain of carbon atoms. These include alanine, cysteine, glycine, iso-leucine, leucine, methionine, serine, threonine, and valine.

ALKALOSIS

A condition where the blood pH rises above 7.4. Metabolic alkalosis may be caused by a loss in body acids; a loss of chloride ion, as occurs in excess vomiting; an excess of antacid intake; or depletion of potassium ion, as occurs with excessive diarrhea.

ALLELE

Any one of a series of different genes that may occupy the same location (locus) on a specific chromosome.

ALLERGENS

Substances capable of eliciting an immunologic response. Allergens in food are either proteins, glycoproteins, or polypeptides. Allergens can also be airborne or can be absorbed through the skin. The allergenicity of a substance is associated with the type of structure of the proteins and peptides: primary, secondary, or tertiary. In the case of tertiary structures, allergenicity often disappears on denaturation. This is not the case with primary structured allergens. The allergen must be of sufficient size to be recognized as "foreign." If the molecular weight is <5000, little immunologic response will be found unless they are bound to an endogenous protein. Dietary substances with a molecular weight of >70,000 are not absorbed because they are too large and therefore do not elicit an allergic response. Food proteins that are not digested and absorbed can elicit an enteric response: diarrhea and/or flatulence. This is not considered an immunologic response (see Figure 2).

ALLERGY

A condition in which body tissues of sensitive people react to specific allergens, while those of non-sensitive people do not. The response is histamine mediated. The reaction can be mild, moderate, or severe depending on the sensitivity of the individual. Symptoms can include headache, urticara, eczema, rash, asthma, hay fever, hemorrhage, gastrointestinal disturbances, nausea, vomiting, and in rare instances, circulatory collapse, shock, and death. In general, there are four different types of immunological hypersensitivity:

1. *Type I hypersensitivity*: After contact with an allergen, B lymphocytes are stimulated to produce immunoglobulin E (IgE) antibodies. These antibodies bind to mast cells and basophils. When there is a subsequent exposure to the same allergen, the allergen becomes bound to two adjacent IgE molecules, resulting in the degranulation of the cell to which the IgE is bound. Several types of (preexisting and/or newly formed) mediators are released. This results in a complex reaction that includes muscle contraction, dilatation, increased permeability of blood vessels, chemotaxis (a mediator-triggered process by which other cells are attracted to the site of the reaction), and release of other immune mediators. The reaction occurs mostly within one hour and is sometimes followed by a so-called late reaction, which starts hours later.
2. *Type II hypersensitivity*: Antibodies of the immunoglobulin M (IgM) class are generated against a cell-surface antigen. This leads to an inflammatory reaction by which the cells are destroyed. Transfusion reactions, due to blood incompatibility, occur according to this mechanism. There is no evidence that this type of allergic reaction plays a role in food allergy.
3. *Type III hypersensitivity*: Antibodies of the type IgG and IgM are formed against antigens that circulate in the blood. This results in the formation of antigen-antibody complexes that

activate the complement system, followed by the release of different mediators from mast cells and basophils. When there is an optimal ratio of antibody to antigen, the complexes may precipitate at different sites in the body, for example, the joints, the kidneys, and the skin. This type of reaction may play a role in some types of food allergic reactions. Type III hypersensitivity reactions may also include hypersensitivity reactions to certain drugs and a few types of vasculitis.

4. *Type IV hypersensitivity*: In contrast to types I, II, and III, no antibodies are involved in this type of reaction. After contact with the antigen, T-lymphocytes are sensitized. These T-lymphocytes then produce cytokines that activate other cells. An example of this type of sensitivity is contact allergy to certain cosmetics. In food allergy, this reaction is seen when the sensitive person comes in contact with a certain food.

ALLICIN

The primary active component of garlic giving it its characteristic aroma.

ALLOGENIC

Referring to the use of tissues or organs from donor humans who have a different genetic background than the recipient.

ALLOPURINOL

A drug useful in the management of gout. It works by inhibiting the enzyme xanthine oxidase. This enzyme is more active in people with gout and results in the production of excess uric acid. Uric acid is normally excreted in the urine, but in excess amounts, it is crystallized and deposited in the fluids around the joints causing inflammation and discomfort. Trade names: Lopurin, Purinol, Zyloprin.

ALLOSTERISM

The binding of an inhibitor or activator to an enzyme at a site other than the active site of the enzyme.

ALLOTRIOPHAGY-PICA

Consumption of nonfood items; deranged appetite.

ALLOXAN

A drug that destroys the insulin-producing β cells of the pancreas. It also can destroy hepatic cells.

ALOPECIA

Loss of hair.

ALUMINUM HYDROXIDE

Common antacid; chronic use is associated with lowering serum phosphorus and excess urinary calcium loss.

ALVEOLI

Cell structures in the lungs responsible for O_2/CO_2 exchange.

ALZHEIMER'S DISEASE

Progressive disease characterized by deterioration of memory and other cognitive functions; major cause of dementia in the elderly.

AMENORRHEA

Cessation of menses. It may be due to the cessation of ovulation as occurs in pregnancy or at the end of the female reproductive period (menopause). It can also be due to inadequate food intake as in anorexia or starvation.

AMIDE BOND (PEPTIDE BOND)

A bond involving an amino group. The peptide bond is the most common amide bond and is formed when two amino acids are joined together as illustrated in Figure 5. (See also Figure 6.)

AMILORIDE HYDROCHLORIDE

An antihypertensive drug that spares potassium. It acts as a diuretic. Trade name: Midamor.

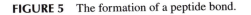

L-alanine + L-serine ⟶ Alanyl-serine (a dipeptide)

FIGURE 5 The formation of a peptide bond.

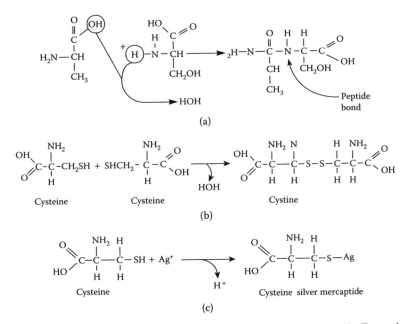

FIGURE 6 Examples of amino acid reactions. (a) Formation of peptide bond. (b) Formation of disulfide bridge. (c) Formation of a mercaptide.

AMINES

Decarboxylated amino acids.

AMINO ACID CATABOLISM

See Metabolic Maps, Appendix 2. Those amino acids in the body's amino acid pool that are not used for peptide or protein synthesis and that are not used to synthesize metabolically important intermediates are deaminated, and the carbon skeletons are either oxidized or used for the synthesis of glucose or fatty acids. There are two general reactions for the removal of NH_3 from the amino acids:

1. Transamination: The amino group is transferred from an amino acid to another carbon chain via aminotransaminases.
2. Oxidative deamination to produce NH_3: The amino group is oxidatively removed through the activity of an amino acid oxidase. The pathways for the catabolism of the amino acids are shown in Appendix 2.

AMINO ACID METABOLISM

See Metabolic Maps, Appendix 2. The use and degradation of amino acids by the body as outlined in the maps found in Appendix 2.

AMINO ACID POOL

The free amino acids present in the cytosol of cells and in the fluids that surround them.

AMINO ACID REACTIONS

Amino acids undergo several characteristic reactions as listed in Table 6. Amino acids can be joined together via peptide bonds, sulfide bridges or can form mercaptides. Examples of these reactions are shown in Figure 6.

AMINO ACID REQUIREMENTS

Specific allowances figures for the intake of the essential amino acids are not available. The recommended daily for protein are shown in Table 7. The assumption is that if the protein consumed is of high quality it will provide the needed amounts of amino acids. Although for most nutrients the Daily Recommended Intake (DRI) is used, figures for protein DRIs have not yet been developed, thus the 1998 RDA is shown. The recommendation shown in Table 7 allows for individual variation

TABLE 6
Characteristic Chemical Reactions of Amino Acids

Reaction Name	Reagent	Use
Ninhydrin reaction	Ninhydrin	To estimate amino acids quantitatively in small amounts
Sanger reaction	1-fluro-2,4-dinitrobenzene	To identify the amino terminal group of a peptide
Dansylchloride reaction	1-deimethylaminonapthalene	To measure very small amounts of amino acids quantitatively
Edmann degradation	Phenylisothiocyanate	To identify the terminal NH_2 group in a protein
Schiff base	Aldehydes	Labile intermediate in some enzymatic reactions

TABLE 7
Food and Nutrition Board, National Academy of Sciences, National Research Council
Recommended Dietary Allowances for Protein (1998 revision) USA

Life Stage	Age	Weight (kg)[a]	Height (cm)[a]	Protein Intake (g/day)[b]
Infant	Birth–6 months	6	60	13
	7–12 months	9	71	14
Child	1–3 years	13	90	16
	4–6	20	112	24
	7–10	28	132	28
Males	11–14	45	157	45
	15–18	66	176	59
	19–24	72	177	58
	25–50	79	176	63
	51+	77	173	63
Females	11–14	46	157	46
	15–18	55	163	64
	19–24	58	164	46
	25–50	63	163	50
	51+	65	160	50
Pregnant				60
Lactating	0–6 months			65
	7–12 months			62

[a] Weights and heights of reference life-stage groups are actual medians for the U.S. population of the designated age, as reported by NHANES II. Use of these measures do not imply that the height to weight ratios are ideal.

[b] These recommendations are expressed as average daily intakes over time and are intended to allow for individual variation and day-to-day variation among normal people living in the United States under usual environmental conditions.

in need. For some life-stage groups the database is very small, and so the recommended intake may change as more information about the protein need for these groups is gathered. See http://www. nap.edu for the latest information about DRIs.

AMINOACIDOPATHY

Mutations in specific genetic sequences for specific gene products resulting in inadequate utilization of one or more amino acids. Common examples include phenylketonuria that results when one or more mutations occur in the gene for the enzyme, phenylalanine hydroxylase. Table 8 lists some of these disorders.

AMINO ACIDS

Simple organic nitrogenous compounds that are the building blocks of proteins. They are divided into those that are essential for adults and those that are not essential because the body can make them in sufficient quantities to meet need. They are listed in Table 5.

Amino acids consist of carbon, hydrogen, oxygen, nitrogen, and occasionally sulfur. All amino acids with the exception of proline have a terminal carboxyl group $\left(-C\begin{smallmatrix}\nearrow O\\\searrow OH\end{smallmatrix}\right)$ and an unsubstituted amino ($-NH_2$) group attached to the α carbon. Proline has a substituted amino group and a carboxyl group. Also attached to the α carbon is a functional group identified as R; R differs for each amino

TABLE 8
Genetic Diseases of Amino Acid Metabolism

Disease	Mutation	Characterisitics
Maple syrup urine disease	Branched chain ketoacid dehydrogenase	Elevated levels of α-ketoacids and their metabolites in blood and urine; mental retardation, ketoacidosis, and early death
Hypermethionemia	Methionine adenosyltransferase	High blood levels of methionine
Homocysteinemia	Cystathionine synthase	Absence of cross-linked collagen; eye malformations, osteoporosis; mental retardation, thromboembolism, and vascular occlusions
Phenylketonuria	Phenylalanine hydroxylase	Mental retardation, decreased neurotransmitter production; shortened life span
Tyrosinemia	Tyrosine transaminase	Eye and skin lesions, mental retardation
Albinism	Tyrosinase	Lack of melanin production; sensitivity to sunlight
Alcaptonuria	Homogentisate oxidase	Elevated homogentisate levels in blood, bones, internal organs; increased susceptibility to viruses and arthritis
Histidinemia	Histidase	Elevated blood and urine levels of histidine; decreased histamine

acid. The general structure of amino acids can be represented as $R-\overset{\displaystyle H}{\underset{\displaystyle NH_2}{C}}-COOH$. While it is convenient to represent amino acids in this manner, in reality the amino acids exist as the dipolar ion $R-\overset{\displaystyle H}{\underset{\displaystyle NH_3^+}{C}}-COO^-$ in the range of pH values (5.0–8.0) found within the body.

Amino acids serve as precursors of several important nonprotein compounds (i.e., thyroxine, epinephrine, serotonin, creatine, creatinine, and ethanolamine). Some amino acids serve as cell signaling molecules and also as regulators of gene expression and protein phosphorylation cascade.

α-AMINOPROPIONIC ACID DERIVATIVES

Nonnutritive natural food components that can elicit a toxicological response. They occur in peas of certain Lathyrus species, notably *Lathyrus sativus*. These substances are known to cause skeletal malformations (osteolathyrism) and neurotoxic effects (neurolathyrism). The peas are easily grown on poor soil and are often used as cattle feed. The peas contain a neurotoxin, N-oxalyl-diaminopropionic acid. Sometimes the pea crop is contaminated with a vetch species (*Vicia sativa*) that also contains a neurotoxin, α-aminopropionic acid derivative, β-cyano-L-alanine. The neurotoxicity of these compounds has been attributed to their similarity to the neurotransmitter, GABA. Both neurotoxins bind irreversibly to the glutamate receptors on specific nerve cells, and this, in turn, results in nerve damage.

AMINOTRANSFERASES (TRANSAMINASES)

Enzymes that catalyze the transfer of an amino group ($-NH_2$ or $-NH_3$) from one carbon chain to another.

AMLODIPINE BESYLATE

An antihypertensive drug that serves as a calcium channel blocker. Trade name: Norvasc.

AMNIOTIC FLUID

The fluid in the uterus that surrounds the unborn child.

AMP

Adenine monophosphate. ATP is broken down to ADP and then to AMP with the release of inorganic phosphate at each step.

AMPHIPATHIC

The characteristic of a compound containing both polar and nonpolar groups. This allows the compound to be soluble in both polar and nonpolar solvents. Water is a polar solvent; chloroform is a nonpolar solvent.

AMPHOTERIC

The characteristic of a compound that allows it to have either an acidic or a basic function depending on the pH of the solution.

AMPK (ADENOSINE MONOPHOSPHATE–ACTIVATED PROTEIN KINASE)

Transduction pathway in the liver that senses amino acids.

AMYLASE

An enzyme that catalyzes the cleavage of glucose molecules from amylose (starch).

AMYLIN

Hormone released by the pancreatic β cells with insulin in response to a glucose signal. It acts in concert with insulin to coordinate the rate of glucose appearance and disappearance in the blood. Amylin is a small peptide having 37 amino acid residues. In healthy adults plasma amylin concentrations range from 4 pmols/L to 25 pmol/L.

AMYLOPECTIN

A branched chain polymer of glucose found in plants.

AMYLOSE

A straight chain polymer of glucose found in plants.

AMYTAL

Amytal is a barbiturate that is an inhibitor of oxidative phosphorylation. It works by inhibiting the passage of electrons from complex I to complex III.

ANABOLISM

The totality of reactions that account for the synthesis of the body's macromolecules.

ANAEROBIC METABOLISM

Metabolic reactions that occur in the relative absence of oxygen.

ANAPHYLACTIC RESPONSE

A systemic allergic reaction to a food or food additive or an exogenous chemical such as bee venom.

ANAPHYLAXIS

Severe immune response that, if untreated, leads to coma and death. The response is due to a massive release of histamine that causes blood vessels to dilate and blood pressure to fall.

ANASTOMOSIS

Joining of two normally separate structures by a surgical procedure.

ANDERSON'S DISEASE

One of the genetic diseases resulting in excess glycogen accumulation. The mutation is in the gene for the glycogen branching enzyme.

ANDROGENS

Male sex hormones.

ANDROID OBESITY

A form of obesity when excess fat stores are found across the shoulders and in the abdominal area.

ANEMIA

A condition characterized by below normal levels of red blood cells and/or hemoglobin due to one or more problems in hemoglobin synthesis and/or red blood cell synthesis or due to loss of blood. Anemia can arise in malnutrition or from nonnutritional causes. The characteristics of nutritional anemia are summarized in Table 9.

TYPES OF ANEMIA

A. Nutritional in Origin

1. *Hemolytic anemia resulting from vitamin E deficiency.*
   Red blood cells have a membrane that makes them extra sensitive to hemolysis. Most often found in premature infants who are given milk formulas containing polyunsaturated fats without adequate vitamin E. An increased rate of destruction of red cells, resulting in anemia, is typical of vitamin E deficiency. Edema and some of its consequences (swollen legs, noisy breathing, and puffy eyelids) are also characteristic of vitamin E deficiency. Severe deficiency of vitamin E in infants may also be accompanied by encephalomalacia.

TABLE 9
Normal Blood Values for Measurements Made to Assess the Presence of Anemia

Measurement	Normal Values	Iron Deficiency	Chronic Disease	B_{12} or Folic Acid Deficiency
Red blood cells (million/mm³);	Males: 4.6–6.2	Low	Low	Low
	Females: 4.2–5.4			
Hemoglobin (g/dL)	Males: 14–18	Low	Low	Low
	Females: 12–16			
Hematocrit (vol %)	Males: 40%–54%	Low	Low	Low
	Females: 37%–47%			
Serum iron	60–280 ug/dL	Low	Low	Normal
TIBC[a]	250–425 ug/dL	High	Low	Normal
Ferritin	60	Less than 12	Normal	Normal
Percent saturation	90%–100%	Low	Normal to high	Normal
Hypochromia	No	Yes	Slight	None
Microcytes	Few	Many	Slight	Few
Macrocytes	Few	Few	None	Many
Red blood cell distribution width (RBC size)	High	High	Normal to low	Very high
Red cell folate	>360 nmol/L	Normal	315–358	<315
Serum folate	>13.5 mg/mL	Normal	Normal	Low (<6.7 mg/mL)
Serum B_{12}	200–900 pg/mL	Normal	Normal	Low
MCV[b]	82–92 cu m	<80	Normal	>80–100

[a] Indirect measure of serum transferrin; iron-binding capacity.
[b] Mean cell volume. When volume increases, the size of the red cell has increased ($\uparrow$ in % of megaloblasts).
TIBC = total iron-binding capacity.

2. *Iron deficiency anemia*
   The most common form of anemia. Red cells are reduced in size (microcytic) and contain a subnormal amount of hemoglobin (hypochromic). Also, the red cell count is low due to a decreased production of hemoglobin. It is most prevalent in infants, children, and pregnant women. Deficiency of hemoglobin and its consequences (paleness of skin and mucous membranes, fatigue, dizziness, sensitivity to cold, shortness of breath, rapid heartbeat, and tingling in fingers and toes) are characteristic of iron deficiency.

3. *Megaloblastic macrocytic anemia*
   Abnormal maturation of red cells resulting in enlarged cells (megaloblasts or macrocytes) with normal concentrations of hemoglobin (normochromic). It is characterized by subnormal cell count and caused by deficiency of folic acid and/or vitamin B_{12}. Blood cells fail to mature

4. *Pernicious anemia*
   Same as above description of megaloblastic anemia. Additionally, there are gastrointestinal disorders (glossitis, achlorhydria, and lack of intrinsic factor for vitamin B_{12} absorption) and neurologic damage (shown by abnormal electroencephalogram).

5. *Pica associated with iron deficiency anemia*
   Abnormal craving for nonfood items leads to the eating of clay, dirt, plaster, paint chips, and ice. Iron deficiency often develops in this disorder. Certain nonfood items (some types of clays) interfere with iron absorption.

6. *Pregnancy anemia*

The added requirements of a developing fetus produce in most cases an iron deficiency anemia. Pregnancy can also increase the need for folic acid so that a folic acid deficiency anemia can develop as well.

7. *Siderotic anemia due to deficiency of pyridoxine (vitamin B$_6$)*

Microcytic, hypochromic anemia similar to that caused by iron deficiency, except that serum iron is normal or at an elevated level. Vitamin B$_6$ deficiency impairs synthesis of hemoglobin. (See effects given above for iron deficiency anemia.)

B. Nonnutritional Anemia

1. *Aplastic anemia*

Cessation of blood cell production in the bone marrow due to toxic agents, reaction to drugs, and unknown causes. Great decrease in all blood cells produced in the bone marrow (red cells, white cells, and platelets). All the complications of anemia plus hemorrhages (due to lack of platelets needed for clotting) are characteristic of aplastic anemia.

2. *Blood loss*

Restoration of the full complement of red cells after blood loss is slower than repletion of other constituents of blood. Effects are the same as those of iron deficiency but may be more severe depending upon the extent of the blood loss.

3. *Familial hemolytic jaundice (spherocytic anemia)*

A hereditary disorder in which red cells are shaped like spheres instead of being toroidal (donutlike) shape. Jaundice, a yellowish color of the skin and whites of the eyes, results from the excessive destruction of the abnormal cells by the spleen. There is a reduction in the number of circulating red cells.

4. *Hemolytic anemia due to deficiency of G6PD enzyme*

Increased hemolysis of red cells due to the effects of drugs, toxic agents, and compounds in foods such as fava beans. It may also be the result of a mutation in the gene for red cell glucose 6-phosphate dehydrogenase (G6PD).

5. *Anemia and jaundice due to excessive hemolysis*

The trait is sexlinked.

6. *Hemolytic anemia of the newborn due to Rh factor incompatibility*

Rh-negative mothers develop antibodies against Rh-positive blood of the fetus. These antibodies are transmitted to the fetus and as a result, the mother gives birth to an infant whose red blood cells are being destroyed, causing anemia. In severe cases, there may be an almost complete destruction of the infant's red cells and damage to the brain by the accumulation of bilirubin (pigment resulting from the breakdown of hemoglobin).

7. *Hookworm or tapeworm infestation*

Infestation of the gastrointestinal tract by parasitic worms which feed on blood (hookworm) or nutrients (tapeworm). Anemia may be due to blood loss, deficiencies of folic acid, iron, and/or vitamin B$_{12}$. Anemia, fatigue, irritability, fever, abdominal discomfort, nausea, or vomiting are characteristic of this infestation.

8. *Infection*

The production of red cells by the marrow is sometimes inhibited by toxins from an infectious agent. Anemia and weakness are observed in this condition.

9. *Leukemia*

A form of cancer in which there is an overproduction of white cells by the body. Normal production of other blood cells (red cells, platelets, and normal white cells) is prevented by the overgrowth of abnormal leukocytes in the bone marrow and other blood-forming organs (liver, spleen, and lymphatic tissues). Grayish-white color of blood with a large excess of leukocytes. Death often results from the acute form of the disease and from the chronic form when it is not treated.

10. *Mediterranean anemia (also called thalassemia and Cooley's anemia)*

A hereditary disease most prevalent in persons whose ancestors came from the Mediterranean basin (Italy, Sicily, Sardinia, Greece, Crete, Cyprus, Syria, and Turkey). Red cells are fragile and contain abnormal hemoglobin. An increased rate of destruction of red cells is observed together with bone abnormalities, enlargement of the spleen, leg ulcers, and jaundice.

11. *Sickle cell anemia*

A hereditary disease in which the red cells have a sickle shape due to the presence of an abnormal hemoglobin. Sickle cells cannot carry as much oxygen as normal red cells, and they have a shorter than normal lifetime. Anemia, pain in the joints and extremities, and limited ability to perform strenuous exercise are features of this disorder. Death may occur if sickle cells clump together and clog blood flow in tissues, such as the brain.

ANERGY

Decreased reaction to specific antigens.

ANEURINE

An old term for the vitamin thiamin.

ANEURISM

A bulge in the vascular tree (usually arterial); if the vessel ruptures, hemorrhage or internal bleeding occurs and, unless treated promptly, death can result.

ANGINA PECTORIS

Sharp chest pain emanating from the breastbone (sternum) to the left arm and fingers due to an inadequate oxygen supply to the heart muscle. If the vascular tree of the heart has lost its elasticity because of atherosclerosis, the circulation of oxygenated blood will be impaired. There are gender differences in where the pain is felt. Females may experience a different pain path; it may emanate from the back or the shoulder blades or travel from the neck rather than from the breastbone. Nitroglycerin is often used to alleviate this pain. Nitroglycerin is a vasodilator.

ANGIOGENESIS

Development of blood vessels; leptin stimulates angiogenesis in the adipose tissue, thereby increasing its blood supply.

ANGIOTENSIN

The natural substrate for renin. It is an α_2-globulin (a glycoprotein) synthesized in the liver and transported to the kidney in an inactive form, angiotensinogen. It is converted to angiotensin I and then to angiotensin II in the kidney. Angiotensin II stimulates the production of aldosterone and also functions as a vasoconstrictor in the circulatory system raising blood pressure. (See Figure 2.)

ANGIOTENSIN CONVERTING ENZYME (ACE)

The enzyme responsible for converting angiotensin I to angiotensin II in the kidney.

ANH (ATRIAL NATRUIRETIC HORMONE)

The hormone that counteracts ADH. This hormone induces water, sodium, and potassium loss, decreases blood pressure, and increases glomerular filtration rate. ANH interferes with the renin-angiotensin system by decreasing the release of renin and aldosterone. It also antagonizes the action of vasoconstrictors such as angiotensin II and norepinephrine.

ANIMAL MODELS FOR HUMAN DISEASE

Numerous small animals have some characteristics in common with diseased humans. These can be used to study the disease process. Some of the more common ones are listed in Table 10.

TABLE 10
Small Animal Analogs for Human Degenerative Diseases

Type 1 Diabetes Mellitus (IDDM)

    Streptozotocin-treated animals of most species; alloxan can be substituted for streptozotocin

    Pancreatectomy will also produce IDDM

    BB rat (autoimmune disease)

    Tuco-tuco (Clenomys tabarum)

Type 2 Diabetes Mellitus (NIDDM)

    db/db mouse

    NOD mouse

    FAT mouse

    NZO mouse

    TUBBY mouse

    Adipose mouse

    Chinese hamster (*Cricetulus griseus*)

    South African hamster (*Mystromys alb icaudatus*)

    WKY rats

    WKY rats

    ob/ob mouse

    KK, yellow KK mouse

    Avy, Ay yellow mouse

    P, PB13/Ld mouse

    db PAS mouse

    BHE/Cdb rat

    Zucker diabetic rat

    SHR/N-cp rat

    Spiny mouse

    HUS rat

    LA/N-cp rat

    Wistar Kyoto rat

Obesity

    Zucker rat

    SHR/N-cp rat

    LA/N-cp rat

    ob/ob mouse

    Ventral hypothalamus lesioned animals

    Osborne–Mendel rats fed high-fat diets

TABLE 10 (*Continued*)
Small Animal Analogs for Human Degenerative Diseases

Hypertension
 SHR rats
 JCR:LA rats
 Transgenic rats

Gallstones
 The rat does not have a gall bladder nor does it have stones
 Gerbil fed a cholesterol-rich, cholic acid-rich diet
 Hamster, prairie dog, squirrel monkey, or tree shrew fed a cholesterol-rich diet

Lipemia
 Zucker fatty rat
 BHE/cdb rat
 NZW mouse
 Transgenic mice given gene for atherosclerosis

Atherosclerosis
 Transgenic mice given gene for atherosclerosis
 NZW mouse
 JCR:LA cp/cp rat

IDDM = insulin-dependent diabetes mellitus, NIDDM = noninsulin dependent diabetes mellitus

ANOMERS

Compounds with identical structures except for the arrangement of atoms around the anomeric carbon. An anomeric carbon has four different atoms or structural groups attached to it.

ANORECTIN

A peptide that serves as a satiety signal.

ANOREXIA NERVOSA

A condition of conscious reduction of food intake that is frequently observed in females in their teens and twenties. It is related to their inaccurate perception of their body fatness. These patients are characterized by little body fat. Because ovulation requires a minimal amount of fat in the body, ovulation ceases. Amenorrhea, hypothermia, hypotension also develop and, if unrecognized and untreated, anorexics may starve to death. Some patients spontaneously correct their condition and resume normal eating patterns. Anorexic people have physiological/biochemical features that are similar to individuals who are starving. Their catabolic hormone levels are high and their body energy stores are being raided as a result. Insulin resistance due to the catabolic hormones is observed. Liver and muscle glycogen levels are low. Severe protein depletion occurs. Fat stores are minimal. As the weight loss proceeds further, these individuals have a reduced bone mass (decreased mineral content of the bone), a decreased metabolic rate, decreased heart rate, hypoglycemia, hypothyroidism, electrolyte imbalance, elevated free fatty acid and cholesterol levels, peripheral edema, and lastly, cardiac and renal failure. When their fat stores fall below 2% of total body weight, they will die. When food intake is restored, there is a preferential deposition of adipose tissue in the abdomen. This is a short-term response to refeeding.

ANOSMIA

Loss of the sense of smell.

ANOXIA

Lack of oxygen in blood or tissues; it may be local due to inadequate oxygen delivery to a localized area or may be global (whole body).

ANTABUSE

Drug used to help alcoholics resist alcohol consumption. When used, the patient will experience severe gastrointestinal upset if alcohol is consumed.

ANTACIDS

Nonabsorbable bases or buffers that combat excessive gastric acidity by neutralizing the acid. Among the more common antacids are aluminum hydroxide, aluminum oxide, calcium carbonate, calcium-magnesium carbonate, dihydroxy aluminum amino acetate, glycine, magnesium carbonate, magnesium phosphate, magnesium trisillicate, sodium bicarbonate, sodium citrate, and urea (carbamide).

ANTAGONIST

A compound that interferes with the action of another compound.

ANTECEDENT EVENTS

Events that precede or are causally linked to an event.

ANTERIOR PITUITARY HORMONES

Hormones produced and released by the anterior pituitary. There are ten hormones released by the anterior portion of the pituitary gland located in the brain. These hormones are growth hormone (GH or somatotropin), prolactin (PRL), thyroid-stimulating hormone (TSH or thyrotropin), follicle-stimulating hormone (FSH), luteinizing hormone (LH), adrenocorticotropic hormone (ACTH), melanocyte-stimulating hormone (MSH), β-lipotropin, β-endorphin, and met-enkephalin. These hormones serve to regulate metabolism, growth, reproduction, mammary gland development, skin color, and the CNS function.

ANTHROPOMETRY

Measurements of body features, such as weight, height, arm circumference, and so on.

ANTIBIOTICS

Drugs that inhibit growth of (or kill) pathogens.

ANTIBODY

A protein synthesized in response to a specific antigen that the immune system recognizes as foreign.

ANTICHOLINERGIC COMPOUNDS

The drug atropine sulfate (a belladonna alkaloid) acts as an anticholinergic compound and is used to control heart rhythm. It is also a vagolytic compound that is used preoperatively to diminish secretions and block vagal reflexes.

ANTICOAGULANTS

Compounds that interfere with blood clotting. Heparin is one such agent.

ANTICODING STRAND

A strand of DNA that is used as a template to direct the synthesis of RNA that is complementary to it.

ANTICODON

A sequence of three bases in the transfer RNA that is complimentary to that in the messenger RNA.

ANTIGEN

A compound that elicits or stimulates the production and release of antibodies.

ANTIHEMORRHAGIC VITAMIN

Vitamin K.

ANTIHISTAMINES

Compounds that inhibit the release and/or synthesis of histamines.

ANTIHYPERTENSIVE DRUGS

Drugs that serve to maintain normal blood pressure. They can block the receptors for the vasoconstrictor hormones, promote water loss by decreasing the renal water reabsorption process, inhibit the activity of the angiotensin converting enzyme (ACE), or interfere with the calcium ion second messenger systems.

ANTI-INFLAMMATORY DRUGS

The two types of anti-inflammatory drugs: steroids and nonsteroids. The steroids, such as hydrocortisone, prednisone, and other similar compounds, are prescription drugs that act by inhibiting the enzyme phospholipase A_2. Phospholipase A_2 stimulates the release of arachidonic acid from the membrane phospholipids. Hence, inhibition of this reaction will result in a decreased supply of arachidonic acid for eicosanoid synthesis. Some eicosanoids act as mediators of inflammation. Nonsteroidal anti-inflammatory drugs are those that inhibit the cyclooxygenase reaction and include common over the counter drugs such as aspirin and ibuprofen.

ANTIMETABOLITE

A compound similar to a naturally occurring metabolite, but which interferes with metabolic processing because it is not identical in all respects to the metabolite.

ANTIMICROBIAL AGENTS

See Antibiotics. Antimicrobial also refers to any treatment that kills microorganisms regardless of where these organisms reside. Cleaning solutions, for example, can be antimicrobial solutions.

ANTIMINERALS

See Type B Antinutritives. Minerals that interfere with the absorption or use of other required minerals or minerals that, in any amount, are toxic. Examples of the former are the zinc, copper, and iron interactions. If any one is in excess, it serves as an antimineral for the others. Examples of the latter are lead, antimony, cadmium, and mercury.

ANTIMYCIN A

An antibiotic; it also is an inhibitor of oxidative phosphorylation blocking the activity of complex III of the respiratory chain.

ANTINEURITIC FACTORS

Factors needed for normal nerve development, usually included are the B vitamins; an antineuritic factor prevents an inflammation of the neuron or axon.

ANTINUTRITIVES

Compounds that are capable of producing nutritional deficiency or interfering in the utilization and function of nutrients. They can interfere with food components before intake, during digestion in the gastrointestinal tract, and after absorption in the body. The conditions under which they may have important effects are malnutrition or a marginal nutritional state.

ANTIOXIDANTS

Agents that prevent or inhibit oxidation reactions; in particular they are agents that prevent the oxidation of unsaturated fatty acids. Vitamins A, E, and C act as antioxidants. Some food additives prolong product freshness by acting as antioxidants.

ANTIPROTEINS

Substances that are type A antinutritives.

ANTIPYRIDOXINE FACTORS

Substances that interfere with the action of pyridoxine. They are type C antinutritives.

ANTIRACHITIC FACTORS

Nutrients that are required for normal bone growth and development; these include vitamins C, K, D, and minerals (calcium, phosphorous, magnesium, manganese, potassium, and some trace minerals).

ANTITHIAMIN FACTORS

Substances that interfere with the action of thiamin. They are type C antinutritives.

ANTIVITAMINS

Substances that interfere with normal vitamin action.

ANURIA

Lack of urine secretion.

ANUS

Opening at the posterior end of the digestive tract.

AORTA

The vessel that carries blood from the left ventricle of the heart to the vessels that serve the rest of the body.

AORTIC ANEURYSM

Aneurysm affecting any part of the aorta.

AORTIC INSUFFICIENCY

Condition in which blood regurgitates into the ventricle through a compromised aortic valve resulting in left ventricle dilation and hypertrophy.

AORTIC STENOSIS

Condition in which the diameter of the aortic valve opening narrows causing left ventricular hypertrophy and leading to congestive heart failure.

APATHY

Indifference.

APHRODISIACS

Substances thought to increase sexual desire as part of a cultural belief about sexual performance. There is little scientific evidence to support these claims.

APOENZYME

The inactive part or "backbone" of an enzyme protein.

APOPTOSIS

Programmed cell death. The half-life of cells varies throughout the body. It depends on a variety of factors including age, nutritional status, health status, and genetics, as well as factors not yet identified. Age is important. Growing individuals are in a phase of life in which cell number is increasing exponentially. Once growth and development are complete this increase in cell number slows down. In contrast, senescence is characterized by a gradual loss in total cell number as well as losses in discrete cell types. Cell turnover has two parts: cell replacement and cell death. Cell death is either a concerted, all at once, event or a programmed, gradual process. If the former, cell death is called necrosis. This occurs if a tissue sustains an injury, whether it be small or large. Necrotic cell death is preceded by cell enlargement and a swelling of all the organelles within the cell. The DNA disintegrates and its nucleotides are degraded.

In contrast, programmed cell death or apoptosis involves a shrinkage of the cell and enzyme catalyzed DNA fragmentation. This fragmentation can be detected as a laddering when the DNA is extracted from the cell and separated by electrophoresis. Apoptosis is a process that is an integral part of living systems. It is part of the growth process as well as the maintenance of cell and tissue function. It is also part of wound healing and recovery from traumatic injury. Adipose tissue remodeling, immune function, epithelial cell turnover, the periodic shedding of the uterine lining are but a few examples of this process. Apoptosis is viewed as a defense mechanism to remove unwanted and potentially dangerous cells such as virally infected cells or tumor cells. The process involves the mitochondria as the "central executioner." The mitochondria produce reactive oxygen (free radicals) as well as other materials that participate in apoptosis. Alterations in mitochondrial function have been observed to occur prior to any other feature of apoptosis. A decrease in mitochondrial membrane potential that in turn affects membrane permeability is an early event. The increase in permeability is followed by a release of cytochrome C that in turn regulates the caspases, which are cysteine proteases. These caspaces stimulate the proteolysis of key cell proteins in various parts of the cell. Altogether the fragmentation of the DNA and the destruction of cell proteins result in the death of the cell via a very orderly process.

Apoptosis is the mechanism used in the thymus to eliminate thymocytes that are self reactive. By doing so the development of autoimmune disease is suppressed. Table 11 lists some of the factors that influence apoptosis.

Many cells can be stimulated to become apoptotic. The p53 protein, for example, can induce apoptosis as one of its modes of protecting the body against tumor cells. The p53 protein is a DNA binding protein. Mutations in tumor cells have been found that inactivate p53. The result of such mutation is that tumor cells grow and multiply. The gene for p53 likewise can mutate and this mutation has been associated with tumor development and growth. Apparently, this gene has several "hot spots" (likely places for mutation to occur), which explains its role in carcinogenesis and its loss in normal function. The Bcl-2 protein, a membrane bound cytoplasmic protein, is another player in this regulation of apoptosis. It is a member of the family of proteins called protooncogenes. Its normal function is to protect valuable cells against apoptosis. It is down regulated when cells are stimulated to die. Inappropriately high Bcl-2 protein levels can provoke cell overgrowth. The cell regulates Bcl-2 protein so as to maintain a normal homeostatic state. Bcl-2 and its homologue, Bcl-xL, blocks apoptosis. Both Bcl-2 and Bcl-xL can heterodimerize with Bax or Bcl-xs and when Bcl-2 or Bcl-xL is over expressed an enhancement of oxidative stress mutagenesis can be observed. This occurs because these proteins suppress the apototic process allowing more exposure of the cell to DNA damage by mutagens.

Nutrients play a role in apoptosis. High levels of zinc (500 μm) have been found to block apoptosis in cultured thymocytes. The zinc blocks the action of glucocorticoids in stimulating apoptosis. Zinc also interferes with tumor necrosis factor (TNF)–induced apoptosis as well as heat-induced death. In contrast, low levels of zinc (0.3–200 μm) have the reverse effect. That is, at low levels of zinc, apoptosis could be stimulated by TNF, glucocorticoid, and heat exposure. The mechanism whereby zinc has these effects must be multifaceted. Zinc has an important role in transcription control as part of the zinc fingers but we do not know how this relates to apoptosis. Manganese, another essential nutrient, also is involved as a cofactor for superoxide dismutase (SOD). In instances where SOD is less active than normal, apoptosis is stimulated coincident with an increase in C2-ceramide, TNFα, and hydrogen peroxide. Peroxides form from unsaturated fatty acids as well as certain of the amino acids. There may be a link therefore between the fatty acid intake of the individual and apoptosis of certain cell types. Manganese, another essential nutrient, also is involved as a cofactor for SOD. In instances where SOD is less active than normal, apoptosis is stimulated coincident

TABLE 11
Factors That Influence Apoptosis

Factor	Effect	
	Suppress	Stimulate
Age		√
Apaf-1 protein		√
p53 protein		√
Bcl-2 protein	√	
Bcl-x$_3$ protein		√
Bcl-x$_L$ protein	√	
Bax protein		√
Bak protein		√
WAF-1		√
ced-3 and 4		√
Glucocorticoids		√
ced 9	√	
High zinc	√	
Low zinc		√
Low retinoic acid	√	
High retinoic acid		√
Interleukin 1β		√
Leptin		√
TNFα		√
Insulin	√	
Low manganese		√
IGF-1	√	
Low SOD activity		√
Peroxidized lipid		√

IGF-1 = insulin-like growth factor.

with an increase in C2-ceramide, TNFα, and hydrogen peroxide. Peroxides form from unsaturated fatty acids as well as certain of the amino acids. There may be a link therefore between the fatty acid intake of the individual and apoptosis of certain cell types. In one study of genetically obese diabetic rats, an increase in fatty acid intake was associated with an increase in β-cell apoptosis.

Retinoic acid (and dietary vitamin A) deficiency stimulates apoptosis. The well-known feature of vitamin A deficiency (suppressed immune function) suggests that vitamin A and its metabolite, retinoic acid, serve to influence the sequence of events leading to cell death. This link is made because it is known that T cell apoptosis is an important defense mechanism and T cells are part of the immune system. Vitamin A is also an antiproliferative agent so its effect on abnormal cell growth is two pronged. One, it stimulates apoptosis, and two, it suppresses proliferation.

Genetic regulation of apoptosis involves not only the transcription factors mentioned above but also specific genes. Already described are the p53 and Bcl-2 DNA binding proteins that, like zinc, retinoic acid and fatty acids, affect gene expression. Add to this list the mitogen activated protein kinases (p42/44) Erk1 and Erk2. When phosphorylated these proteins suppress apoptosis in brown adipocytes. Apoptosis is also suppressed by certain of the cytokines (IL6, IL3, interferon γ) and stimulated by others (leptin). Lastly, the gene Nedd 2 encodes a protein similar to the nematode cell death gene ced 3 and the mammalian interleukin 1β converting enzyme. Overexpression of this gene induces apoptosis.

With the understanding of apoptosis comes the understanding of how and why the body changes in its composition as it ages from conception to death. The young animal has little fat while the older one has gained fat sometimes at the expense of body protein. Clearly, the body is continually being remodeled and quite clearly this remodeling is the result of a combination of many factors including the apoptotic process.

APOPROTEINS

Proteins that are complexed with other materials such as lipids, carbohydrates, or specific minerals, and so on. The term apoprotein can also refer to proteins that are components of transport or enzyme systems.

APPARENT DIGESTED ENERGY (DE)

Energy in food consumed (IE) less the energy in the feces (FE). (DE = IE-FE).

APPESTAT THEORY

Also referred to as the set-point theory, which hypothesizes that the body establishes a preferred weight and defends that weight under varying food intake conditions.

APPETITE

Desire for food.

ARACHIDONIC ACID

Long chain fatty acid having four double bonds and 20 carbons.

ARACHIS OIL

Peanut oil.

ARCHIMEDES' PRINCIPLE

An object's volume when submerged in water equals the volume of the water it displaces. If the mass and volume are known, the density can be calculated. This principle underlies the determination of body fatness through underwater weighing.

ARGINASE

An enzyme that catalyzes the cleavage of arginine to urea and ornithine.

ARGINEMIA

A rare genetic disease where a mutation in the gene for arginase has occurred and is characterized by high blood levels of arginine.

ARGININE

An essential amino acid for growing animals. Precursor of nitric oxide, a vasoactive compound; precursor of urea in the urea cycle.

ARM CIRCUMFERENCE

See Mid-Arm Circumference.

AROMATIC AMINO ACIDS

Amino acids that have a ring structure. Included are phenylalanine, tyrosine, and tryptophan.

ARRHYTHMIA

Condition resulting from abnormal cardiac impulse initiation and/or conduction causing the heart to pump irregularly.

ARS

Autonomously replicating sequence; the origin of replication in yeast.

ARSENIC

A metabolic poison. Arsenic is a mineral that may be essential in ultra-small amounts and is regarded by some scientists as a possible essential ultra trace element.

ARTERIAL BLOOD GAS (ABG) STUDIES

Group of laboratory tests used to reflect the acid-base balance of the body. Included in arterial blood gas analysis are tests that provide information on pH, partial pressure of carbon dioxide ($PaCO_2$), partial pressure of oxygen (PaO_2), oxygen saturation (SaO_2), bicarbonate (HCO_3), and base excess.

ARTERIOGRAPHY

A method of examining the arteries using X-rays and an infusion of a radio-opaque dye solution.

ARTERIOSCLEROSIS

General term for degeneration of the arteries due to thickening and hardening of the arterial wall; referred to as "hardening of the arteries." There is a loss of elasticity when plaques are formed.

ARTERIOSCLEROSIS OBLITERANS

Proliferation of the intima of an artery resulting in complete blockage of that artery.

ARTIFICIAL SWEETENERS

Substances that elicit a sweet taste but which have little or no energy value.

ASCITES

Characterized by accumulation of fluid in the abdomen.

ASCORBIC ACID

Vitamin C; dehydroascorbic acid is the oxidized form of ascorbic acid. The chemical name is 2,3-didehydro L-threo-hexano-1,4-lactone. The compound can readily donate or accept hydrogen ions and thus exists in either state as shown in Figure 7. Because of this feature, it serves as a good antioxidant. In order for the compound to have vitamin activity it must have a 2,3-endiol structure and be a six-carbon lactone. Vitamin C is soluble in water, glycerol, and ethanol but insoluble in fat solvents such as chloroform and ether. It exists in both D and L forms but the L form is the biologically active form.

Citrus fruits, strawberries, melons, raw cabbage, and related vegetables are good sources of the vitamin. In the human, ascorbate is absorbed in the small intestine by an active transport system that is sodium and energy dependent and requires a carrier protein. Any excess vitamin consumed beyond need is excreted in the urine. There is a very efficient reabsorption mechanism in the kidneys which serves to conserve ascorbic acid in times of need.

Ascorbic acid readily converts between the free and dehydro form. Thus, it functions in hydrogen ion transfer systems and aids in the regulation of redox states in the cells. Since it is a powerful water soluble antioxidant it helps to protect other naturally occurring antioxidants which may or may not be water soluble. For example, polyunsaturated fatty acids and vitamin E are protected from peroxidation by ascorbic acid. Ascorbic acid protects certain proteins from oxidative damage and, in addition to its role as an antioxidant, it serves to maintain the unsaturation:saturation ratio of fatty acids. Ascorbic acid aids in the conversion of folic acid to folinic acid and facilitates the absorption of iron by maintaining it in the ferrous state. Ascorbic acid plays a role in the detoxification reactions in the microsomes by virtue of its role as a cofactor in hydroxylation reactions. Ascorbic acid is also found in the brain uniformly distributed, where it serves as a cofactor for an enzyme which converts dopamine to norepinephrine.

Table 12 provides a list of those enzymes in which ascorbate is a coenzyme. Many of these are dioxygenases. Again this is due to the ascorbate-dehydroascorbate interconversion. A number of these enzymes are involved in collagen synthesis. This explains the poor wound healing found in deficient subjects.

Ascorbic acid deficiency signs are listed in Table 13. Although vitamin C is a water-soluble vitamin and is not usually stored, toxic states can develop if long term large intakes are maintained. Oxalate is an end product of ascorbate metabolism and is excreted in the urine. As the dose consumed increases, the urinary oxalate does not increase and some investigators have suggested that megadoses of vitamin C may be a risk factor in renal oxalate stores. Massive doses of vitamin C have been shown to reduce serum vitamin B_{12} levels. In part, this may be due to an effect of ascorbic acid on vitamin B_{12} in food. Ascorbic acid destroys B_{12} in food. Ascorbic acid also inhibits the utilization of β carotene.

ASCORBIC ACID OXIDASE

See Type C Antinutritives. An enzyme present in food that catalyzes the oxidation of ascorbic acid.

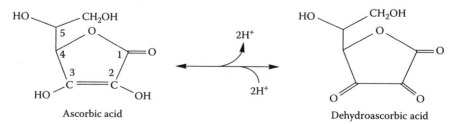

Ascorbic acid   Dehydroascorbic acid

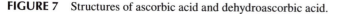

FIGURE 7   Structures of ascorbic acid and dehydroascorbic acid.

TABLE 12
Enzymes Using Ascorbate as a Coenzyme

Cytochrome P450 oxidases (several)
Dopamine-α-monooxygenase
Peptidyl glycine α-amidating monooxygenase
Cholesterol 7α-hydroxylase
4-hydroxyphenylpyruvate oxidase
Homogentisate 1,2-dioxygenase
Proline hydroxylase
Procollagen-proline 2-oxoglutarate 3-dioxygenase
Lysine hydroxylase
γ-butyrobetaine, 2-oxoglutarate 4-dioxygenase
Trimethyllysine-2-oxoglutarate dioxygenase

TABLE 13
Signs of Ascorbic Acid Deficiency

Hyperkeratosis
Congestion of follicles
Petechial and other skin hemorrhages
Conjunctival lesions
Sublingual hemorrhages
Gum swelling, congestion
Bleeding gums
Papillary swelling
Peripheral neuropathy with hemorrhages into nerve sheaths
Pain, bone endings are tender
Epiphyseal separations occur with subsequent bone (chest) deformities

---

ASEPTIC

Sterile; absence of pathogens.

ASPARAGINE

A nonessential amino acid containing two amino groups, four carbons, and two carboxy groups.

ASPARTAME

A nonnutritive sweetener composed of two amino acids, aspartate, and phenylalanine. (See also Nonnutritive Sweeteners.)

ASPARTATE (ASPARTIC ACID)

A nonessential amino acid containing two carboxyl groups.

ASPIRATION

The process of withdrawing fluids by suction. Can also refer to the inspiration of food, food particles or fluids into the trachea.

ASPIRIN (ACETYLSALICYLIC ACID)

Anti-inflamatory drug that is an over the counter (OTC) medication. Useful in managing pain, suppressing inflammation, and reducing the formation of blood clots. Aspirin reduces the clotting of blood through its inhibition of the cyclooxygenase reaction, one of the main pathways for eicosanoid synthesis. The thromboxanes (eicosanoids) are involved in blood clotting. Trade names: Aspirin, Bufferin, Ecotrin, and so on.

ASSIMILATION

See Absorption.

ASTHMA

Complex disease of the airways of the lungs. Involves an inflammation of the air passages and bronchial obstruction. The disease origin is unclear but seems to be associated with airborne allergens. It may also be due to an infection of the respiratory tract. Susceptibility to asthma may have some genetic links.

ATAXIA

Lack of coordination of muscle movement.

ATENOLOL

An antihypertensive drug that serves as a beta blocker. Trade names: Apo-Atenolol, Nu-Atenol, Tenormin.

ATHEROGENIC

Athersclerosis producing.

ATHEROSCLEROSIS

A progressive degenerative condition occurring within the vascular tree and resulting in occlusions and loss of vascular elasticity. Vessels are occluded when deposits of sterols and minerals (plaques) attach to the interior aspect (the intima) of the vessels. When these occur within the heart vascular system, the disease is cardiovascular disease or atherosclerosis. When these deposits occur elsewhere the disease is arteriosclerosis.

ATORVASTATIN CALCIUM

A member of the statin group of drugs that lower blood cholesterol by inhibiting HMG CoA reductase, the rate limiting enzyme in the pathway for cholesterol synthesis. Used to lower blood cholesterol levels in hypercholesterolemic patients. Trade name: Lipitor.

ATP (ADENOSINE TRIPHOSPHATE)

The energy-rich compound that serves as the energy coinage of the cell.

ATPASE

A group of enzymes that catalyze the removal or addition of a single phosphate group to the high-energy compound containing adenine. In the direction of cleavage $ATP \rightarrow ADP + Pi$; in the reverse, $ADP + Pi \rightarrow ATP$.

ATRIAL FIBRILLATION

An arrhythmia characterized by a rapid atrial rate of 350–600 beats/min, with the ventricular rate 160–200 beats/min.

ATROPHY

Reduced size or shrinkage of an organ, tissue, or cell.

ATTENTION DEFICIT HYPERACTIVITY DISORDER (ADHD)

Term used to describe behavior involving short attention span, impulsiveness, hyperactivity, or restlessness.

ATTENUATED

Weakened; lessened.

ATTRIBUTABLE PROPORTION (AP)

An effect parameter, indicating the proportion of diseased persons (cases) which can be attributed to exposure. This proportion (AP_c) is obtained by dividing the rate difference by the rate among the exposed: $AP_c = (I_1 - I_0)/I_1$. This is also a parameter for the proportion of cases in the total population which can be attributed to exposure. The total population can be divided in a proportion unexposed individuals (P_0) and a proportion of exposed individuals (P_1). The incidence rate in the total population (I_1) can be calculated from $I_1 = P_0 I_0 + P_1 I_1$. The attributable proportion among the total population (AP_1) is defined as $AP_1 = (I_1 - I_0)/I_1$.

ATTRIBUTABLE RATE

See Rate Difference.

AUTOCRINE SYSTEM

A variation of the paracrine system where the hormone secreting cell and the target of the hormone are located in the same cell.

AUTOIMMUNE DIABETES MELLITUS (TYPE 1 DIABETES MELLITUS)

Diabetes mellitus due to autoimmune destruction of the insulin-producing pancreatic islet cells. The prevalence of type 1 diabetes appears to be approximately 0.12% of the U.S. population. This prevalence is a far smaller number than that for type 2. In autoimmune disease, the insulin-producing pancreatic islet cell is destroyed because the immune system has sensed the presence of an antigen that it recognizes, not as a self-made protein, but as a foreign protein. It then destroys this protein. The interleukins are involved in the autoimmune process and so too is apoptosis.

Autoimmune diabetes can be accompanied by a number of other diseases and multiple endocrine failure. This means that autoimmune diabetes can be found in a person who also develops psoriasis, rheumatoid arthritis, or thyroiditis (inflammation of the thyroid gland). In autoimmune diabetes, there may be an immune tolerance that is particularly difficult to break. This is because the body may lack antibody specificity. Antibodies can be raised that will react to a group of closely related compounds in an instance of "mistaken identity." Usually, an antibody reacts to a single antigen rather than to a group of closely related antigens. In autoimmune disease, the body tolerates a range of exposures to these antigens before it reacts. Thus, the term *immune tolerance* means that the individual will tolerate a wide range of exposures to an antigen or group of antigens before a systemic immunologic reaction is elicited. This is not the same thing as food allergies, skin allergies, or localized reactions to allergens nor should this term, *immune tolerance*, be confused with diseases of the immune system per se.

Autoimmunity is characterized by an increase in the number of T cells. The T cell originates in the thymus and is a type of cell that is an essential component of the immune system. It recognizes antigens and produces antibodies to them. In some instances, the recognition is nonspecific. That is, antibodies are produced that react to a group of related antigens. This occurs in autoimmune disease. There is a loss in specificity with the result of a progressive autoimmunologically mediated destruction of the islet cells. Immunosuppression can interfere with this destruction but the use of such drugs has its own set of problems such as kidney disease or increased susceptibility to infectious disease. The immunologic response is initiated when the T cell receptor recognizes an antigen on the correct histocompatability complex on the surface of antigen-presenting cell. Transmission of this signal to the nucleus of the cell involves the calcium ion, a complex of related proteins, and the phosphatidylinositol cycle, which is responsible for the movement of the calcium ion from the intracellular store to where it is needed. Antigens are then produced.

Several cell surface proteins have been found to stimulate antibody production in susceptible individuals. In autoimmune diabetes, the destruction of the β cell in the islets of Langerhans appears to be associated with one or more mutations in the genes that encode the major histocompatibility complex (MHC). More than 100 genes are involved. These genes have been mapped to the short arm of chromosome 6 and comprise approximately 2×10^6 nucleotides. Mutations in these genes have been divided into two classes (I and II) and are further identified by letter designations. There are so many genes that it would be impossible to list them all. Suffice to say that the class II HLA genes are more closely linked to autoimmune diabetes than are the class I HLA genes. The development of autoimmune diabetes is associated with an inflammation of the pancreatic islet cells (insulitis). In insulitis, CD4 and CD8 T cells, B cells, macrophages, and killer T cells have been found. The presence of these marker cells indicates that an immunologic reaction is taking place.

In humans with autoimmune diabetes, islet cell antibodies to cytoplasmic antigens can be detected. One of these is glutamic acid decarboxylase (GAD), an enzyme found in β cells that catalyzes the synthesis of the neurotransmitter, gamma aminobutyric acid (GABA). Islet β cells, like neuronal cells, possess a mechanism for hormone release that depends on a specific trophic stimulus. GABA and GAD are components of this secretion signaling system as is the glucose transporter, the enzyme, glucokinase, and the mitochondrial oxidative phosphorylation system that produces ATP. ATP and the calcium ion are major players in the insulin release mechanism. Autoantibodies to GAD have been observed prior to the development of the clinical state, and the presence of these antibodies has been suggested as an early indication of the disease.

AUTOIMMUNITY

The destruction of self through the development of antibodies to the body's own proteins. It is the result of a loss in antigen recognition specificity. The body produces antibodies to closely related proteins. A number of diseases are thought to be autoimmune diseases. These include thyroiditis, autoimmune type 1 diabetes mellitus, psoriasis, rheumatoid arthritis, and lupus.

AUTONOMIC NERVOUS SYSTEM

The system that includes portions of the brain, spinal cord, and adrenals and that serves to regulate the synthesis and release of epinephrine, the enkephalins, and norepinephrine.

AUTOPHAGY

Consumption of self as occurs when cells regenerate; some cell structures are destroyed, and the components of these structures are reused or catabolized. It can also refer to self-destructive behavior, as in nail-biting.

AUTORADIOGRAPHY

Detection of radioactive molecules by visualization on photographic film.

AUTOSOMAL RECESSIVE TRAIT

A genetic trait that will express itself only if the individual inherits two identical copies of the same gene (one from each parent). It refers (usually) to a mutated gene on any chromosome except the X or Y chromosomes (the sex chromosomes).

AUTOSOMAL TRAIT

A genetic trait or characteristic carried on any of the chromosomes except the sex chromosomes.

AUTOSOMES

All chromosomes except for the X and Y sex chromosomes; a diplod cell contains two copies of each autosome.

AUTOXIDATION

Reaction of an organic compound with elemental oxygen under mild conditions. Compounds such as polyunsaturated fatty acids, alcohols, phenols, and amines may undergo autoxidation. Free fatty acids are more susceptible to autoxidation than the fatty acids attached to glycerol as part of triacyglycerides.

AVIDIN

A glycoprotein found in raw egg white that binds biotin rendering this vitamin unavailable to the consumer. If the egg is cooked, the avidin is denatured and no longer binds biotin. Avidin is an antinutrient.

AVITAMINOSIS

Vitamin deficient state.

AZO DYES

Additives involved in idiosyncratic food intolerance reactions. Tartrazine, a yellow azo dye, is frequently associated with these reactions. In Europe, it is used in lemonades, puddings, ice cream, mayonnaise, sweets, and preservatives. Urticaria and angioedema sometimes are associated with the ingestion of this dye.

AZOTEMIA

Elevation of urea and other nitrogenous waste products in the blood due to renal failure.

B

β ADRENERGIC BLOCKERS

Drugs used to control blood pressure.

β-ALANINE

A naturally occurring form of alanine that is not incorporated into protein but is an essential component of coenzyme A, pantothenic acid, and carnosine.

β-CAROTENE

Precursor of active vitamin A. β-carotene provides some of the rich yellow and orange color of vegetables rich in this substance. Carrots are an example.

β CASMORPHIN

A component of milk with opioid activity.

B CELLS

Lymphocytic cells produced in the bone marrow that are not processed further by the thymus gland.

β CELLS

Cells in the islets of Langerhans in the endocrine pancreas that release insulin upon a glucose signal. When these cells are destroyed either through autoimmune destruction, viral-mediated destruction, or through chemicals such as alloxan or streptozotocin, insulin-dependent diabetes mellitus results.

β-HYDROXYBUTYRATE, β-HYDROXYBUTYRIC ACID

Included in the group of compounds called ketone bodies. It is actually an acid. It is synthesized by the reduction of acetoacetate via β-hydroxybutyrate dehydrogenase with NAD^+ as the hydrogen acceptor.

β OXIDATION

Process in the mitochondria for the oxidation of fatty acids. (See Metabolic Maps, Fatty-acid Oxidation, Appendix 2.)

B VITAMINS

A group of vitamins that generally are water soluble. These include thiamin (B_1), riboflavin (B_2), niacin (B_3, nicotinic acid, nicotinamide), pyridoxine (B_6, pryridoxal, pyridoxamine), folacin (folate, folic acid), vitamin B_{12} (cobalamin), pantothenic acid (pantothenate), and biotin.

BABY BOTTLE SYNDROME

Extensive dental caries that form in children allowed to nurse on bottles of fluid that contain carbohydrate. Usually the syndrome is noted in children less than two years of age who have been habitually put to bed with a bottle of milk or juice.

BACLOFEN

An γ-aminobutyric acid (GABA) analog that serves as a muscle relaxant. Trade names: Lioresal, Lioresalintrathecal.

BACTERIAL TOXINS

Toxins produced by bacteria. According to the mechanisms underlying the effects of bacterial toxins, they can be classified as follows:

- Subunit bacterial toxins
- Membrane-affecting bacterial toxins
- Lesion-causing bacterial toxins
- Immunoactive bacterial toxins

BACTERIOPHAGE

Bacteria eater.

BAKING SODA

Leavening agent that releases CO_2 when wet. The gas is trapped in the dough mix, giving volume and fragility or tenderness to the mix when baked.

BALANCE METHOD

A method that quantitates intake versus excretion of a given nutrient. When balance is positive, intake exceeds excretion; when negative, excretion exceeds intake.

BALSALAZIDE DISODIUM

An anti-inflamatory drug especially useful in the treatment of gastrointestinal tract ailments. Trade name: Colazal.

BARBITURATES

Sedatives that can be habit forming if misused.

BARDET-BIEDL SYNDROME

A genetic disorder characterized by obesity, mental retardation, polydactyly (extra fingers or toes), and hypogonadism.

BARIATRIC SURGERY

Surgical technique that reduces the size of the stomach and partially ablates the small intestine with the goal of reducing the absorptive capacity of the gastrointestinal system. Other surgical techniques can also be included in this group of techniques designed to help the obese individual reduce their fat stores. Removal of a portion of the omental fat pad, cosmetic surgery to reduce the skin folds after fat is lost, and other procedures can be included in the techniques used by the bariatric surgeon.

BARIATRICS

A medical term referring to the management of people who are overfat or obese.

BARIUM

A radiopaque mineral used in the X-ray examination of the gastrointestinal tract.

BARORECEPTORS

Sensory nerve endings in the walls of the auricles of the heart, carotid artery sinus, vena cava, and aortic arch that respond to changes in pressure.

BASAL ENERGY EXPENDITURE (BEE)

Estimated energy used by the body at rest in a fasting state to maintain essential body functions. The BEE is then adjusted for activity, injury or disease, and the thermic effect of food to predict the total daily energy expenditure. This is then used to estimate the energy intake requirement.

BASAL METABOLISM (BASAL METABOLIC RATE, BMR)

The minimum activity of metabolic processes occurring in the body. With reference to energy, it is the least amount of energy used by the body to sustain itself. When measured, the individual is at rest (not asleep), in a comfortable environment (neither shivering nor sweating), free of emotional, mental, and physical stress, and at sexual repose. The basal metabolic rate can be measured as the heat produced or as the oxygen consumed by the body under these conditions. Oxygen consumption is considered the indirect measure of basal metabolism under the assumption that energy consuming reactions which produce heat also use oxygen. Other indirect measures have been devised that relate to either heat production or oxygen use. Table 14 lists some of these methods.

BASE PAIRS

A partnership of adenosine with thymidine or cytosine with guanine in a double helix.

BASEDOW'S DISEASE

Excess thyroid hormone production. Also called Graves' disease or hyperthyroidism.

BASIC AMINO ACIDS

Amino acids whose side chains have positively charged amino groups. These are histidine, lysine, and arginine.

TABLE 14
Methods and Equations Used for Calculating Basal Energy Need

Method

1. Heat production, direct measurement (calorimetry); kcal (kJ)/m² (surface area)
2. Oxygen consumption; indirect; O_2 cons/$w^{0.75}$
3. Heat production; indirect;
   Insensible water loss (IW) = Insensible weight loss (IWL) + (CO_2 exhaled − O_2 inhaled)
   Heat production = IW × 0.58 (0.58 = kcal to evaporate 1 g water)
4. Estimate (energy need not be measured)
   BMR = 66.4730 + 13.751W + 5.0033L − 6.550A (men)
   BMR = 655.0955 + 9.463W + 1.8496L − 4.6756A (women)
5. Estimate (energy need not be measured)
   BMR = $71.2W^{0.75}[1 − 0.004(30 − A) + 0.010(L/W^{0.33} − 43.4)]$ (men)
   BMR = $65.8W^{0.75}[1 + 0.004(30 − A) + 0.018(L/W^{0.33} − 42.1)]$ (women)

Source: From Berdanier, C. D., and J. Zempleni. 2009. *Advanced Nutrition: Macronutrients,*
            Micronutrients and Metabolism. 6. Boca Raton, FL: CRC Press. With permission.
Note: W = weight in kilograms; L = height in centimeters; A = age in years.

BASIC LIFE SUPPORT (BLS)

Resuscitation techniques involving the mechanical support of respiration and heart action.

BAT (BROWN ADIPOSE TISSUE) THERMOGENESIS

Heat produced by BAT located at the base of the neck, beneath the sternum, and under the shoulder blades. Brown adipose tissue is brown because its cells contain many more mitochondria than white fat cells. BAT mitochondria produce heat when stimulated by catecholamines.

BCAA

Branched chain amino acids. These are valine, leucine, and isoleucine.

BECLOMETHASONE DIPROPIONATE

A synthetic glucocorticoid that acts as an anti-inflammatory, antiasthmatic medication. Trade name: QVAR.

BEE

Basal energy expenditure.

BEEF TEA

Beef broth.

BEHAVIOR MODIFICATION

Self-monitoring techniques useful in weight control that provides individuals with new methods to apply to current overeating situations.

BENAZEPRIL HYDROCHLORIDE

An antihypertensive drug that is an ACE inhibitor. Trade name: Lotensin.

BENZEDRINE

A member of the amphetamine family of drugs that are stimulants and appetite suppressants.

BENZMALACENE

A compound that blocks sterol synthesis between isopentyl pyrophosphate and farnesyl phosphate.

BEPRIDIL HYDROCHLORIDE

A drug that acts as a calcium channel blocker and is used as an antianginal medication. Trade name: Vascor.

BERI BERI

Thiamin deficiency disease characterized by neural disorders, accumulation of fluid in the heart sac, impaired heart action, anorexia, and muscle pain. Table 15 gives the characteristics of this disease. It is often seen in alcoholism. The most serious form of thiamin deficiency in alcoholics is Wernicke's syndrome. It is characterized by ophthalmoplegia, sixth nerve palsy, nystagmus, ptosis, ataxia, confusion, and coma, which may terminate in death. Often the confusional state persists after treatment of the acute thiamin deficiency. This is known as Korsakoff's psychosis.

TABLE 15
Clinical Features of Thiamin Deficiency

Wet and dry beri beri	Malaise
	Heaviness and weakness of legs
	Calf muscle tenderness
	"Pins and needles" and numbness in legs
	Anesthesia of skin, particularly at the tibia
	Increased pulse rate and palpitations
Wet beri beri	Edema of legs, face, and trunk and serous cavities
	Tense calf muscles
	Fast pulse
	Distended neck veins
	High blood pressure
	Decreased urine volume
Dry beri beri	Worsening of polyneuritis of early stage
	Difficulty walking
	Wernicke-Korsakoff syndrome; encephalopathy may occur
	Disorientation
	Loss of immediate memory
	Nystagmus (jerky movements of the eyes)
	Ataxia (staggering gait)

BETAINE

Precursor of choline.

BETEL NUTS

Nuts from the areta palm; when chewed, these nuts have a stimulant effect.

BIAS

A measure of inaccuracy or departure from accuracy.

BICARBONATE

Any salt containing HCO_3; bicarbonate in the blood is indicative of the alkali reserve.

BIFIDUS FACTOR

Compound in human milk that inhibits growth of particular bacteria in the digestive tract.

BIGUANIDES

Antihyperglycemic drugs useful in controlling elevated blood glucose levels in type 2 diabetes mellitus. One such drug is metformin. Trade name: Glucophage.

BILE

Fluid produced by the liver and stored in the gall bladder which releases this fluid in response to a variety of gut hormonal signals (primarily cholecystokinen). Bile contains bile acids that exist as salts.

BILE ACID SEQUESTRANTS

Group of medications used to treat hypercholesterolemia.

BILE ACIDS

Cholic and chenodeoxycholic acid are synthesized by the liver from cholesterol. These acids are present as anions and are referred to as bile salts. At pH values above 7.4, bile salts form aggregates with fats at concentrations above 2–5 mM. These aggregates are called micelles. The primary bile acids are secreted into the intestine, and the intestinal flora convert these acids to their conjugated forms by dehydroxylating carbon 7. Further metabolism occurs at the far end of the intestinal tract where lithocholate is sulfated. The dehydroxylated acids can be reabsorbed and sent back to the liver via the portal blood, whereas the sulfated lithocholate is not and appears in the feces. All four of the bile acids, the primary and dehydroxylated forms, are recirculated via the enterohepatic system such that very little of the bile acids is lost. It has been estimated that the bile acid lost in the feces (~0.8 g/day) equals that newly synthesized by the liver such that the total pool remains between 3–5 g. The amount secreted per day is in the order of 16–70 g. Since the pool size is only 3–5 g, this means that these acids are recirculated as much as 14 times a day. The function of the bile acids is thus quite similar to that of enzymes. Neither are "used up" by the processes they participate in and facilitate. In fat absorption, the bile acids facilitate the formation of micelles, which in turn facilitate the uptake of the dietary fatty acids, monoglycerides, sterols, phospholipids, and other fat-soluble nutrients by the enterocyte of the small intestine.

BILE PIGMENTS

Breakdown products of the heme portion of hemoglobin, myoglobin, and the cytochromes (bilirubin, biliverdin, and heme).

BILE SALTS

Anionic forms of bile acids. Glycocholate is a combination of cholyl CoA with glycine; taurocholate is a combination of cholyl CoA with taurine.

BILIARY CALCULI

Stones in the biliary tree. If vessels are blocked by these stones, biliary cirrhosis results.

BILIRUBIN

A bile pigment resulting from the breakdown of heme, the nonprotein, iron-containing portion of hemoglobin. In excessive hemoglobin breakdown, bilirubin may spill into the blood and produces a deep yellow color in the skin. This is called jaundice. Excess billirubin in the blood is called bilirubinemia.

BILIVERDIN

The product of the first step in heme catabolism.

BIOAVAILABILITY

Quantity of nutrient available to the body after absorption. Bioavailability is a particular concern in the absorption of essential minerals. In this setting, bioavailability is defined as the percent of the consumed mineral that enters via the intestine and is used for its intended purpose.

BIOELECTRICAL IMPEDENCE

The measure of resistance to an alternating current in a body. Used to estimate percent body fat and body water.

BIOFLAVONOIDS (FLAVONOIDS)

A group of yellow pigments in plants that have biological activity but are not considered essential nutrients. These are compounds that are phenolic derivatives of 2-phenyl-1,4benzopyrone and that assist vitamin C as an antioxidant. They also act to suppress inflammatory mediators. Common flavonoids in human foods are quercetin, (-)-epicatechin, epigallocatechingallate. Increases in dietary flavonol intake may lower stroke risk.

BIOGENIC AMINES

Formed in the body by decarboxylation of amino acids. They can be found in food plants. Large dietary intakes of foods containing these amines can pose some risk of harm. Biogenic amines in food can originate from fermentation of that food or from bacterial contamination. The main producers of biogenic amines in foods are Enterobacteriaceae and Enterococci. Examples of biogenic amines include ethylamine (precursor: alanine), putrescine (precursor: ornithine), histamine (precursor: histidine), cadaverine (precursor: lysine), tyramine (precursor: tyrosine), phenylethylamine (precursor: phenylalanine), and tryptamine (precursor: tryptophan). Symptoms of biogenic amine intoxication, persisting for several hours, include burning throat, flushing, headache, nausea, hypertension, numbness, and tingling of the lips, rapid pulse, and vomiting. Factors stimulating the formation of biogenic amines include the following: presence of free amino acids, acting as precursors; low pH of the product; high NaCl concentration; and microbial decarboxylase activity. Occurrence of biogenic amines has been reported in lactate-fermented products, in particular wine, cheese, fish, and meat, and in fermented vegetables. Natural occurrences of biogenic amines (produced by microbial decarboxylase activity) have been reported in fruits, vegetables, and fish. Pasteurization of cheese and milk, good hygienic practices, and selection of bacterial cultures having low decarboxylase activity can prevent the accumulation of biogenic amines.

BIOLOGICAL VALUE OF PROTEINS

A measure of the nutritional quality of a dietary protein. It takes into consideration its availability and its amino acid composition in terms of the amino acid needs of the consumer. Foods containing high-quality proteins are usually from animal sources (milk, eggs, meat, cheese, etc.), while poor-quality proteins are usually (but not always) from plants.

BIOMARKER

A measurement of a particular enzyme, substrate, or specific characteristic of cells, tissues, or whole animals that characterizes and identifies that particular biological system.

BIOPSY

The removal of a very small amount of tissue from a selected site.

BIOTIN

A water-soluble member of the B family of vitamins. An important coenzyme in fatty acid synthesis and in pyruvate metabolism. Carboxylases require biotin attached to a lysine residue for activity. The oxidation of odd-chain fatty acids also requires biotin, as does gluconeogenesis. Biotin is the trivial name for the compound, cis-hexahydro-2-oxo-1H-thieno (3,4-d) imidazole-4-pentanoic acid. Its structure is shown in Figure 8. In order to have vitamin activity, the structure must contain a conjoined ureido and tetrahydro-thiophene ring and the ureido $3^{l}N$ must be sterically hindered, preventing substitution. The ureido $1^{l}N$ is a poor nucleophile.

BIOTINASE

An enzyme that will cleave protein-bound biotin. Biotinase has been cloned and sequenced and its distribution throughout the body determined. Although it is active in the intestinal tract, its activity

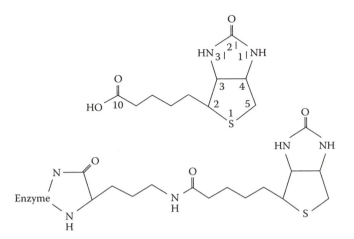

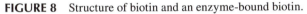

FIGURE 8   Structure of biotin and an enzyme-bound biotin.

is not sufficient to catalyze all of the bound biotin found in food. It is an enzyme needed for biotin recycling.

Biotin occurs in eight isomeric forms, but only D-biotin has vitamin activity. Several biotin analogs have been synthesized or isolated from natural sources. Among these are oxybiotin or biotinol, biocytin, dethiobiotin, and biotin sulfoxide. The latter two are inactive as vitamins, whereas the first two have some vitamin activity albeit less than that of D-biotin.

Biotin is a white crystalline substance that in its dry form is stable to air, heat, and light. Its molecular weight is 244.3 and melting point is 167°. It decomposes at 230°C–232°C. It has a limited solubility in water (22 mg/mL HOH) and is more soluble in ethanol. In solution, it is unstable to oxygen and strong acid or alkaline conditions and will be gradually destroyed by ultraviolet light.

SOURCES

There are numerous food sources for biotin. Biotin is found in every living cell in minute amounts, where it exists either in its enzyme-bound form or as a biotin ester or an amide. Rich sources include organ meats, egg yolk, brewer's yeast, and royal jelly. Soy flour or soybean, rice polishings, various ocean fish, and whole grains are good sources of the vitamin.

ABSORPTION AND METABOLISM

Biotin in food exists in the free and enzyme-bound form. The protein-bound form can be digested, which in turn yields biocytin, a combination of biotin and lysine. Biocytin is hydrolyzed via the action of biotinase to its component parts. The resultant biotin is then available for absorption. Biotin is absorbed via a carrier-mediated process that is shared with pantothenic acid and lipoate. The jejunum is the major site for this absorption. Once absorbed, it circulates as free biotin. There may be some species differences in absorptive mechanism. In addition, there is synthesis of the biotin by the gut flora. Biotinidase cleaves biotin from its protein-bound form. Instances of mutation in the gene for this enzyme have been reported. Such a mutation is an autosomal recessive disorder that results in a secondary biotin deficiency. The effects of the mutation can be overcome if large quantities of supplemental biotin are provided. The clinical symptoms of this genetic disorder are the same as those of the biotin deficient state, and they relate to the function of biotin as a coenzyme in intermediary metabolism, especially the carboxylase reactions.

Biotin can be rendered unavailable by avidin, a protein found in raw egg white. Once the egg is cooked, the avidin is denatured and no longer binds the biotin. This binding is the explanation of the disorder "egg white injury." Other proteins, particularly membrane and transport proteins, bind biotin and are responsible for its entry into all cells that use the vitamin.

FUNCTION

Biotin influences transcription in all living organisms. Biotinylation of lysine-12 in histone H4 represses long-term terminal repeat retrotransposons. This brings stability to the nuclear genome. Biotin is part of a ligase that catalyzes post transcriptional biotin addition to the biotin-dependent carboxylase and to the histones. Biotin serves as a mobile carboxyl carrier, as it is attached to enzymes that catalyze carboxyl group transfer. A number of enzymes require biotin as a prosthetic group for their function. These are listed in Table 16.

Biotin is involved in the reactions of inflammation. Biotin-deficient animals are more susceptible to stimulators of inflammation than are normal animals.

DEFICIENCY

In man, the symptoms of severe deficiency include dermatitis, skin rash, hair loss (alopecia), developmental delay, seizures, conjunctivitis, visual and auditory loss, metabolic keto lactic acidosis, hyperammonemia, and organic acidemia. These symptoms have been reported in persons lacking normal biotinase activity through a genetic error. In a genetically normal human population, a true biotin deficiency is extremely rare. Only a few instances have been reported. In one, the deficient state was caused by the chronic consumption of 30 raw eggs/day for several months. In this individual, the symptoms were primarily related to the skin. Teratogenic effects of biotin deficiency have been reported in mice.

RECOMMENDED INTAKE

At present, there is no recommended intake for biotin. Because the vitamin is present in a wide variety of foods and because it can be synthesized by the intestinal flora, a fixed intake figure has been difficult to determine. However, the National Academy of Sciences, Food and Nutrition Board has published a safe and adequate dietary intake for this vitamin. These suggested intakes are shown in Table 17.

TABLE 16
Biotin-Dependent Enzymes in Animals

Enzyme	Role	Location
Pyruvate carboxylase	First reaction in pathway that converts 3-carbon precursors to glucose (gluconeogenesis)	Mitochondria (rate limiting step in gluconeogenesis)
	Replenishes oxaloacetate for citric acid cycle	
Acetyl-CoA carboxylase	Commits acetate units to fatty acid synthesis by forming malonyl-CoA	Cytosol (rate limiting step in fatty acid synthesis)
Propionyl-CoA carboxylase	Converts propionate to succinate, which can then enter citric acid cycle	Mitochondria
β-methylcrotonyl-CoA carboxylase	Catabolism of leucine and certain isoprenoid compounds	Mitochondria

TABLE 17
Safe and Adequate Dietary Intake of Biotin (µg/day)

Infants	0–6 months	35 µg
	7–12 months	50 µg
Children	1–3 years	65 µg
	4–6 years	85 µg
	7–10 years	120 µg
Adolescents, adults		100–200 µg

See http://www.nap.edu.

BISACODYL

Laxative. Trade names: Correctol, Dulcolax, Feen-a-mint.

BISMUTH SUBSALICYLATE

An antidiarrheal agent and an adsorbent. Trade names: Bismatrol, Pepto-Bismol, Pink Bismuth.

BISOPROLOL FUMARATE

An antihypertensive agent that acts as a beta blocker. Trade name: Zebeta.

BITOT'S SPOTS

Shiny foam-like spots on the white of the eye; often observed in malnutrition.

BIVALIRUDIN

Anticoagulant. Trade name: Angiomax.

BLACK TONGUE

A disease seen in dogs due to niacin deficiency; the canine equivalent of pellagra.

BLANCHING

A processing technique involving brief exposure of foods to boiling water. Blanching wilts the leaf structure of plants, inhibits the peroxidation of fats and oils, and results in inactivation of a variety of enzymes that contribute to food spoilage.

BLAND DIET

Diet designed to potentially avoid irritation of the gastrointestinal tract and to decrease peristalsis. Considerable variability exists among diet manuals for foods allowed on a bland diet; many health care facilities do not use a bland diet because the diet does not decrease gastric acid secretion or increase healing rate of peptic ulcers. Peptic ulcers have been found to be the result of a bacterial infection and are usually treated with antibiotics.

BLEPHARITIS

Inflammation of the eyelids.

BLIND LOOP SYNDROME

Condition resulting from an undesirable change in the anatomy of the small intestine where a loop is formed in which intestinal contents enter but cannot leave.

BLOOD CLOTTING

See Vitamin K. Blood clotting occurs in response to injury. The formation of the clot is a cascade of reactions involving both intrinsic and extrinsic factors. A deficiency of vitamin K prolongs the blood clotting time. Blood clots can also occur internally within the vascular system. The initiation signal for these clots is not completely known.

BLOOD COMPOSITION

The composition of blood in addition to water includes a number of proteins, metabolites, minerals, and vitamins. Some of these components are shown in Table 18.

BLOOD GLUCOSE

Normal fasting level ranges between 80 and 120 mg/dL or 4 and 6 mmol/L.

BLOOD PRESSURE

The pressure exerted on the vascular tree by the pumping action of the heart. Normal blood pressure is 120 (systolic) over 80 (diastolic) mm mercury. Pressure is measured by a sphygmomanometer.

- Hypotension—low blood pressure
- Hypertension—high blood pressure

TABLE 18
Composition of Serum and Cell Fluid in Normal Human Blood

	Serum mM/Kg	mEq/L	Cell Fluid mM/Kg	mEq/L
Urea	7	–	7	–
Glucose	4	–	4	–
Other organic compounds	Variable	–	Variable	–
Sodium	150	150	27	27
Potassium	4	4	135	135
Calcium	3	5	0	0
Magnesium	1	2	3	5
Chloride	111	111	74	74
Bicarbonate	28	28	27	27
Inorganic phosphate	2	3	2	3
Organic phosphate	Trace	–	21	–
Sulfate	1	1	–	–
Protein	1	18	7	62
Total milliosmoles	312		307	
Total mEq/L	322		333	

BLOOD UREA NITROGEN (BUN)

Biochemical test used to evaluate renal excretory capacity and to diagnose renal disease. The level of urea in the blood is 8–20 mg/dL or 2.86–7.14 mmol/L.

BLUNT-ENDED DNA

Two strands of a DNA duplex having ends that are flush with each other.

BMI

Body mass index = body weight (kg)/height (cm)^2. Used as a general index of body fatness; however, it does not apply to persons with high muscle mass such as elite athletes.

BMR

Basal metabolic rate. The minimal amount of energy needed to sustain the body's metabolism. Frequently expressed in terms of the amount of oxygen used to sustain this metabolism because of the constancy between energy flux and oxygen use.

BODY CELL MASS

The metabolically active, energy requiring mass of the body.

BODY COMPOSITION

The body consists of fat, protein, water, and ash (minerals). Normal bodies usually consist of 16%–20% protein, 3%–5% ash (mineral matter), 10%–12% fat, and 60%–70% water. Age, diet, genetic background, physical activity, hormonal status, and gender can affect not only the proximate composition of the whole body, that is, the magnitude of each of these components, but also their distribution.

Lean body mass can be predicted from skeletal measurements and from bone weight. Sophisticated techniques using ultrasound, neutron activation analysis, infrared interactance, dual energy X-ray absorptiometry, computer-assisted tomography, magnetic resonance imaging, or bio-electrical impedance are available for the determination of body composition. As the instrumentation improves, these methods may become practical in the clinical setting. These methods are noninvasive and allow for the sequential determination of changes in one or more of the major body components as a result of dietary change, activity change, age, or a change in endocrine status. Dual energy X-ray absorptiometry (DEXA) is one method in common use. It can estimate bone density and soft tissue composition. Bone density as a fraction of the fat free mass can be distinguished and quantitated as can the fat mass. The remaining tissue is the lean body mass. One can then distinguish and quantitate the muscle mass using its creatine content.

If one assumes that the major component of the lean is the muscle, one can determine the muscle mass using the dilution of radioactive creatine or creatine labeled with a heavy nonradioactive isotope. This has been used successfully in rats and may be applicable to humans because creatine is almost exclusively located in the muscle. Labeled creatine must be infused, and after a set interval, a muscle biopsy is obtained. The total muscle mass can be calculated using the $C_1/C_2 = V_2/V_1$ equation as follows:

$$\frac{\text{Total }^{14}\text{C creatine infused}}{[^{14}\text{C creatine}] \text{ in sample}} = \frac{\text{Muscle sample size}}{\text{Total muscle mass}}$$

Based on the assumption that lean body mass has a constant potassium content and that neutral fat does not bind the electrolyte, lean body mass can also be estimated by measuring the body content of the heavy potassium isotope ^{40}K or by measuring the dilution of ^{42}K (the radioactive isotope) in the body cells. The former requires a whole body scintillation counter, whereas the latter can be determined in a small tissue (muscle biopsy) sample. The formula for calculating lean body mass is as follows:

$$ LBM = \frac{Total\ K\ content}{Concentration\ of\ K/kg\ tissue} $$

Either of these methods may underestimate the lean body mass because of the lack of corrections for the small amounts of potassium in the extracellular fluids.

Lean body mass and percent fat can be estimated using measures of body density or specific gravity of the individual. The fat-free body will have a specific gravity of 1.1000. This will decrease as the body increases its fat content since fat has a lower (~0.92) specific gravity than the fat free body mass. Thus, the fatter the subject, the lower the specific gravity or density. The body density can be determined in the adult using Archimedes' principle. The subject is weighed in air and again when immersed in water. The difference in the two body weights is the weight of the body that is water. Since water has a density of 1 (1 mL of water weighs 1 g), the volume of the water displaced represents both the volume of the body immersed and its density. The immersion weight/unit volume of water displaced then is diluted by the air weight/unit volume of water displaced, which in turn is the specific gravity of the subject. Corrections for the residual air in the lungs and intestines must be made. There are a number of reports on body density and body fat using this technique. Age affects body density and percent body fat. In one study of women of different ages, it was found that young (16–40 years of age) women had body densities ranging from 1.0342 g/mL to 1.0343 g/mL and percent body fats of 28.69–28.75. Older women (50–70 years of age) had body densities which ranged from 1.0095 g/mL to 1.0050 g/mL and percent body fats of 41.88–44.56. Body fat can be estimated using the Siri et al. equation:

$$ fat\ \% = \frac{2.118 - 1.354 - 0.78}{density} \cdot \left(\frac{\%\ TBW}{body\ weight} \right) $$

where 2.118, 1.354, and 0.78 are constants, and the density (g/cm^3), body weight (kg), and total body water (TBW) in kg are determined.

Other prediction equations for percent fat from specific gravity are available. One devised by Siri et al. allows one to calculate % fat = 100 (5.548 – 5.044)/Specific gravity. The Pace-Rathbun method calculates percent fat using the formula:

$$ \%\ fat = 100 - TBW/0.732 $$

The Pace-Rathbun method is based on TBW only and compensates for the structural lipids (those in cell membranes, etc., as contrasted to the depot lipids) by adding 3%. This gives a lean body mass that is somewhat different from that of Siri et al. Another technique for estimating body fatness is the measurement of skinfold thicknesses at different locations of the body. Table 19 gives the general formulas for calculating body fatness from these measurements.

For population surveys where close estimates of body fat, protein, lean body mass, and so on, are not critical, simpler estimates of body fatness are frequently used. Using the patient's body weight and height, one can compare these values to those considered desirable for men and women.

A broader database using subjects of all ages, economic status, both sexes, and from minority and majority cultural or ethnic groups was obtained by the National Health and Nutrition Examination

---

TABLE 19
General Formulas for Calculating Body Fatness from Skinfold Measurements

Males:

% Body fat $= 29.288 \times 10^{-2}(X) - 5 \times 10^{-4}(X)^2 + 15.845 \times 10^{-2}(\text{age})$

Females:

% Body fat $= 29.699 \times 10^{-2}(X) - 43 \times 10^{-5}(X)^2 + 29.63 \times 10^{-3}(\text{age}) + 1.4072$

where X = sum of abdomen, suprailiac, triceps, and thigh skinfolds and age is in years.

Source: From Jackson, A. S., and M. L. Pollack. 1985. *Physician Sports Med* 13:76–90. With permission.

Survey (NHANES). These surveys have been conducted at intervals by the Centers for Disease Control of the U.S. Department of Health and Human Services. The surveys have collected data not only from young adult men and women but also from children and aging adults. The weights and heights have been used to create tables giving weight ranges for males and females. In addition, NHANES made detailed measurements of skinfold thickness, skeletal size and density, and a variety of biochemical and physiological features using a representative subset of the population assessed. The NHANES tables are useful in comparing population groups.

Perhaps more popular now is the use of body mass index (BMI). This is a useful term in that it is an index of the body weight (kg) divided by the height (meters) squared (wt/ht^2). BMI correlates with body fatness and with the risk of obesity-related disease or diseases for which obesity is a compounding factor. Overweight is defined as BMI between 25 and 30 and obesity as BMI over 30. The BMI varies with age. A desirable BMI for people aged 19–24 is between 19 and 24, while that for people aged 55–64 is between 23 and 28. While simple in concept, this term does not assess body composition per se. It only provides a basis for assessing the health risks associated or presumed to be associated with excess body fatness. BMI applies only to normal individuals not the super athlete or the body builder who may be quite heavy yet have little body fat.

While total body fatness is an important risk factor for several degenerative diseases, the distribution of the stored fat may impact upon these disease states as well. Males and females differ in the pattern of body fat stores. Males tend to deposit fat in the abdominal area, while females tend to deposit fat in the gluteal area. Measuring the waist and hip circumference allows one to compute the waist to hip ratio (WHR), and as this ratio increases so too does the risk for cardiovascular disease, diabetes mellitus, and hypertension. In men, if the WHR is greater than 0.90 and in women if the WHR is greater than 0.80, the risk for cardiovascular disease increases.

BODY DENSITY

Weight (mass) per unit volume.

BODY FRAME SIZE

Determined by measuring wrist circumference at the smallest circumference distal to the styloid process of the radius and ulna and comparing to established classifications as small, medium, or large body frame.

BODY-ORIENTED FOOD CHEMICALS

Food chemicals in the form of nutrients, which are necessary for growth, maintenance, and reproduction of living organisms. They are divided into two groups: (1) macronutrients (fats, carbohydrates, and proteins), and (2) micronutrients (vitamins and minerals, including trace elements).

BOLUS

Single large dose of a substance sometimes administered as a pill and sometimes as a solution.

BOMB CALORIMETER

The bomb calorimeter is an instrument used to measure heat production when a known amount of food is completely oxidized. It is a highly insulated box-like container. All the heat produced during the oxidation of a dried sample of food is absorbed by a weighed amount of water surrounding the combustion chamber. A thermometer registers the change in the chamber temperature. The instrument's name is derived from the design of the combustion chamber, which is a small bomb. The energy value of protein foods obtained in this manner is higher than the actual biologic value because in biologic systems, the end products of oxidation must be excreted as urea, a process that costs energy. For instance, in a bomb calorimeter, the combustion or oxidation of protein yields 5.6 calories (23.5 kJ)/g; the energy yield from the oxidation of protein after correction for urea formation and digestive loss by the body is about 4 calories (16.8 kJ)/g. Corrections for digestive losses are also applied to the values obtained for the combustion of lipids and carbohydrates. The value of 4.1 calories (17.22 kJ)/g is rounded off to 4 (16.8 kJ) for carbohydrates and the value of 9.4 (39.5 kJ) for lipids is rounded off to 9 (37.8 kJ). See http://www.nal.usda.gov/fnic/foodcomp/Data/foods.82nutrients for an extensive list of foods and their energy value.

BOMBESIN

A 14-amino acid peptide hormone found in the CNS, the thyroid gland, lung, adrenal, and skin. It raises blood glucose level, lowers body temperature, increases locomotor activity, and raises the pain threshold. It also signals satiety and thus plays a role in food intake regulation. As a neuropeptide, bombesin is found in all neurons of the CNS. It is found in large quantities in the hypothalamus where it functions as a modulary agent altering dopamine metabolism. Bombesin is also known as gastrin-releasing peptide. In the intestinal tract, the action of bombesin opposes that of somatostatin. It directly stimulates pancreatic enzyme release and gastric acid secretion.

BORON

A mineral needed in very small amounts. Found in the bone mineral.

BOSENTAN

Drug that is an endothelin antagonist and thus serves as an antihypertensive drug. Trade name: Tracleer.

BOTULISM

One of the diseases caused by "food poisoning." (See Foodborne Disease.) A bacterial intoxication caused by ingestion of food contaminated by toxins of *Clostridium botulinum* or *Clostridium parabotulinum*.

BOWEL

Synonym for large intestine; sometimes includes the small intestine as well.

BOWMAN'S CAPSULE

The capsule surrounding the glomerulus, the filtration unit of the kidney.

BRADYCARDIA

A slow heart rate characterized by a pulse less than 60 beats per minute.

BRANCHED CHAIN AMINO ACIDS

A group of amino acids (leucine, isoleucine, valine) metabolized by muscle tissue rather than the liver.

BRIGHT'S DISEASE

Kidney disease.

BROMOCRIPTINE MESYLATE

A dopamine receptor agonist that is a semisynthetic ergot alkaloid. It is used in the treatment of Parkinson's disease. It is also an inhibitor of prolactin release and growth hormone release. Trade name: Pariodel.

BROWN ADIPOSE TISSUE (BAT)

Highly vascularized adipose tissue with mitochondria-rich adipocytes. (See BAT Thermogenesis.)

BTU

British thermal unit. Amount of energy needed to raise the temperature of 1 lb of water 1°F.

BUDESONIDE

A glucocorticoid-like compound that acts as an anti-inflamatory drug. Trade name: Entocort EC.

BUFFER

A compound that resists a change in hydrogen ion concentration in solution.

BULIMIA

Habitual self-induced vomiting. It frequently accompanies anorexia nervosa and may follow binge eating. It is associated with abnormal signaling of hunger and satiety.

BUPROPION HYDROCHLORIDE

An antidepressant drug. Trade name: Wellbutrim. Also used as a nicotine replacement. Trade name: Zyban.

BUTYLATED HYDROXYANISOL (BHA)

A food additive similar in function to BHT.

BUTYLATED HYDROXYTOLUENE (BHT)

A food additive that serves as an antioxidant, particularly useful in preventing the autoxidation of unsaturated fatty acids.

C

CACHETIN

A mediator of toxic shock; a macrophage hormone with a short (6 minutes) half-life. Also called TNF.

CACHEXIA

Tissue wasting, as in a disease or overwhelming trauma or starvation.

CACOGEUSIA

The presence of a bad taste in the mouth.

CADMIUM

A mineral that is toxic.

CAFFEIC ACID

A type C antinutritive.

CAFFEINE

An alkaloid present in coffee. Has diuretic properties as well as stimulatory effects on circulation and respiration. Can also stimulate bowel movements in sensitive people.

CALBINDINS

Members of a family of tight calcium-binding proteins that are produced in response to vitamin D $(1,25 (OH)_2D_3)$ binding to its receptor in the cell. Other members of this family include calmodulin, troponin C, and parvalbumin.

CALCIDIOL

A metabolite of vitamin D; 25-hydroxyvitamin D is used to make the active form, 1,25 dihydroxy vitamin D. Synthesis of the active form takes place in the kidney.

CALCIFEROL

Synonym for vitamin D.

CALCIFICATION

Deposition of calcium as a salt of phosphate in the ground substance of bone.

CALCITONIN

Hormone secreted by the thyroid gland; functions in the maintenance of calcium homeostasis by opposing the calcium-mobilizing action of parathormone. It can also serve as a satiety signal.

CALCITROL

A vitamin D-dependent calcium absorption protein active in the intestinal tract.

CALCIUM

An essential mineral; important as a second messenger for a variety of hormones; essential in the regulation of intermediary metabolism and oxidative phosphorylation and for bone mineralization. May play a role in the control of food intake as well as in the regulation of fat synthesis and degradation (energy balance).

CALCIUM CARBONATE

Calcium supplement. Trade names: Alka-mints, Calci-chew, Chooz, Os-cal 500, Tums 500.

CALCIUM CHANNEL BLOCKERS

Drugs used to increase the pumping action of the heart.

CALCIUM GLUCONATE

Water-soluble salt of calcium.

CALCIUM POLYCARBOPHIL

Hydrophilic bulk laxative that can also be used as an antidiarrheal agent. Trade names: Equalactin, FiberCon, Fiber-Lax, FiberNorm, Mitrolan.

CALCIUM TETANY

Muscle spasms that occur when muscle calcium is deficient. Occurs in high-producing milk cows as their lactation surges after the birth of a calf. Sometimes called "milk fever," it is treated with an intravenous infusion of calcium.

CALCULUS

Synonym for gallstones or kidney stones; complex mineral precipitants.

CALMODULIN (CAM)

Calcium-dependent regulatory protein. It has four calcium-binding sites, and full occupancy of these sites leads to a marked conformational change, which in turn is related to the ability of the protein to activate or inactivate enzymes. Calmodulin is a calcium transport protein within the cell that carries calcium from the endoplasmic reticulum (where calcium is stored) to sites for its use. It is a delta subunit of phosphorylase kinase.

CALORIE (KILOCALORIE)

A unit of energy. Classical nutritionists use the term Calorie or kilocalorie (kcal) to represent the amount of heat required to raise the temperature of 1 kg of water by 1°C. The international unit of energy is the joule. One Calorie or kilocalorie is equal to 4.184 kJ or 4.2 kJ. There are cogent reasons to express energy in terms of kilojoules. Nutritionists have realized that the energy provided by food is used for more than heat production. It is also used for mechanical work (muscle movement) and for electrical signaling (vision; neuronal messages) and is stored as chemical energy. The joule is 107 ergs where 1 erg is the amount of energy expended in accelerating a mass of 1 g by 1 cm/s. The international joule is defined as the energy liberated by one international ampere flowing through a resistance of one international ohm in 1 second. Even though the use of joules or kilojoules is being urged by international scientists as a means to ease the confusion in discussions about energy, students will still find the term Calorie or kcal in many texts and references. In some texts, the term calorie, spelled with a lower case "c," is used. This heat is actually 1/1000 of the heat unit spelled with an upper case "C." Physicists use the term calorie to represent the amount of heat required to raise the temperature of 1 g of water by 1°C. Note that this definition uses 1 g, not 1 kg as stated above. Even though it is not correct, the term calorie is used in some nutrition literature when in fact Calorie or kcal is intended.

CALORIMETRY

The measurement of heat produced by the body or by food.

CALPAIN

A calcium-dependent protease involved in the degradation of protein within the cell. Also called cathepsin.

cAMP

Cyclic 3'5' adenosine monophosphate. An activator of protein kinase; serves as a second messenger for certain hormones.

CANCER

A group of diseases characterized by abnormal growth of cells which, because the growth is uncontrolled, subsumes the normal functions of vital organs and tissues.

CANDESARTAN CILEXETIL

A selective angiotensin II receptor antagonist that is an effective antihypertensive agent. Trade name: Atacand.

CANDIDATE GENE

A gene, if mutated, that is suspected to play a causal role in a clinical syndrome.

CANOLA OIL

An oil extracted from a variety of the rapeseed plant renamed canola; good source of α-linolenic acid, an unsaturated fatty acid of the omega 3 family.

CAP

The structure at the 5′ end of eukaryotic mRNA, introduced after transcription by linking the terminal phosphate of 5′GTP to the terminal base of the messenger RNA. The added G (and sometimes other bases) is methylated.

CAPTOPRIL

An ACE inhibitor that serves as an antihypertensive agent. Trade names: Apo-Capto, Capoten, Novo-Captopril.

CARBAMAZEPINE

An anticonvulsant. Trade names: Ago-Carbamazeprine, Carbatrol, Tegretol, Epitol, Novo-Carbamaz, Tegretol-XR, Teril.

CARBAMIDE PEROXIDE

A topical antiseptic. It is also useful in ear wax removal. Trade name: Debrox.

CARBOHYDRATE

Polyhydroxy aldehydes or ketones and their derivatives. The carbohydrates are divided into three major classes: monosaccharides, oligosaccharides, and polysaccharides.

STRUCTURE AND NOMENCLATURE

Monosaccharides

Monosaccharides, called simple sugars, have the empirical formula $(CH_2O)_n$, where n is 3 or more. Although monosaccharides may have as few as three or as many as nine carbon atoms, the ones of interest to the nutritionist have five or six carbon atoms. The carbon skeleton is unbranched, and each carbon atom, except one, has a hydroxyl group and a hydrogen atom. At the remaining carbon atom, there is a carbonyl group. If the carbonyl function is on the last carbon atom, the compound is an aldehyde and is called an aldose; if it occurs at any other carbon, the compound is a ketone and is called a ketose.

The simplest monosaccharide is the three-carbon aldehyde or ketone, triose. Glyceraldehyde is an aldotriose; dihydroxyacetone is a ketotriose. Successive chain elongation of trioses yields tetroses, pentoses, hexoses, heptoses, and octoses. In the aldo-series, these are called aldotriose, aldotetrose, aldopentose, aldohexose, etc., and in the keto-series ketotriose, ketotetrose, ketopentose, ketohexose, and so on.

Hexoses are white crystalline compounds, freely soluble in water but insoluble in such nonpolar solvents as benzene and hexane. Most of these have a sweet taste and are by far the most abundant of the monosaccharides in the human diet. Of these, glucose, fructose, and galactose are most often found in foods. Mannose is occasionally found but only in complexes that are poorly digested. Aldopentoses are important components of nucleic acid; derivatives of triose and heptose are intermediates in carbohydrate metabolism.

The monosaccharides in the body undergo a number of reactions. (See Metabolic Maps, Appendix 2.) These reactions produce five general groups of products, as shown in Table 20.

Oligosaccharides

Oligosaccharides consist of 2–10 monosaccharides joined with a glycosidic bond. The bond is formed between the anomeric carbon of one sugar and any hydroxyl function of another sugar. If

TABLE 20
Characteristic Reaction Products of Carbohydrates in the Body

Product	Example
Phosphoric acid esters	Glucose 6 phosphate
Polyhydroxy alcohols	Sorbitol
Deoxy sugars	Deoxyribose
Sugar acids	Gluconic acid
Amino sugars	Glucosamine

two monosaccharides are bonded in this manner, the resulting molecule is a disaccharide; if three, a trisaccharide; if four, a tetrasaccharide, and so on.

Disaccharides

Of the oligosaccharides, by far the most prevalent in nature are the disaccharides. Of dietary significance are the disaccharides lactose, maltose, and sucrose. Lactose, the sugar found in the milk of most mammals, consists of a D-galactose and D-glucose joined with a glycosidic linkage at carbon 1 of galactose and carbon 4 of glucose. Lactose promotes the growth of certain beneficial lactic acid-producing bacteria in the intestinal tract. These bacteria can displace some of the undesirable putrefactive bacteria in the tract. Lactose also enhances the absorption of calcium.

Maltose, also known as malt sugar, contains two glucose residues. Cellobiose, the repeating disaccharide unit of cellulose, and gentiobiose are two other disaccharides that have as their repeating units D-glucose. All have free anomeric carbons and are reducing sugars.

Sucrose, also known as table sugar, cane sugar, beet sugar, or grape sugar, is a disaccharide of glucose and fructose linked through the anomeric carbon of each monosaccharide. Because neither anomeric carbon is free, sucrose is a nonreducing sugar. When sucrose is used in the preparation of acidic foods, some inversion (hydrolysis of sucrose to glucose and fructose) takes place. Inverted sugar is sweeter than sucrose. Invertase occurs in the bee and inverts the sucrose in the nectar the bees collect from the flowers they visit. The bees make honey from this nectar, and it contains glucose, fructose, sucrose, water, and small quantities of flavor extract unique to the flower from which the nectar was obtained.

Dietary disaccharides are hydrolyzed into their component monosaccharides in the enterocyte and converted to glucose which is the body's primary metabolic fuel.

A few oligosaccharides with more than two monosaccharide moieties are of nutritional significance. Stachyose, a tetrasaccharide composed of two molecules of D-galactose, one of D-glucose, and one of D-fructose, is found in certain foods, particularly those of legume origin. It is usually found with raffinose (fructose, glucose, and galactose) and sucrose. The human digestive tract does not possess an enzyme which can hydrolyze stachyose or raffinose. These carbohydrates are fermented in the lower intestinal tract by the intestinal flora. This further metabolism produces some short-chain fatty acids and gas that become part of the flatus associated with the consumption of foods rich in these carbohydrates.

Polysaccharides

Polysaccharides (also known as glycans) are compounds consisting of large numbers of monosaccharides linked by glycosidic bonds. Some have as few as 30–90 monosaccharides. Others contain several hundred or even thousands of monosaccharide units. Polysaccharides differ from one another in the nature of their repeating monosaccharide units, in the number of such units in their chain, and in the degree of branching.

The polysaccharides which contain only a single kind of monosaccharide or monosaccharide derivative are called *homopolysaccharides*; those which have two or more different monomeric units are called *heteropolysaccharides*. Often homopolysaccharides are given names which indicate the nature of the building blocks: for example, those which contain mannose units are mannans; those which contain fructose units are called fructans. The important biological polysaccharides are the storage polysaccharides, the structural polysaccharides, and the mucopolysaccharides.

Storage Polysaccharides

Among plants the most abundant storage polysaccharide is starch. It is deposited abundantly in grains, fruits, and tubers in the form of large granules in the cytoplasm of cells; each plant deposits a starch characteristic of its species. Starch exists in two forms: α-amylose and amylopectin. α-Amylose makes up 20–30% of most starches and consists of 250–300 unbranched glucose residues bonded by α $(1 \rightarrow 4)$ linkages. The chains vary in molecular weight from a few thousand to 500,000. The molecule is twisted into a helical coil. The remainder of the starch in a plant is highly branched and is called amylopectin. Its backbone consists of glucose residues with α $(1 \rightarrow 4)$ glycosidic linkages; its branch points are α $(1 \rightarrow 6)$ glycosidic bonds and exists as a helical coil.

When amylose is broken down in successive stages by either the enzyme amylase or by the action of dry heat, as in toasting, the resulting polysaccharides of intermediate chain length are called dextrin. Amylopectin, when broken down by the same methods, does not cleave at its branch points. This end product is a large, highly branched product called limit dextrin.

Other homopolysaccharides are found in plants, bacteria, yeast, and mold as storage polysaccharides. Dextrans, found in yeast and bacteria, are branched polysaccharides of D-glucose with their major backbone linkage α $(1 \rightarrow 6)$. Inulin, found in artichokes, consists of D-fructose monomers with β $(2 \rightarrow 1)$ glycosidic linkages. Mannans are composed of mannose residues and are found in bacteria, yeasts, mold, and higher plants.

Among animals, the storage polysaccharide is glycogen. Glycogen is stored primarily in the liver and muscles. Like amylopectin, glycogen is a branched polysaccharide of D-glucose with a backbone glycosidic linkage of α $(1 \rightarrow 4)$ and branch points of α $(1 \rightarrow 6)$. However, its branches occur every 8–10 residues, as compared to every 12 for amylopectin. For muscle glycogen, the molecular weight has been estimated to be about 106; for liver, 5×106 (corresponding to about 30,000 glucose residues). Glycogen is of no importance as a dietary source of carbohydrate. The small amount of glycogen in an animal's body when it is slaughtered is quickly degraded during the postmortem period.

Structural Polysaccharides

Cellulose is the most abundant structural polysaccharide in the plant world. Of the carbon in vegetables, 50% is cellulose; wood is about one-half cellulose, and cotton is nearly pure cellulose. It is a straight chain polymer of D-glucose with β $(1 \rightarrow 4)$ glycosidic linkages between the monosaccharides. Cellobiose, a disaccharide, is obtained on partial hydrolysis of cellulose. The molecular weight of cellulose has been estimated to range from 50,000 to 500,000 (equivalent to 300–3000 glucose residues). Cellulose molecules are organized in bundles of parallel chains, called fibrils, which are cross-linked by hydrogen bonding; these chains of glucose units are relatively rigid and are cemented together with hemicelluloses, pectin, and lignin.

Hemicellulose bears no relation structurally to cellulose. It is composed of polymers of D-xylose with β $(1 \rightarrow 4)$ glycosidic linkages and side chains of arabinose and other sugars. Pectin is a polymer of methyl D-galacturonate. Pectin is found in fruits and is the substance needed to make jelly out of cooked fruit. The juice plus sucrose plus the pectin form a gel that is stable for many months at room temperature. Pectin is a nonabsorbable carbohydrate that has pharmacological use as well. It is a key component, together with kaolin, of an antidiarrheal remedy, kaopectate.

There are other structural polysaccharides found in nature. Chitin is a polysaccharide which forms the hard skeleton of insects and crustaceans and is a homopolymer of N-acetyl-D-glucosamine. Agar, derived from sea algae, contains D- and L-galactose residues, some esterified with sulfuric acid, primarily with 1 → 3 bonds; alginic acid, derived from algae and kelp, contains monomers of D-mannuronic acid; and vegetable gum (gum arabic) contains D-galactose, D-glucuronic acid, rhamnose, and arabinose. These are used as food stabilizers by the food processing industry. Algin derivatives, for example, are used to stabilize the emulsions made in salad dressings; gum arabic is frequently used to stabilize processed cheese products, where it acts to retard the separation of the solids from the fluid component in such products.

Mucopolysaccharides

The mucopolysaccharides are heteropolysaccharides, which are components of the structural polysaccharides found at various places in the body. Mucopolysaccharides consist of disaccharide units in which glucuroic acid is bound to acetylated or sulfurated amino sugars with glycosidic (1 → 3) linkages. Each disaccharide unit is bound to the next by a β (1 → 4) glycosidic linkage. Thus, they are linear polymers with alternating β (1 → 3) and β (1 → 4) linkages. Hyaluronic acid is the most abundant mucopolysaccharide. It is the principal component of the ground substance of connective tissue and is also abundant in the synovial fluid in joints and the vitreous humor of the eye. The repeating unit of hyaluronic acid is a disaccharide composed of D-glucuronic acid and N-acetyl-D-glucosamine; it has alternating β (1 → 3) and β (1 → 4) glycosidic linkages. The molecular weight is several million.

Another mucopolysaccharide which forms part of the structure of connective tissue is chondroitin. It differs from hyaluronic acid only in that it contains N-acetyl-D-galactosamine residues rather than N-acetyl-D-glucosamine residues. The sulfate ester derivatives of chondroitin, chondroitin sulfate A and chondroitin sulfate C, are major structural components of cartilage, bone, cornea, and connective tissues. Types A and C have the same structure as chondroitin except for a sulfate ester at carbon atom 4 of the N-acetyl-D-galactosamine residue on type A and one at carbon atom 6 of type C. Heparin (β-heparin), an anticoagulant, is a mucopolysaccharide which is similar in structure to hyaluronic acid because it contains residues of D-glucuronic acid, sulfate, and acetyl groups. Its structure is not entirely known.

Carbohydrate Digestion

Once a carbohydrate-rich food is consumed, digestion begins. As the food is chewed it is mixed with saliva. Saliva contains α amylase. This amylase begins the digestion of starch by attacking the internal α 1,4-glucosidic bonds. It will not attack the branch points having α 1,4 or α 1,6-glucosidic bonds, hence the salivary α amylase will produce molecules of glucose, maltose, α-limit dextrin, and maltotriose. The α amylase in saliva is an isozyme with the same function as that in the pancreatic juice. The salivary α amylase is denatured in the stomach as the food is mixed and acidified with the gastric hydrochloric acid. As the stomach contents move into the duodenum, it is called chyme. The movement of chyme into the duodenum stimulates cholesystokinin release. This gut hormone acts on the exocrine pancreas stimulating it to release pancreatic juice into the duodenum and on the gall bladder to release bile. Cholesystokinin is secreted by the epithelial endocrine cells of the small intestine, particularly the duodenum. Its release is stimulated by amino acids in the lumen and by the acid pH of the stomach contents as it passes into the duodenum. The low pH of the chyme also stimulates the release of secretin which, in turn, stimulates the exocrine pancreas to release bicarbonate and water so as to raise the pH of the chyme. This is necessary to maximize the activity of the digestive enzymes located on the surface of the intestinal luminal cell. Starch digestion begins in the mouth with salivary amylase. It pauses in the stomach as the stomach contents are acidified but resumes when the chyme enters the duodenum and the pH is raised. The amylase of the pancreatic juice is the same as that of the saliva. It attacks the same bonds in the same locations and produces the same products, maltose, maltotriose, and the small polysaccharides (average of eight glucose molecules) called α-limit dextrins. The limit dextrins are further hydrolyzed by glucosidases on the surface of the luminal cells. The hydrolyses of the bonds not attacked by α amylase, α glucosidase, or the disaccharidases, maltase, lactase, or sucrase, are passed to the lower part of the intestine where they are attacked by the enzymes of the intestinal flora. Most of the products of this digestion are used by the flora themselves; however, the microbial metabolic products may be of use. The flora can produce useful amounts of short-chain fatty acids and lactate as well as methane gas, carbon dioxide, water, and hydrogen gas. The carbohydrates of legumes typify the substrates these flora use. Raffinose, which is a galactose $1 \rightarrow 6$ glucose $1 \rightarrow 2$ β fructose, and trehalose, an α glucose $1 \rightarrow 1$ α glucose, are the typical substrates from legumes for these flora. The flora will also attack portions of the fibers and celluloses that are the structural elements in fruits and vegetables. Again, some useful products may be produced, but the bulk of these complex polysaccharides having β linkages and perhaps other substituent groups as part of their structure is largely untouched by both intestinal and bacterial enzymes. These undigested unavailable carbohydrates serve very useful functions in that they provide bulk to the diet, which in turn helps to regulate the rate of food passage from mouth to anus. They act as adsorbants of noxious or potentially noxious materials in the food, and they assist in the excretion of cholesterol and several minerals, thereby protecting the body from overload.

The disaccharides in the diet are hydrolyzed to their component monosaccharides by enzymes also located on the surface of the luminal cell. Lactose is hydrolyzed to glucose and galactose by lactase, sucrose is hydrolyzed to fructose and glucose, and maltose is hydrolyzed to two molecules of glucose. Table 21 lists these enzymes together with their substrates and products.

CARBOHYDRATE LOADING (GLYCOGEN LOADING)

A technique used by endurance athletes to increase their muscle glycogen content. This technique dictates the exhaustion of the muscle glycogen store followed by rest and glycogen repletion just prior to the competitive event. The rest/repletion routine results in an increased store of glucose as glycogen within the muscle.

CARBONYL GROUP

An aldehyde (–CH=O) group or ketone (–C=O) group; a group which characterizes aldehydes and ketones.

CARBOXYLASE

An enzyme which catalyzes the addition of a carboxyl group to a carbon chain. This enzyme class usually requires thiamin as thiamin pyrophosphate (TPP) as a coenzyme.

TABLE 21
Enzymes of Importance to Carbohydrate Digestion

Enzyme	Substrate	Products
α amylase	Starch, amylopectin	Glucose, maltose, maltotriose, α-limit dextrin
α glucosidase	α-limit dextrin	Glucose
Lactase	Lactose	Galactose, glucose
Maltase	Maltose	Glucose
Sucrase	Sucrose	Glucose, fructose

Source: From Berdanier, C. D., and J. Zempleni. 2009. *Advanced Nutrition: Macronutrients, Micronutrients and Metabolism*. Boca Raton, FL: CRC Press. With permission.

CARBOXYLATION

The addition of a carboxyl (–COOH) group to a carbon chain.

CARCINOGEN

An agent that damages DNA sufficient to induce a mutation that in turn leads to uncontrolled cell growth (cancer).

CARCINOGENESIS

The process of developing cancer.

CARDAMON

A spice derived from a plant native to India and Ceylon. The oil extracted from the fruit is used as a flavoring agent.

CARDIAC CATHETERIZATION

Procedure used to identify coronary artery blockage. A catheter is introduced into the vascular system, and a radiopaque dye is infused. The heart is then visualized such that occluded vessels are apparent.

CARDIAC FAILURE

Heart ceases to pump or pumps inadequately. In congestive heart failure, there is a buildup of fluid in the lungs and in the extremities.

CARDIAC HYPERTROPHY

Enlarged heart.

CARDIAC OUTPUT

The quantity of blood discharged from the left ventricle per minute. Normal cardiac output at rest is 3.0 L/m^2 of body surface per minute.

CARDIOMYOPATHY

Structural or functional disease of the heart muscle (the myocardium).

CARDIOPULMONARY ARREST

Sudden cessation of ventilation and circulation.

CARDIOPULMONARY BYPASS

A procedure used to divert blood from the heart and lungs while maintaining perfusion and oxygenation to the rest of the body through the use of a heart-lung machine.

CARDIOVASCULAR DISEASE

A group of degenerative diseases characterized by a diminution of heart action. The oxygen and nutrient supply to the heart may be impeded because the coronary vessels are partially or fully occluded and/or the heart muscle degenerated or the vascular tree, which supplies the heart has degenerated. Frequently, cardiovascular disease is associated with elevated blood lipids as well as with elevated blood pressure (hypertension) and with diabetes mellitus. Management of these conditions can reduce the risk of a mortal event; however, people with diabetes have five times the risk of heart disease even when their diabetes is well managed. Cardiovascular disease has a strong genetic component. (See http://www.omim.com for heart disease.)

CARDIOVASCULAR TESTS AND THERAPIES

Cardiovascular Bypass

Surgical correction of occluded vessels in the heart. Donor vessels are taken from the leg or mammary veins and attached to the heart vessel such that the occluded portion is "bypassed."

Electrophysiological Studies

Various techniques that record electrical activity from the body surface and the surface of the heart.

Intravascular Stents

Procedure in which a stainless steel stent, attached to a balloon-tipped catheter, is placed in a blocked area of a coronary artery to open it.

Laser Angioplasty

Procedure in which a laser is used to open a partially occluded coronary artery. Laser angioplasty is often followed by balloon angioplasty to further open the artery.

Mechanical Atherectomy

The process of mechanically removing a coronary artery blockage, usually with the aid of a drill-type catheter.

Percutaneous Transluminal Coronary Angioplasty (PTCA)

A procedure in which an inflated balloon-tipped catheter is used to dilate a blocked coronary artery.

CARIOGENESIS

The process of tooth decay.

CARNITINE

An essential component of fatty acid oxidation; participates in the transport of fatty acids into the mitochondrion prior to oxidation. Carnitine (see Figure 9) also functions as an acyl group acceptor

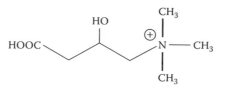

FIGURE 9   Structure of carnitine.

that facilitates mitochondrial export of excess carbons in the form of acylcarnitines. Carnitine is synthesized from lysine and methionine. (See Metabolic Maps for the pathways of fatty acid transport and for carnitine synthesis, Appendix 2.) Diminished carnitine synthesis has been noted as a feature of aging. There may be some justification in supplementing the aged with this compound. However, since carnitine is synthesized in the body, there does not seem to be a need to include this in normal diets.

CARNOSINE

A dipeptide synthesized from β alanine and histidine. Found in muscle, where it activates myosin ATPase. Carnosine also serves to buffer the acidic state that develops in working muscle.

CAROTENES, CAROTINOIDS

A group of yellow-orange pigments some of which can be hydrolyzed to active vitamin A. (See Vitamins and Table 49.) α, β, and γ carotene are considered provitamins because they can be converted to active vitamin A. The carotenes have an antioxidant function.

CARRIER

A substance, usually a protein, which binds to a substrate and transports it from its point of origin to its point of use.

CARVEDIOL

A beta blocker, vasodilator, and antihypertensive drug. Trade name: Coreg.

CASE-CONTROL STUDIES

Nonexperimental studies in which cases of a particular disease are selected and the patient's exposure in the past is compared with that of people without the disease. This type of study is suitable for studying rare diseases. The numbers of subjects needed are small compared to those needed in cohort studies. Since the cases are selected without knowing the size of the source population at risk from which they arose, no information on the incidence rate of the disease in the population is obtained in these studies. Consequently, the relative risk cannot be calculated but is approximated by calculating an odds ratio. The advantage of this study design is that exposure and disease are both measured at the same time, and therefore one does not have to wait as long as in the cohort design. In this type of study, however, valid assessment of exposure may be a problem, since exposure in the past is measured after the disease has occurred. The disease may have affected recollection of the exposure by the subject. For diseases with a long latency period information on exposure in the distant past is needed. This may be impossible.

CASPASE

A heterotetrameric cysteine protease that hydrolyzes cellular proteins including caspase zymogens as part of the apoptotic cascade.

CASSAVA

A starchy root that is a primary food source in tropical countries.

CATABOLISM

The totality of those reactions that reduce macromolecules to usable metabolites, carbon dioxide, and water.

CATALASE

An enzyme which catalyzes the conversion of peroxide to water and oxygen; this is a key enzyme in the cytoplasmic free radical suppression system.

CATALYST

A substance, usually a protein, in living (or nonliving) systems that enhances or promotes a chemical reaction without being a reactant. Enzymes are catalysts.

CATARACT

Loss of transparency of the lens of the eye.

CATARRH

Simple inflammation of the mucous membranes of the respiratory tract. Also called chronic rhinitis. If it occurs in the pollen season, it is called hay fever.

CATECHOLAMINES

Neurotransmitters (epinephrine, dopamine, and norepinephrine) which are produced in the adrenal medulla from tyrosine. These hormones are instrumental in orchestrating the "fight or flight" response to stress conditions.

CATHEPSIN

A calcium-dependent protease involved in the degradation of cellular protein.

CATION

A positively charged ion.

CAUTERIZATION

The process of burning or scarring the skin or tissues.

cDNA

A single-stranded DNA molecule that is complimentary to an mRNA and is synthesized from it by the action of reverse transcriptase.

CDP

Cytidine diphosphate. A nucleotide consisting of cytosine (a pyrimidine), ribose, and two high-energy phosphate groups.

CECUM

A blind appendage of the intestinal tract located at the juncture of the small and large intestine. Also called the appendix.

CELECOXIB

A COX-2 inhibitor that is a nonsteroid anti-inflamatory drug. Used in the treatment of arthritis. Trade name: Celebrex.

CELIAC DISEASE

A group of disorders characterized by diarrhea and malabsorption. Included is the disorder gluten-induced enteropathy.

CELL ANATOMY

The location of the various organelles of a eukaryotic cell is shown in Figure 10. The function of each component is listed in Table 22.

CELL CULTURE

A technique for studying cells from specific tissues. After isolation, the cells are grown in media containing all the known ingredients essential for their support. Different cell types may have different requirements.

CELL CYCLE

The sequence of events between eukaryotic cell divisions; it includes mitosis and cell division (M phase), a gap stage (G_1 phase), a period of DNA synthesis (S phase), and a second gap stage (G_2 phase) before the next M phase.

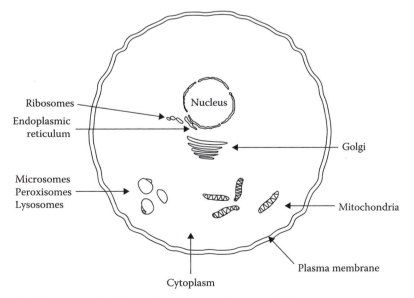

FIGURE 10   Typical eukaryotic cell showing representative intracellular structures.

TABLE 22
Functions of the Organelles/Cell Fractions of the Typical Eucaryotic Cell

Organelle/Cell Fraction	Role in Cell	Processes Found
Plasma membrane	Cell boundary holds receptors for hormones/substrates	Processes, exports, and imports substrates, ions, hormones
Cytoplasm	Medium for a variety of enzymes, substrates, products, ions	Glycolysis, glycogenesis, glycogenolysis, lipogenesis, pentose shunt, urea synthesis (part), protein synthesis (part)
Nucleus	Contains DNA, RNA	Protein synthesis starts here with DNA transcription
Endoplasmic reticulum	Ca^{2+} stored here	Has role in many synthetic processes
Golgi apparatus	Sequesters and releases proteins	Export mechanism for release of macromolecules
Mitochondria	Powerhouse of cell	Krebs cycle, respiratory chain, ATP synthesis, fatty acid oxidation; first step of urea synthesis
Ribosomes	Site for completion of protein synthesis	Protein synthesis
Lysosomes	Intracellular digestion	Protein and macromolecule degradation
Peroxisomes	Suppression of oxygen-free radicals	Antioxidant enzymes
Microsomes	Drug detoxification	Detoxification

CELL DIFFERENTIATION

Although all nucleated cells possess the same DNA, some of the specific DNA regions (genes) are not transcribed or translated. If translated, some gene products are not very active. Thus, not all cells have the same processes with the same degree of activity. Cellular differentiation has taken place such that muscle cells differ from fat cells that, in turn, differ from brain cells and so forth. In each cell type, there are processes and metabolic pathways that may be unique to that cell type. An example is the great lipid storage capacity of the adipocyte, a feature not found in a bone cell or a brain cell or a muscle cell, although each of these cells do contain lipid. Similarly, the capacity to form and retain a mineral appetite (a mixture of different minerals) is characteristic of a bone cell, and the synthesis of contractile proteins by muscle cells are also examples of cell uniqueness. Cells differ in their choice of metabolic fuel. Hepatic and muscle cells make, store, and use significant amounts of glycogen. Adipocytes and hepatocytes make, store, and sometimes use triacylglycerols. All of these special features have an impact on the composition of specific organs and tissues in the body that collectively comprise and contribute to body composition. One must consider the function of each organ and tissue in the context of the whole body. Similarly, the determination of the activity of a single process in a single cell type or organ may not necessarily predict the activity (and cumulative result) of that process in the whole body.

CELLULAR IMMUNITY

Immunity mediated by the T lymphocytes. (T cells, cells originating from the thymus.)

CELLULOSE

A structural polysaccharide found primarily in plants and composed of glucose units linked together with β 1,4 bonds. (See Carbohydrates.)

CENTRAL STIMULANTS

Substances increasing the state of activity of the nervous system. An example of a class of stimulants is the methylxanthines, which have effects on the peripheral and central nervous system. Caffeine, theophylline, and theobromine are methylxanthines.

CENTROMERE

The eukaryotic chromosomal region that attaches to the mitotic spindle during cell division; it contains high concentrations of repetitive DNA.

CEPHALIN

A phospholipid, similar to lecithin, present in the brain.

CERAMIDE

A sphingosine derivative with an acyl group attached to its amino group.

CEREBROSIDE

A ceramide with a sugar residue as a head group. This is a complex lipid in nerve and other tissues. A cerebroside is a sphingolipid.

CEREBROVASCULAR ACCIDENT

Also referred to as a stroke; sudden circulatory impairment in the vasculature system of the brain.

CEREBROVASCULAR DISEASE

Similar to cardiovascular disease in that the vascular tree of the brain has developed atherosclerotic lesions, which restrict or occlude the blood supply to this organ.

CERULOPLASMIN

A copper-containing globulin in blood plasma with a molecular weight of 150,000 and eight copper atoms. It catalyzes the oxidation of amines, phenols, and ascorbic acid. It is reduced in amount in Wilson's disease (hepatolenticular disease).

CETOLIC ACID

$(CH_3(CH_2)_9CH=CH(CH_2)_9COOH)$. A toxic monounsaturated fatty acid, which occurs in herring oil. Its toxic effects are similar to those of erucic acid.

CHARGAFF'S RULE

Applies to DNA in that there are equal numbers of adenine and thymine residues and equal numbers of guanine and cytosine residues in this genetic material.

CHEILOSIS

Cracks at the corners of the mouth. Associated with inadequate riboflavin intake; however, it can also occur in the presence of adequate vitamin intake.

CHELATE, CHELATION

A combination of metal ions chemically held within a ring of heterocyclic structures by bonds from each of these structures to the metal. Iron is held by heme in this fashion as part of the hemoglobin structure.

CHEMICAL POTENTIAL

The partial molar free energy of a substance.

CHEMIOSMOTIC THEORY

The postulate that the free energy of electron transport in the mitochondrial respiratory chain is conserved in the formation of a transmembrane proton gradient. The electrochemical potential of this gradient is used to drive ATP synthesis.

CHEMOTHERAPY

Treatment of illness using medication; however, the term usually means the treatment of cancer.

CHIARI-FROMMEL SYNDROME

The occurrence of galactorrhea (nonnursing lactation) and amenorrhea during the postpartum period; the disease may be due to a prolactin-secreting tumor.

CHIMERIC MOLECULE

A molecule of DNA or RNA or protein containing sequences from two different species.

CHINESE RESTAURANT SYNDROME

In sensitive people, this term refers to the headache that follows the consumption of large amounts of monosodium glutamate (MSG, a key ingredient in soy sauce).

CHLORIDE

A major anion in the extracellular fluid. The major dietary source is table salt (NaCl). The normal concentration of chloride ions in serum is about 100 meq/L.

CHLORIDE SHIFT

Part of the system which maintains the blood acid-base balance. Chloride and bicarbonate ions exchange across the erythrocyte plasma membrane, "the shift."

CHLOROPHYLL

A heterocyclic iron/copper-containing green pigment in plants.

CHOLECALCIFEROL

A metabolite of cholesterol formed in the pathway for vitamin D activation. Cholecalciferol is hydroxylated in the kidney to 1,25 dihydroxy-cholecalciferol, the active vitamin D.

CHOLECYSTITIS

Inflammation of the gallbladder.

CHOLECYSTOKININ (CCK)

A hormone released from duodenal cells and which stimulates the gall bladder to contract and release bile into the duodenum. It also serves as a satiety signal.

CHOLEDOCHOLITHIASIS

Obstruction of the common bile duct; presence of a stone in the duct.

CHOLELITHIASIS

Presence or formation of gallstones.

CHOLERA

A severe gastrointestinal disease caused by an organism called *vibrio cholera*. This organism produces a toxin that binds to specific receptors on the intestinal cell wall. The toxin activates adenylate cyclase by causing ADP-ribosylation of the GαS protein involved in regulating the cyclase. This results in an elevation in cAMP levels, which turns on electrolyte secretion and thereby inhibits the active transport processes necessary for the absorption of nutrients from the gut. While water can pass freely from the intestine, other materials cannot and, as such, create an osmotic pull on the water. In turn, the water and unabsorbed nutrients fill the intestine stimulating peristalsis and evacuation of the colon. If the massive fluid and electrolyte losses are not replaced, the cholera victim does not survive and recover.

CHOLESTASIS

Arrest of bile excretion.

CHOLESTATIC JAUNDICE

Jaundice resulting from an abnormality (obstruction) in the flow of bile from the liver to the gall bladder to the intestine.

CHOLESTEROL

A four-ringed structure in the nonsaponifiable lipid class that is an important substrate for steroid hormone synthesis. (See Metabolic Maps for cholesterol synthesis pathway, Appendix 2.)

CHOLESTYRAMINE

An ion exchange resin that is used to adsorb cholesterol in the gastrointestinal tract. It also serves as a bile acid sequestrant. Trade names: LoCholest, LoCholest Light, Prevalite, Questran, Questran Light.

CHOLESYSTECTOMY

Surgical removal of gall bladder (and gallstones) from a patient whose bladder has become inflamed; the bile duct from the liver is connected directly to the small intestine.

CHOLINE

An amine. An essential nutrient that can be synthesized by the carboxylation of serine. Choline (see Figure 11) is a part of the phospholipid, lecithin. It is also an important component of the neurotransmitter, acetylcholine. Essential to the developing brain, hence there is a critical need to assure that pregnant and lactating women consume sufficient choline to support the growth of the fetus and young child. A DRI has been published with suggested intakes that are age and gender dependent (see http://www.nap.edu). Pregnant females should consume 450 mg/day, lactating females 550 mg/day, and males 550 mg/day. Eggs, meat, and milk are good sources of choline.

CHONDROCYTES

Cartilage precursor cells or cartilage cells.

CHORIONIC GONADOTROPIN

A heterodimeric glycoprotein hormone of 57 kDa consisting of a noncovalent bound α (92 amino acid residues) and a distinctive β (134 amino acid residues) subunits found in the blood of pregnant females. The major function of this hormone is to stimulate the production of progesterone by the corpus luteum. This ensures a continuous supply of ovarian progesterone until the placenta has developed to the point when it can generate its own supply of progesterone.

CHORIONIC SOMATOMAMMOTROPIN

A 190 amino acid hormone that is similar to growth hormone. It plays a role in mobilizing maternal fat stores to support the developing fetus and also has a role in the regulation of glucose homeostasis in the pregnant female.

CHORIONIC THYROTROPIN

Hormone produced by the placenta; an analog of thyroid-stimulating hormone.

CHROMAFFIN CELLS

Cells in the adrenal medulla and also the kidney, ovary, testis, heart, and gastrointestinal tract. Similar cell types are found in the carotid and aortic bodies. In the adrenal medulla, these cells produce epinephrine.

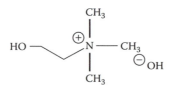

FIGURE 11 Structure of choline.

CHROMATIN

A complex of DNA and protein in the nucleus of the interphase cell. It is a protein-DNA complex that comprises the chromosomes.

CHROMIUM

A trace mineral; may or may not be essential to the optimal use of glucose.

CHROMOSOME WALKING

The sequential isolation of clones carrying overlapping sequences of DNA, allowing large regions of the chromosomes to be spanned. Walking is often performed to reach a specific area of interest.

CHROMOSOMES

When DNA is extracted from the cell nucleus, it is not one continuous strand. Rather, it breaks up into fairly predictable arrangements called chromosomes. The chromosomes exist in pairs and have been numbered. Those determining the sex of the individual (the sex chromosomes) are labeled as X or Y. If the individual has one X and one Y, he is a male. If the individual has two X chromosomes, she is a female. All the other chromosomes are autosomes. Many characteristics have been localized to particular chromosomes. There are species differences in the number of chromosomes. There are 23 sets of chromosomes (46 total) in the human.

CHRONIC DISEASE

A disease which takes years to develop.

CHRONIC LEAD INTOXICATION

Accumulation of lead in soft tissue and bone as a result of continuous exposure to this metal either in the air or in food or beverages.

CHRONIC OBSTRUCTIVE PULMONARY DISEASE (COPD)

Descriptive term characterized by chronic or recurring obstruction of air flow in the lungs resulting from chronic bronchitis, bronchial asthma, emphysema, or bronchiectasis.

CHRONIC RENAL DISEASE (CHRONIC KIDNEY DISEASE)

Kidney damage or degenerative change that results in a loss of filtration function. Filtration rates of less than 60 mL/min/1.73 m^2 define the disease state. Complications include anemia, cardiovascular disease, and poor growth. Patients can be sustained through dialysis several times a week; however, dialysis can result in a loss of essential trace minerals such as zinc. Other nutritional disturbances may also develop. The irreversible loss of kidney function develops in four progressive stages. The first stage is characterized by diminishing renal reserve as indicated by a 50% decrease in glomerular filtration rate. Progression to the second stage occurs when the glomerular filtration rate decreases further to between 20% and 50% of normal and azotemia, polyuria, and nocturia develop. The third stage, described as renal failure, occurs when the glomerular filtration rate drops below 20% of normal and uremia is present. In the final stage, referred to as end-stage renal disease, the glomerular filtration rate has decreased to less than 5% of the normal value and the individual is terminally uremic.

CHYLE

A turbid white or yellow fluid, taken up by the lacteals in the process of lipid digestion and absorption.

CHYLOMICRON

Fat-protein complex formed to carry absorbed dietary fats from the intestine to other tissues; not normally found in the blood of a fasting individual.

CHYME

The semifluid mass of partly digested food extruded from the stomach into the duodenum of the small intestine.

CIGUATERA POISONING

A disease resulting from the consumption of contaminated fish, in which the toxin has accumulated via a food chain. The alga involved (the photosynthetic dinoflagellate *Gambierdis custoxicus*) is consumed by a small herbivorous fish. Larger fish feeding on the smaller fish concentrate the toxin further in the chain. This kind of intoxication is found in the South Pacific and the Caribbean. The various ciguatera toxins do not all contribute to poisoning to the same extent. The main cause is ciguatoxin. Symptoms of ciguatera poisoning are paresthesia in lips, fingers, and toes, vomiting, nausea, abdominal pain, diarrhea, bradycardia, muscular weakness, and joint pain. The mechanism underlying these symptoms may be based on the neuroactivity of ciguatoxin. It increases sodium permeability, leading to depolarization of nerves.

CILIA, CILIUM

Hair-like processes extending out from the surface of epithelial cells.

CIMETIDINE

H_2-receptor antagonist that serves as an antiulcerative. Trade names: Tagamet, Tagamet HB.

CIRRHOSIS

Chronic liver disease in which fatty deposits and fibrous connective tissue have replaced functioning liver cells. Cirrhosis may lead to loss of hepatic function and death.

CIS CONFORMATION

An arrangement of carbon atoms on the same side of either a double bond or a peptide bond.

CITRATE

An intermediate in the citric acid cycle; the essential starting metabolite for fatty acid synthesis in the cytosol.

CITRIC ACID CYCLE (KREBS CYCLE)

A cycle found in mitochondria which produces reducing equivalents for use by the respiratory chain and which also produces carbon dioxide. (See Metabolic Maps, Appendix 2.)

CITRULLINEMIA

Excessive, high levels of citrulline in the blood. Citrulline is a metabolite formed from ornithine and carbamyl phosphate. Citrulline accumulates in a genetic disease caused by the mutation in the gene for arginosuccinate synthetase.

CLATHRIN

A three-part protein that polymerizes to form a polyhydral structure defining the shape of membrane vesicles that travel between the plasma membrane and intracellular organelles such as the Golgi apparatus.

CLEAR LIQUID DIET

Therapeutic diet providing foods and beverages that are transparent and liquid at room temperature.

CLINICAL NUTRIENT DEFICIENCY SIGNS

Poor growth, skin lesions, lethargy, tissue wasting and/or malfunction, anemia.

CLINICAL TRIAL

An experiment using human subjects. Usually these are conducted in three phases to test a drug's safety, its effectiveness, and whether it has side effects in humans.

CLONE

A large number of cells or molecules that are identical with a single parental cell or molecule.

CLONIDINE, CLONIDINE HYDROCHLORIDE

A drug that is a centrally acting adrenergic and antihypertensive. Trade names: Catapres-TTS; Catapres, Dixarit.

CLOPIDOGREL BISULFATE

An ADP-induced platelet aggregation inhibitor; antiplatelet drug. Trade name: Plavix.

CMP

Cytidine monophosphate. A nucleotide consisting of cytosine (a pyrimidine), ribose, and one high-energy phosphate group.

CoA (COENZYME A)

Coenzyme A is a pantothenic acid containing coenzyme important in the activation of acyl compounds. CoA forms a thioester bond with acetyl and acyl groups and with amino acids and facilitates their metabolism. Its structure is shown in Figure 12.

COALESCENCE

Irreversible destabilization of an emulsion.

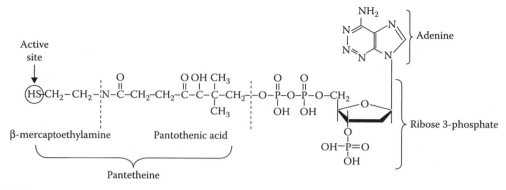

FIGURE 12   Structure of coenzyme A.

COATED VESICLE

A membranous intracellular transport vesicle that is encased by clathrin or another coat protein.

COBALAMIN

See Vitamin B_{12}.

COBALT

An essential mineral needed as a component of vitamin B_{12}.

CODON

A sequence of three bases (triplet) which specifies a particular amino acid in the sequence of reactions which comprise protein synthesis. The codons of the messenger RNA are matched by the anticodon of the transfer RNA, which brings the amino acids to the ribosome for incorporation into the protein being synthesized.

CODING STRAND

A strand of DNA with the same sequence as mRNA.

COEFFICIENT OF DIGESTIBILITY

The percentage of a consumed food that is digested and absorbed and which does not appear in the feces.

COENZYME

A small organic molecule, usually a vitamin, that is required for the catalytic activity of an enzyme.

COFACTOR

A small molecule needed for the activity of an enzyme. Many of the essential minerals serve as cofactors.

COHORT STUDIES

See Follow-Up Studies.

COLCHICINE

A drug useful in the treatment of gout.

COLIC

Condition characterized by excessive flatus and belly pain.

COLITIS

Inflammation of the colon. (See Crohn's Disease.)

COLLAGEN

The principle structural protein of bones, teeth, skin, cartilage, tendons, cornea, and blood vessels. Rich in proline and hydroxyproline. The synthesis of collagen in vivo is dependent on adequate intakes of vitamin C. Collagen, when boiled, becomes partly soluble. The soluble portion can be separated from the insoluble portion and when separated is known as gelatin. Gelatin is deficient in tryptophan and thus is a poor-quality dietary protein.

COLORINGS

See Additives (Tables 3 and 4).

COLOSTOMY

Procedure in which a part of the colon is brought through the abdominal wall. The feces are then collected in an artificial collection container instead of being eliminated through the anus.

COLOSTRUM

The first milk of the lactating mother; rich in antibodies. This milk provides passive immunity to the newborn child.

COMPARTMENTATION

The division of a cell into smaller functionally discrete systems.

COMPETITIVE INHIBITION

Inhibition of an enzymatic reaction which occurs when a substance, closely related to the substrate, binds to the active site of the enzyme yet is not catalyzed by it.

COMPLEMENT 3 POLYMORPHISMS

Variants in the base sequence for complement 3; some of these associate with an increased risk for metabolic syndrome. Polyunsaturated fatty acids can bind to complement 3 DNA, affecting its expression.

COMPLEMENTARY BASE PAIRS

The pairing of purine and pyrmidine bases of the DNA. Adenine is paired with thymine and cytosine with guanine. These pairs are linked together via hydrogen bonds, which form the cross-links between the two strands of DNA for the double helix typical of the nuclear genetic material. In RNA, adenine pairs with uracil. Figure 13 illustrates this pairing.

COMPLETE PROTEIN

A dietary protein which contains all of the essential amino acids in amounts needed by the consumer.

COMPLEX CARBOHYDRATES

Polymers of simple sugars (monosaccharides) that are branched and which may contain lipid or protein or other substituents (SH groups, etc.). See Carbohydrate.

COMPLEX SIMILAR ACTION

Combination of substances with common sites of main action and interaction between the components. An example is the protection against goitrogens of the thiocarbamate type (e.g., goitrin) by iodine treatment. The goitrogens prevent the incorporation of iodine into tyrosine, the first step in thyroid hormone biosynthesis.

COMPONENT PUREEING

Meal preparation technique in which each menu item is individually pureed and then presented either separately or in a casserole.

CONCORDANCE

The chance that an identical disease will occur in related family members. This is particularly important in studies of the occurrence of a disease in identical twins. In type 1 diabetes mellitus for example, studies of identical twins have reported a concordance of 30%–60%. This means that if one twin develops type 1 diabetes, the other has a 30%–60% chance of developing diabetes as well.

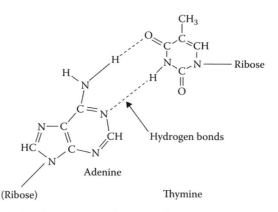

FIGURE 13   Hydrogen bonds form between complementary bases—adenine complements thymine; guanine complements cytosine.

CONDENSATION REACTION

The formation of a covalent bond between two molecules during which the elements of water are lost; condensation is the reverse of hydrolysis.

CONFOUNDING

The combined effect of the factor under investigation and other factors. A factor can only be a confounder if the occurrence of the disease as well as the exposure under investigation is associated with it. There is an essential difference between confounding and information or selection bias. If information on the confounder is collected during the study, it can be adjusted for in the statistical analyses. Sometimes, however, an unknown or not measured confounder is present. Such a confounder cannot be adjusted for in the statistical analyses and gives rise to bias in the study results.

CONGENITAL HEART DISEASE

Heart disease present at birth.

CONGESTIVE HEART FAILURE

Heart failure accompanied by venous congestion, or edema, noted in the lungs and peripheral venous system.

CONJUGATED LINOLEIC ACID (CLA)

Linoleic acid with two double bonds separated by a single bond. There are a number of cis and trans isomers of this 18 carbon fatty acid with the double bonds at 9 and 11 or at 10 and 12 or 11 and 13. Common in dairy fat is the cis 9–trans 11 conjugated linolenic acid.

CONSENSUS SEQUENCE

An idealized sequence in which each position represents the bases most often found when many actual sequences are compared.

CONSERVATIVE SUBSTITUTION

A change in amino acid residue in a protein to one with similar properties. For example, the substitution of isoleucine for leucine or aspartate for glutamate.

CONSTIPATION

Condition resulting in difficulty with expelling feces, typically from prolonged retention of feces in the colon.

CONSTITUTIVE ENZYME

An enzyme that is synthesized at a more or less steady rate and that is required for basic cell function.

CONSTITUTIVE GENES

Genes that are expressed as a function of the interaction of RNA polymerase with the promoter, without additional regulation; sometimes called "housekeeping" genes in the context of describing functions expressed in all cells at a low level.

CONTAMINANT

A chemical contaminant in a food is a substance which is not normally present in that food in its natural form or which is present in concentrations not normally found or which is not permitted under the food regulations to be present, or, being an additive as defined under the regulations, exceeds the concentration permitted.

CONTAMINATION OF FOOD

Contamination of food with inorganic contaminants, including the corresponding organometallic complexes. The most important contaminants are mercury, cadmium, and lead. The major types of food involved are cereal grains (bread, flour), meats (beef, pork, beef liver, canned meats, sausages), fish (canned salmon, shellfish, whitefish), dairy products (milk, cheese, butter), fruits, vegetables (fresh and canned), eggs (white and yolk), and beer. Fish and other seafoods are particularly affected, as the mercury in fish occurs in its most toxic form, the methyl form. Mercury can be observed in various forms: the elemental form ($Hg0$), the inorganic or ionic form (Hg^{2+}), or the organic complex form ($R–Hg^+$). Elemental mercury can be oxidized to the inorganic form in the blood and other animal tissues, a process which is mediated by the enzyme catalase. Outside the body, such as in sediments, the oxidation can take place nonenzymatically in the presence of oxygen and organic matter. The formation of organic mercury (by methylation) can occur under a variety of conditions, both in environmental systems and in the animal body. Exposure to organic complexes of mercury, especially methylmercury, is more toxic than exposure to elemental or inorganic mercury. The clinical signs of methylmercury poisoning in humans include numbness and tingling of the extremities, mouth, and lips; loss of hearing and coordination; gross narrowing of the visual fields; reflex changes; progressive psychologic and mental deterioration; sweating and salivation; and muscle fasciculation and atrophy. The total daily intake of mercury per individual in the United States and in Western Europe is estimated at 1–20 mg. The tolerable weekly intake is 300 mg, of which not more than 200 mg should be in the form of methylmercury.

The extensive technological uses of cadmium have resulted in a widespread contamination of the soil, air, water, vegetation, and food supply. Sewage sludge, which is used as fertilizer and soil conditioner, is an important source of soil pollution with cadmium. The major types of food involved are dairy products; meat, fish, and poultry; grains and cereals; potatoes; vegetables (leafy vegetables, legumes, root vegetables); garden and other fruits; oils and fats; sugars and adjuncts; and beverages. In foodstuffs, only inorganic salts of cadmium are present. Factors affecting the absorption and retention of cadmium include the following:

- Calcium deficiency (increases absorption and retention)
- Pyridoxine deficiency (decreases absorption)
- Iron deficiency (increases absorption)
- Milk (increases absorption)
- Age (infants absorb and accumulate more cadmium than adults, whereas retention of cadmium in the kidneys increases with age)

Cadmium has a remarkably low turnover rate in human tissues. The principal organs involved in cadmium accumulation are the kidneys and the liver, although it has also been found in the pancreas and the lungs. Two forms of cadmium poisoning can be observed: (1) acute poisoning (symptoms: nausea, vomiting), and (2) chronic poisoning (symptoms: hypertension, lumbar pains and myalgia in the legs, skeletal deformation, reduced body height, multiple fractures, proteinuria, glaucoma). The intake of cadmium is estimated at 0.14–0.21 mg per week, of which 90% is attributed to the diet. The tolerable weekly intake of cadmium is 0.4–0.5 mg.

The principal source of the total body burden of lead is considered to be the diet, including drinking water. The major types of food involved in lead contamination include cereal grains, seafood (raw and canned), meats, whole eggs, vegetables (leafy vegetables; raw, dried, frozen, or canned legumes), and milk. In foodstuffs, lead exists exclusively as salts, oxides, or sulfhydryl complexes. Most lead salts and oxides are quite insoluble; this property has a significant relationship to the oral toxicity of lead. Since most lead compounds have very low water solubility, only 10% of the ingested lead is absorbed. Absorbed lead can be distributed into three compartments: (1) the freely diffusible lead, which probably includes blood lead and freely exchangeable lead of soft tissues; (2) the more firmly bound but exchangeable soft tissue lead; and (3) the hard tissue lead, such as in bones, teeth, hair, and nails. Blood and soft tissue lead are most likely to be responsible for the symptoms of poisoning. However, hard tissue lead may be an important source of blood and soft tissue lead. Lead poisoning in humans is associated with deficits in the central and peripheral nervous system function, anemia, hemolysis of red blood cells, acute abdominal colic, constipation, vomiting, and progressive renal failure. The average lead intake in the United States varies from 0.7–3.5 mg per week. The tolerable weekly intake through food is 3 mg for adults and 25 mg per kg body weight for children.

CONTAMINATION OF MILK WITH PLANT TOXINS

Milk is readily contaminated when lactating animals or women ingest toxins. Contamination of milk with plant toxins (white snakeroot or rayless goldenrod, for example) has been observed in the United States in rural areas, where the inhabitants depend on the local milk supply. Especially during periods of drought, when grazing plants are scarce and the weeds are in flower, the milk may contain sufficient toxin (tremetone) to give rise to outbreaks of "milk sickness." Symptoms include weakness, followed by anorexia, abdominal pain, vomiting, muscle tremor, delirium, coma, and eventually death. A characteristic accompanying phenomenon is the presence of acetone in the expired air.

CONTAMINATION WITH ORGANIC CHEMICALS

Major types of organic substances occurring as food contaminants are pesticides, industrial chemicals such as halogenated aromatic hydrocarbons, and antibiotics. Pesticides are biocidal substances or mixtures of such substances together with so-called inert ingredients, which are used to control or eliminate unwanted species of insects, ascarids, rodents, fungi, higher plants (weeds), unwanted birds, and other pests. Any substance remaining on foodstuffs together with their degradation products, other derivatives or metabolites, and other types of contaminants of toxicological significance arising from the use of a pesticide is called a pesticide residue. Common classes of pesticides include organochlorines (e.g., aldrin/dieldrin; captafol; captan; 4,4-dichlorodiphenyltrichloroethane [DDT]; 2,3,7,8-tetrachlorodibenzo-p-dioxin [TCDD]), organophosphorus compounds (e.g., malathion; [methyl] parathion), and carbamates (e.g., carbaryl; thiram). Among the types of food involved in contamination with pesticide residues are dairy products, fruits, vegetables, cereals, grains and grain products, fish, meat and meat products, poultry, wines, and honey. The major health hazards of pesticide residues in foodstuffs include carcino-genicity (pesticides which are carcinogenic after conversion to proximate carcinogenic metabolites, or pesticides which become carcinogenic by transformation into nitrosocompounds outside the body or in the alimentary tract in the presence of nitrites), mutagenicity, and teratogenicity. Other toxic effects caused by pesticides are immunosuppression, allergenicity, photosensitivity, estrogenicity, and neurotoxicity. Many of the techniques presently in use for the processing of food give a considerable reduction of pesticide residue levels. Many types of residues can be degraded to harmless products during processing due to heat, steam, light, and acid or alkaline conditions. Furthermore, major reduction of residue levels results from their physical removal by peeling, cleaning, or trimming of foods such as vegetables, fruits, meat, fish, and poultry.

Halogenated aromatic hydrocarbons acting as food contaminants include polychlorinated biphenyls, polychlorinated dibenzodioxins, and polychlorinated dibenzofurans. Polychlorinated biphenyls (PCBs) consist of eight types of compounds, depending on the number of chlorine substituents. They are characterized by their high chemical stability to water, acids, alkalis, and temperatures up to 650°C. Furthermore, they are nonflammable, nonconductors of electricity, and have very low vapor pressures, making them well suited for several industrial uses. Some well-known PCBs are 2,4,3′,4′-tetra-chlorobiphenyl, 2,3,5,3′,4′-penta-chlorobiphenyl, and 2,4,5,2′,4′,5′-hexachlorobi-phenyl. PCBs have been reported to be present in the total diet in many countries and especially in dairy products, meat, fish, poultry, and cereals. Even though production and importation of PCBs have been terminated in the United States and other countries, their health hazard remains because of their persistence in the body and the environment. PCB poisoning has been shown to cause chloracne, induction of phase I (i.e., oxidases, reductases) and phase II (i.e., conjugases) xeno-biotic-metabolizing enzymes, cancer, teratogenic effects, and neurotoxic effects. The most prominent effect in humans is persistent chloracne on the skin of head and chest. The mechanism of the carcinogenicity of PCBs involves promotion rather than initiation. They stimulate the growth of tumors (induced) in the liver, skin, and lungs. Although PCBs have been reported to be carcinogenic in animals, there are only a few reports suggesting that these compounds are also carcinogenic in man. Polychlorinated dibenzodioxins (PCDDs) and polychlorinated dibenzofurans (PCDFs) originate from several sources. PCDD/PCDF emission can result from the incineration of domestic waste containing low-molecular chlorinated hydrocarbons and PCBs. PCDDs and PCDFs are also formed during the production of organochlorine compounds such as polychlorobenzenes, polyc-hlorophenols, and PCBs. The most toxic polyhalogenated aromatic hydrocarbon is 2,3,7,8-tetrachlorodibenzo-p-dioxin (TCDD). Many TCDD-induced effects are similar to those caused by PCBs and other structurally related compounds (e.g., enzyme induction). Other effects of PCDDs and PCDFs include teratogenic effects, immunosuppression, and thymic atrophy.

An important concern of veterinary toxicology is the possible transmission of harmful substances from meat, milk, and other foodstuffs to the human population. This concerns the use of antibiotics as feed additives. These include tetracyclines, nitrofurans, and sulfonamides. Oxytetracycline and furazolidone are suspected of being carcinogens. Oxytetracycline has been reported to react with nitrite to yield (carcinogenic) nitrosamines. In addition, the majority of the antibiotics in use as feed additives pose a serious (indirect) health hazard to humans. Ingestion of these antibiotics may lead to an increased resistance to bacteria, resulting in transfer of antibiotic-resistant bacteria to humans via food intake, originating from animals treated with antibiotics or infected by resistant bacteria, and transfer of the resistance factor (R-factor) from resistant nonpathogenic bacteria to other bacteria which will lead to widespread resistance.

CONTINUOUS SUBCUTANEOUS INSULIN INFUSION (INSULIN PUMP)

Provision of insulin 24 hours daily via a small pump worn by an individual that contains a needle attached under the skin.

COPPER

An essential mineral important as an antioxidant, as a component of the cytochromes, and is essential to the use of iron and the synthesis of hemoglobin.

COPRA, COCONUT OIL

Copra is ground coconut meal from which coconut oil is extracted. Coconut oil is rich in medium-chain saturated fatty acids but does not contain the essential fatty acids. It is one of the group of fats called tropical oils. While solid at 70°F they are liquid at 85°F.

CoQ (COENZYME Q)

Coenzyme Q, also called ubiquinone, is a carrier of hydrogen ions and electrons in the mitochondrial electron transport chain. It transfers electrons between the flavoproteins and the cytochromes. It is nonpolar and can diffuse through the mitochondrial membrane. It is the only component of the respiratory chain that is not fixed. All the other components are proteins.

The synthesis of this compound follows the pathway for cholesterol synthesis. When cholesterol synthesis is inhibited, as happens with the use of the statin drugs, this compound becomes a required nutrient.

COREPRESSOR

A small molecule that triggers repression of transcription by binding to a regulator protein or transcription factor.

CORI CYCLE

A cycle which occurs between the red blood cell, kidneys, muscle, platelets, and the liver and which helps maintain a normal blood glucose level in the face of changes in lactate production. Cori cycle activity is particularly important during exercise as the working muscle is unable to oxidize all the lactate it produces. The muscle does not have gluconeogenic activity. Thus, it must export the accumulating lactate via the blood to the liver, which in turn uses it to make glucose. Figure 14 illustrates this cycle.

CORI DISEASE

Glycogen storage disease, type III, an inherited disease where a mutation has occurred in the gene for the glycogen debranching enzyme (amylo 1,6 glucosidase). It is characterized by excess stored branched glycogen.

CORONARY ARTERIOGRAPHY

The openness of the coronary vasculature is evaluated using an infused radiopaque dye and X-ray pictures.

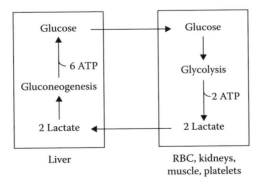

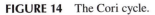

FIGURE 14   The Cori cycle.

CORONARY ARTERY BYPASS GRAFT (CABG)

A common type of cardiac surgery involving the use of the leg's saphenous vein or the internal mammary artery to bypass blockages in one or more coronary arteries.

CORONARY ARTERY DISEASE

Condition in which one or more coronary arteries are occluded, providing decreased blood supply to the heart and resulting in myocardial damage. (See Atherosclerosis.)

CORONARY HEART DISEASE

A disease of the heart resulting from inadequate circulation of blood to the heart muscle.

CORPUS LUTEUM

When the ovary releases an egg via follicle rupture, the cells comprising the follicle enlarge and differentiate, giving rise to the corpus luteum whose function is to produce progesterone and estrogen after ovulation. If the egg is not fertilized this structure will first enlarge and then completely disappear. If the egg is fertilized the corpus luteum will continue to grow and function for the first three months of pregnancy. After this, it will again disappear once the placenta is capable of producing the needed progesterone.

CORTICOSTEROIDS

See Adrenocortical Hormones.

COSMID

A plasmid into which the DNA sequences from bacteriophage lambda that are necessary for the packaging of DNA (cos sites) have been inserted; this permits the plasmid DNA to be packaged in vitro.

COUMARIN

A chroman derivative, occurring in many flavoring agents, such as cassie, woodruff, lavender, and lovage. These flavoring agents are extensively used in sweets, liqueurs, and certain wines. Coumarin is a minor constituent of certain edible fruits, for example, strawberries, cherries, apricots, and a major constituent of tonka beans. Trace quantities of coumarin are also found in citrus oils and carrotseed oil. Coumarin has moderate acute toxicity in animals including man. About 5 g is fatal to sheep; about 4 g produces mild toxic effects in humans; and about 40 g is lethal to horses. Coumarin, which can also be made synthetically, is still allowed for food use in Europe. It is prohibited in the United States as it has been found to cause liver damage in rats.

COUMARIN, DICOUMAROL

A drug that is useful as an anticoagulant in patients with heart disease.

COUPLED REACTION

Two reactions that have a common intermediate which transfers electrons or reducing equivalents or some other element from one set of reactants to another.

COW'S MILK ALLERGY (CMA)

An immunologic response to milk consumption. Cow's milk contains 30–35 g protein per liter. The main antigens are β-lactoglobulin, casein, α-lactalbumin, serum lactalbumin, and the immunoglobulins. β-Lactoglobulin and α-lactalbumin are referred to as the whey proteins. Casein and β-lactoglobulin are the most heat-resistant. Cow's milk allergy is most frequently seen in babies. In 10% of the cases, the symptoms appear in the first week of life, 33% in the second to fourth week, and in 40% during the following months. The main symptoms are eczema and gastrointestinal complaints such as diarrhea, cramps, vomiting, and constipation. Also, rhinitis, asthma, and rash may develop. An often obvious feature is irritability and restlessness. If the diagnosis is cow's milk allergy, a few alternatives for cow's milk are available. Goat's milk and soy milk are sometimes used as are synthetic formulas using purified proteins and/or amino acids.

C-PEPTIDE

A fragment of proinsulin that is cleaved when insulin is active.

C-REACTIVE PROTEIN

A cytokine that is produced by the liver and that circulates in the blood. It is a biomarker for inflammation. The levels of C-reactive protein are inversely related to dietary flavonoid intake. High levels of C-reactive protein are associated with obesity, insulin resistance, and heart disease.

CREAM

The fat-rich layer of nonhomogenized milk that rises to the top of the container.

CREATINE

A metabolite in muscle which is synthesized from glycine and arginine and which can be phosphorylated to form creatine phosphate.

CREATINE PHOSPHATE

A high-energy compound in muscle which has a higher phosphate group transfer potential than ATP. It acts as a reservoir for phosphate so that the muscle can maintain a steady level of ATP to support muscle contraction. It also serves this function in nerve so that a steady supply of ATP for nerve conduction is provided. Creatine phosphate synthesis is shown in Figure 15.

CREATINE PHOSPHOKINASE (CREATINE KINASE)

Enzyme in skeletal muscle, in cardiac muscle, and in brain tissue that catalyzes the transfer of high-energy phosphate from phosphocreatine to ADP to make ATP.

CREATININE

The urinary excretion product of creatine breakdown. The conversion of creatine to creatinine is irreversible. Figure 15 shows the conversion of creatine to creatinine.

CREATININE CLEARANCE

A test for renal function which measures the degree to which creatinine is cleared from the blood.

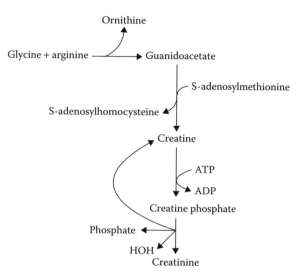

FIGURE 15 Formation of creatine phosphate.

CRETINISM

A disease in children which results from too little thyroxine production by the thyroid gland. It is characterized by poor growth and development and mental retardation.

CRISTAE

The invaginations of the inner mitochondrial membrane.

CRITICAL CONCENTRATION

The target cell/organ concentration at which adverse (reversible/irreversible) functional changes occur. These changes are called critical effects.

CRITICAL ORGAN

The organ in which the critical concentration is reached first under specified conditions for a given population.

CROHN'S DISEASE

A type of inflammatory bowel disease characterized by diarrhea, malabsorption, and ulcers in the gastrointestinal tract, usually in the terminal ileum and colon. Also known as regional enteritis. The malabsorption that is characteristic of this disease leads to malnutrition.

CROSS-SECTIONAL STUDIES

Nonexperimental studies in which data on exposure as well as biological effects are collected at the same time. This kind of study is often used to describe the prevalence of certain exposures or diseases in a population. From an etiological point of view, an essential disadvantage of these studies is the problem of discerning effect from cause.

CRUCIFEROUS VEGETABLES

Vegetables that are members of the cabbage family. Included are various types of cabbage, brussels sprouts, broccoli, kohlrabi, and kale.

CRUDE FIBER

The residue of plant food left after extraction by dilute acid and alkali. The term crude fiber does not include all the undigested material, which may prove to have nutritional value to man. While cellulose, plant fibers, and other so-called nondigestible carbohydrates are not digestible by the enzymes located in the upper portion of the intestine, the intestine contains flora which can partially degrade some of these food components. This degradation provides fatty acids and other useful compounds which are then absorbed by the lower small intestine and colon. (See Fiber.)

CRYPTORCHIDISM

One or both testes do not descend from the abdominal cavity at birth. If undescended the male could be infertile.

C-TERMINUS

The end of an amino acid chain having a carboxyl group.

CTP

Cytidine triphosphate. A nucleotide consisting of cytosine (a pyrimidine), ribose, and three high-energy phosphate groups.

CURCUMIN

A component of the seasoning turmeric; it is a polyphenol that serves as an inhibitor of the NFκB signaling pathway and thus serves to reduce the inflammatory response by modulating T-cell nuclear factor (NFκB) activation. Curcumin inhibits adipogenesis and T-cell proliferation as well as interleukin-2 production.

CURD

The coagulum of milk from which cheese can be made.

CUSHING'S SYNDROME

A disease due to overproduction of glucocorticoids by the adrenal cortex. The syndrome is characterized by abnormal glucose tolerance, excess muscle protein degradation, fatigue, osteoporosis, excess hair growth, excess fat deposition on shoulders and abdomen, and skin discoloration.

CYANIDE

A metabolic poison. It blocks the transport of reducing equivalents from complex III to complex IV of the respiratory chain in the mitochondria and blocks complex IV of oxidative phosphorylation.

CYANOCOBALAMIN

See Vitamin B_{12}.

CYANOGENIC GLYCOSIDES

Glycosides from which cyanide is formed by the activity of hydrolytic enzymes. More than 1000 plant species from 90 families and 250 genera have been reported to be cyanophoric. The cyanogenic glycoside molecule consists of a monosaccharide (glucose) or disaccharide (vicianose or gentiobiose) and an aglycone in the form of a β-hydroxynitrile. The glycoside is hydrolyzed in the presence of β-glucosidase; the nitrile undergoes further degradation by a lyase, generating hydrogen cyanide and other metabolites.

CYANOSIS

A dark bluish or purplish skin color due to inadequate oxygenation of the blood in the lungs or to an obstruction to blood flow through the capillaries. The color is due to the accumulation of reduced hemoglobin.

CYCLAMATE

Nonnutritive sweetener; sodium cyclamate. When fed to rats in very high amounts, sodium cyclamate was found to produce bladder tumors. On the basis of this finding, the Delaney Clause of the U.S. Pure Food and Drug Act was exercised, and this sweetener was withdrawn from use in foods in the United States.

CYCLIC AMP (cAMP)

A second messenger for catabolic hormone effects. The hormone binds to a membrane receptor which in turn stimulates adenyl cyclase which acts on ATP to produce cyclic AMP.

CYCLIN

A member of a family of proteins that participate in regulating the stages of the cell cycle and whose concentrations change dramatically over the course of the cell cycle.

CYCLOBENZAPRINE HYDROCHLORIDE

A drug that is used as a muscle relaxant. Trade name: Flexeril.

CYCLOOXYGENASE (COX)

Two forms exist, COX I and COX II. It is the enzyme responsible for the formation of eicosanoids, particularly those that act as inflammatories. COX I is a constitutive enzyme present in most cell types and works under noninflammatory conditions. COX II is inducible in cells as part of an inflammatory response to injury or irritation. COX II is the target of several prescription anti-inflammatory drugs useful in the treatment of arthritis.

CYCLOPROPENE FATTY ACIDS

Fatty acids occurring in the oils or fat of every plant of the order Malvales, except for cocoa butter from *Theobroma cocoa*. From a food toxicological point of view, only the acids in the oils of cottonseed and kapok seed are of significance. The most important acids are sterculic and malvalic acids; both are toxic monounsaturated fatty acids.

CYSTATHIONINURIA

A high level of cystathionine in the urine caused by a mutation in the gene for cystathionase which catalyzes the production of cysteine from cystathionine.

CYSTEINE

A nonessential 3 carbon amino acid containing sulfur; can be made from methionine.

CYSTIC FIBROSIS

A genetic disease in which the body fails to conserve the chloride ion.

CYSTINE

A molecule containing two cysteines joined through the terminal sulfur atoms.

CYSTINURIA

An inherited disease characterized by excessive amounts of cystine in the urine. The disease is due to a mutation in the gene for the renal carrier of cystine, lysine, and arginine.

CYTIDINE

A nucleotide consisting of cytosine (a pyrimidine) and ribose.

CYTOCHROMES

Electron carriers in the respiratory chain and elsewhere. All cytochromes have a heme prosthetic group which contains iron. The iron fluctuates between the +2 and +3 states. The cytochrome P-450 enzymes are important to the detoxification processes in the body.

CYTOKINES

Small peptides that have regulatory properties or hormone-like actions. Table 23 provides a list of these compounds. Cytokines are produced by macrophages, lymphocytes, brain, adipocytes, and other cell types.

TABLE 23
Cytokines, Their Receptors, and Their Signaling Mechanisms

Cytokine	Receptor Distribution	Signaling Mechanism
IL-2	T cells, B cells, monocytes, myeloid precursors, NK cells	High-affinity binding induces phosphorylation of tyrosine kinase
IL-1	T cells, B cells, fibroblasts, endothelial cells, keratinocytes	A GTP-binding motif suggests G protein activity. May involve cAMP and PLC activation
IL-5	B cells, eosinophils, basophils	Cellular tyrosine kinase induces phosphorylation of several proteins, and this proline-rich receptor protein may be one of them
IL-4	T cells, B cells, monocytes, macrophages, granulocytes, megakaryocytes, erythroid products, NK cells, fibroblasts, endothelial cells	Cellular tyrosine kinase induces phosphorylation of this serine and proline-rich receptor protein
IL-6	T cells, B cells, monocytes, fibroblasts, megakaryocytes, hepatocytes, keratinocytes, mesangial cells	Tyrosine kinase-mediated signaling system
IL-8	Neutrophils, basophils, monocytes, T cells (3 types of receptors)	Tyrosine kinase-mediated signaling system
IL-3	Myeloid precursors, basophils, mast cells, macrophages, megakaryocytes	Involves tyrosine kinase protein kinase C
IL-7	Two types: high and low affinity, B-cell progenetors, thymocytes	Tyrosine kinase
IL-3	Basophils, myeloid precursors, mast cells, macrophages, megakaryocytes	Tyrosine kinase
SCF	Pluripotent stem cells, lymphoid precursors, myeloid precursors, megakaryocyte precursors, erythroid precursors	SCF binding initial dimerization of receptors. Also involves the tyrosine kinase, phosphorylation of PLC γ, c-raf, and PI-3 kinase. Ca^{++} is also involved as a second messenger
LIF	Hematopoietic stem cells, megakaryocyte progenitors, osteoblasts, neurons, myoblasts, adipocytes, embryonic stem cells, hepatocytes, kidney epithelial cells, placental cells	Involves the tyrosine kinase system
G-CSF	Granulocytes, pluripotent stem cells, myeloid progenitors, T cells, fibroblasts, endothelial cells	Involves G proteins and the tyrosine kinase
EPO	Erythoid precursors, megakaryocytes	?
GM-CSF	Myeloid precursors, monocytes, macrophages, eosinophils, neutrophils, megakaryocytes, endothelial cells, osteoblasts, Langerhans cells	Involves the tyrosine kinase system
M-CSF	Monocytes, macrophages	Involves the tyrosine kinase system
TGF α, β	Several related cytokines and receptors. Found in most cells	Involves the tyrosine kinase system
NPY	Found in most neural cells	Involves the tyrosine kinase system
TGF α, β	Found in many cell types	?
Leptin	Found in brain cells as well as other cell types	?

CYTOKINESIS

The splitting of the cell into two following mitosis.

CYTOPLASM (CYTOSOL)

Cell sap; the medium in which the organelles of the cell are suspended.

CYTOSINE

A pyrimidine base found in the genetic materials DNA and RNA.

CYTOSKELETON

The network of intracellular fibers that gives a cell its shape and structural rigidity.

CYTOTOXIC AGENTS

Chemicals that destroy specific cells; streptozotocin is an example. This agent destroys the insulin-producing β cells of the pancreas.

D

D5W SOLUTION

An isotonic solution containing 50 g of glucose per liter of solution.

D-ARM

A conserved stem-loop structure in a tRNA molecule that usually contains the modified base dihydrouridine.

DAILY RECOMMENDED INTAKE (DRI)

A recent revision of the Recommended Dietary Allowance (RDA) by the Food and Nutrition Board (National Academy of Sciences) that provides guidance in assessing the dietary intakes of selected population groups. Many of the DRI values for minerals are different from the RDAs in that ranges are provided rather than set figures. The population is also divided differently with respect to the age or sex groupings. Current DRIs can be found online at http://www.nap.edu.

DAILY REFERENCE VALUES (DRVS)

Desirable intakes of specific nutrients.

DALTEPARIN SODIUM

A low molecular weight heparin that is useful as an anticoagulant. Trade name: Fragmin.

DALTON (DA)

A unit of molecular mass; 1/12 the mass of a $_{12}C$ atom.

DARBEPOETIN ALFA

A drug that can stimulate hematopoiesis and is therefore useful in combating anemia. Trade name: Aranesp.

DARK ADAPTATION

Adaptation of the visual cycle to changes in light intensity. The process is dependent on adequate vitamin A intake. Failure to adapt to changing light intensity is one of the first symptoms of vitamin A deficiency.

DAWN PHENOMENON

Early morning hyperglycemia thought to result from decreased sensitivity to insulin.

DE

Digestive energy. The energy of food after the costs (and losses) of digestion are subtracted.

DEAMINASE

An enzyme which catalyzes the removal of an amino group from a carbon chain.

DEAMINATION

The process of amino group removal.

DEBRANCHING

The enzymatic removal of side chains from a branched polymer such as glycogen.

DEBRIDEMENT

Removal of necrotic tissue.

DECARBOXYLASE

An enzyme that catalyzes the removal of a carboxyl group from a carbon chain.

DECARBOXYLATION

The reaction in which a carboxyl group is removed.

DECIDUOUS TEETH

The first teeth of the young. These teeth are replaced by permanent teeth as the individual matures.

DECUBITUS ULCER

Term used to describe a pressure ulcer.

DEEP FRYING

A food preparation method consisting of immersing the food totally in hot fat. This method may result in the formation of small amounts of stable peroxides.

DEFIBRILLATION

Ceasing heart fibrillation with drugs or physical means.

DEGRADE

To reduce large molecules to smaller ones.

DEHYDRATASES

Enzymes that catalyze the removal of a molecule of water from a carbon chain. These enzymes frequently require pyridoxine as a coenzyme.

DEHYDRATION

The process of water removal.

DEHYDROASCORBIC ACID

A form of ascorbic acid (vitamin C) in which two hydrogens have been removed.

DEHYDROEPIANDOSTERONE (DHEA)

A metabolic intermediate in the pathway for testosterone synthesis. It is produced by the adrenals and the gonads.

DEHYDROGENASES

Enzymes that catalyze the removal of reducing equivalents (hydrogen ions) from carbon chains.

DEHYDROGENATION

Removal of hydrogen ions. It is catalyzed by a group of enzymes called dehydrogenases.

DELANY CLAUSE OF THE U.S. FOOD, DRUG, AND COSMETC ACT

Law that prohibits the use of any chemical in foods that can be shown to cause cancer at any level of intake.

DELIRIUM TREMENS

A condition characterized by agitation, anorexia, hallucinations, and uncontrollable movement.

DELTA (Δ)

Change. The Greek symbol is Δ.

$\Delta G°$

Free energy that is available to do work.

$\Delta G°'$

Standard free energy of biochemical reactions.

$\Delta \Psi$

Membrane potential

DEMENTIA

Condition characterized by a reduction in cognitive function.

DENATURATION

See Protein Denaturation.

DENATURE

To disrupt the native conformation of a polymer.

DENSITOMETRY

Measurement of body density.

DENTIN

The major portion of a tooth; about 20% is organic matrix (collagen with some elastin), while 80% is hydroxyapatite containing calcium, phosphorous, magnesium, carbonate, and fluoride.

DEOXY SUGAR

A saccharide (sugar) produced by replacement of an OH group by H.

DEOXYADENOSINE

A nucleoside containing adenine (a purine) and deoxyribose.

DEOXYCYTIDINE

A nucleoside containing cytosine (a pyrimidine) and deoxyribose.

DEOXYGUANINE

A nucleoside containing guanine (a purine) and deoxyribose.

DEPENDENT ACTION

Combination of substances with different sites of action and interaction between the components.

DEPOLARIZATION

The loss of membrane potential that occurs during electrical signaling in cells such as neurons.

DEPRESSION

Condition characterized by extreme sadness, helplessness, and social isolation. Part of the condition is known as bipolar disease.

DERMATITIS

Inflammation of the skin. Red, scaly, itchy skin characterizes dermatitis.

DESATURASE

An enzyme that introduces double bonds into a newly synthesized fatty acid.

DESLORATADINE

A selective H_1-receptor antagonist that serves as an antihistamine. Trade name: Clarinex.

DETOXIFICATION

Removal of toxic properties of a substance; metabolic conversion of pharmacologically active compounds to nonactive compounds.

DEUTERIUM

A hydrogen isotope having twice the mass of the common hydrogen atom.

DEUTERIUM OXIDE

Heavy water contains two molecules of deuterium and one molecule of oxygen.

DEXA

Dual energy X-ray absorptiometry (DEXA) is used to estimate bone density and soft tissue composition. Bone density as a fraction of the fat free mass can be distinguished and quantitated using this method.

DEXAMETHASONE

A synthetic glucocorticoid that is four times stronger than natural cortisol. It is sold as a sodium salt, as an acetate, or as a sodium phosphate. Both tablet and solutions are marketed. It serves as an anti-inflammatory and as an immunosuppresant. Trade names: Decadron, Hexadrol, Cortestat, Decaject, Dexone, Dexasone, Delalone, Maxidex.

DEXTRAN

A glucose polymer.

DEXTROSE

Synonymous with glucose.

DHHS

U.S. Department of Health and Human Services.

DIABETES INSIPIDUS

A disease of the pituitary that results in excessive urination and thirst due to a lack of ADH.

DIABETES KETOACIDOSIS

Abnormal (greater than 20 mg/L) levels of ketones in blood, which cannot be neutralized by the body's buffering system. If untreated can cause coma and death.

DIABETES MELLITUS

A group of genetic diseases characterized by an inappropriate glucose-insulin relationship. The number of genetic mutations thought to be responsible is in excess of 300 depending on the definitions used for the disease (see http://www.omim.com). Not all of the genetic mutations that cause the diabetic state have been found. Furthermore, there are twice as many people with mutations that associate with diabetes than there are people with the disease. This indicates that factors in addition to genetic ones may be involved in the development of the disease. The disease is divided into two major groups: (1) type 1 diabetes mellitus, and (2) type 2 diabetes mellitus. The division is based on the therapy needed upon diagnosis, and there is some blurring of this separation. Of the total population with diabetes mellitus, about 10% have the disease as a result of pancreatic insulin production failure, while 90% develop the disease as a response to one or more failures in the target tissues such as liver, muscle, and/or adipose tissue.

Diabetes mellitus in its most severe form is characterized by the symptoms of excessive thirst, excessive urination, rapid weight loss, and if not recognized and treated promptly, coma and death can occur. Less severe forms of the disease have less striking symptoms. The American Diabetes Association has identified several criteria for the diagnosis of the disorder. These are listed in Table 24.

Uncontrolled diabetes is characterized by tissue wasting. The fat stores and body protein are raided. Proteolysis is enhanced, and the amino acids thus liberated are used for energy or as substrates for intracellular glucose synthesis. The ammonia released as a product of the deamination of these amino acids assists in the buffering of the accumulating ketones. However, this ammonia is in itself cytotoxic, so the body must increase its capacity to convert it to urea. Humans with uncontrolled diabetes thus are characterized by a loss in body protein, an increase in blood and urine levels of ammonia, an increase in urea synthesis, a negative nitrogen balance, a loss in fat store, elevated blood and urine levels of glucose, and elevated levels of fatty acid oxidation products. Some of these metabolic products are also excreted via the lungs in the expired air. The breath of an uncontrolled diabetic has the aroma of the ketones.

Several explanations for pancreatic insulin production failure have been offered. The two most generally accepted are (1) failure due to autoimmune destruction of the insulin-producing islet cells in the pancreas, and (2) failure due to viral destruction of the islet β cells. In each of these instances, the genetic heritage of the individual plays a role and the immune system is involved. Other causes of diabetes mellitus include genetic errors in insulin structure, insulin receptor structure, downstream signaling, and genetically determined problems in glucose metabolism. Insulin resistance is observed in that the target tissues are resistant to the glucose-lowering effect of insulin. Diabetes

---

TABLE 24
Criteria for the Diagnosis of Diabetes Mellitus[1]

1. A1C (a measure of the amount of glucose associated with hemoglobin) of less than 6.5%. This test should be performed in a laboratory that is NGSP certified and standardized to the DCCT assay.

OR

2. Fasting blood glucose ≥126 mg/dL (7.0 mmol/L). Fasting is defined as no food intake for at least 8 hours.[2]

OR

3. 2-hour plasma glucose ≥200 mg/dL (11.1 mmol/L) during an oral glucose tolerance test.[2] The test should be performed as described by WHO using a glucose load containing the equivalent of 75 g anhydrous glucose dissolved in water.

OR

4. In a patient with classic symptoms of hyperglycemia or hyperglycemic crisis, a random plasma glucose greater than 200 mg/dL (11.1 mmol/L). Casual is defined as any time of day without regard to time since the last meal. The classic symptoms of diabetes include polyuria, polydipsia, and unexplained weight loss.

NGSP = National Glycohemoglobin Standardization Program; DCCT = Diabetes Control and Complications Trial.

[1] These criteria are updated periodically by an expert panel of the American Diabetes Association. Table 24 can be found in the January 2010 issue of *Diabetes Care*, Supplement 1, 100 pgs.

[2] These measures should be repeated on a different day to confirm diagnosis.

can develop secondary to the accretion of excess fat stores. This condition can also be genetically determined as well as by an interaction of genetic predisposition and lifestyle choices.

When the fat cell becomes enlarged, it becomes insulin resistant. For decades, it has been known that overly fat people who are insulin resistant can reverse their condition by restricting their energy intake, thereby reducing their excess fat store. When the adipocyte returns to its normal size it becomes normally responsive to the action of insulin. Both obesity and type 2 diabetes are associated with chronic inflammation. There is an abnormally high level of tumor necrosis factor alpha (TNFα) as well as abnormal levels of biomarkers of inflammation (c-reactive protein, cytokines, lipid peroxides, etc).

Insulin resistance can be observed in muscle and adipose tissue. By definition, insulin resistance means that it takes abnormally large amounts of insulin to regulate or control blood glucose within normal limits. A person with insulin resistance may not develop abnormal glucose tolerance if the pancreas is able to sustain an abnormally high insulin output. In this circumstance, the individual may be insulin resistant and hyperinsulinemic but not hyperglycemic or have abnormal glucose tolerance. Eventually, the islet β cells may not be able to sustain this high insulin output and the insulin resistance will then progress to abnormal glucose tolerance and subsequently to the diabetic hyperglycemic state. Insulin resistance can also be attributed to postreceptor defects. Errors in the codes for the glucose transporter genes and in the genes for the downstream signaling molecules can result in diabetes. Errors in the codes (either in the mitochondrial genome or the nuclear genome) for components of the mitochondrial oxidative phosphorylation system are associated with the development of diabetes.

DIABETES MELLITUS CARE

Upon diagnosis, glucose management through exercise, diet control, blood glucose assessment, and regular physician assessment can optimize the health status of the patient. Glucose management may include insulin replacement and/or the use of hypoglycemic drugs. Exercise will assist glucose use by the muscles. Weight control, if necessary, will also promote normalization of blood glucose. Physician assessment should include regular examination of eyes, renal function, and the function of the vascular system. The latter should include assessment of blood pressure, blood lipids, and cardiovascular function. Medications to help normalize these functions may be needed.

DIABETIC NEPHROPATHY

Renal disease that is a secondary complication of diabetes mellitus and involves degenerative changes in the glomerulus and thickening of the basement membrane.

DIABETIC NEUROPATHY

Degenerative changes in the peripheral nerves attributed to the diabetic state. Such changes are associated with circulatory failure and are characterized by losses in sensation in the affected area. Loss in perception of pain or other sensations can result in losses of tissue through infection.

DIABETIC RETINOPATHY

Degenerative changes in the capillaries in the retina, which in turn progress to blindness.

DIACYLGLYCEROL

A lipid having two fatty acids esterified to glycerol; it is also called diglyceride.

DIAGNOSIS-RELATED GROUPS (DRGS)

Classes of medical diagnoses in a system devised to control health care costs and used to establish reimbursement for hospital care.

DIALYSIS

Process of removing toxic compounds from blood and body fluid using instrumentation, which allows for diffusion and filtration between solutions separated by a semipermeable membrane.

DIAPHORESIS

Excessive perspiration.

DIARRHEA

Excessive loss of feces and water through the intestine. The most frequent cause of diarrhea is that of food-borne illness. A variety of pathogens can cause food-borne illness. Diarrhea can result when the individual develops an irritable colon. A hyperirritable intestine may be the result of a particular medication, or it may be permanent due to a genetic error. Genetic errors resulting in the absence of a particular digestive enzyme will result in an accumulation of that substrate in the gut. This in turn will "pull" water into the intestine and diarrhea will result. Lactose intolerance due to the absence of the enzyme lactase is an example of a genetic disorder characterized by diarrhea. Gluten-induced enteropathy is another example. In this instance, the patient is unable to digest the wheat protein gluten. Diarrhea is characteristic of this condition and if allowed to continue untreated, the intestinal villi will be abraded and the absorption of nutrients in addition to the gluten will be seriously impaired. Treatment for these types of diarrhea is fairly straightforward. If the offending nutrient is eliminated from the diet, the patient will gradually rebuild the absorptive surface of the intestine and will recover.

DIARRHEIC SHELLFISH POISONING

Characterized by gastrointestinal complaints, including diarrhea, vomiting, nausea, and abdominal spasms. Recently, toxins involved in this poisoning have been chemically identified. They constitute a group of derivatives of a C38 fatty acid, okada acid. These shellfish poisons are produced by the dinoflagellate species, Dinophysis and Prorocentrum.

DIBASIC AMINO ACID

Amino acids having two amino groups. Lysine and arginine are dibasic amino acids.

DICOUMAROL

Vitamin K antagonist; it interferes with normal blood clotting; produced when sweet clover spoils. Other names are dicoumarin, dicumol, dufalone, and melitoxin. Active ingredient in warfarin, a rat poison.

DICLOFENAC

A drug useful in the treatment of arthritis; it is a nonsteroidal anti-inflammatory drug. It is offered as either a sodium or potassium salt. Trade names: Solaraze, Voltarin, Cataflam.

DICYCLOMINE HYDROCHLORIDE

A drug that is an antispasmodic and antimuscarinic. It is particularly useful as an antispasmodic in the gastrointestinal tract. Trade names: Antispas, Bentyl, Neoquess, Spasmoban.

DIET-INDUCED THERMOGENESIS

A rise in heat production associated with the consumption of food. This energy loss represents the energy cost of the processing of food for metabolic use.

DIET THERAPY

Modification of a normal diet to manage the symptoms of a disease.

DIETARY BEHAVIOR

Includes a multitude of behaviors and can refer to food choice, food preparation, food preservation, and (actual) food consumption.

Attempts have been made to change certain dietary behaviors of the population for reasons of health. These nutritional interventions are aimed at groups of patients, high-risk groups, healthy people, or intermediaries, such as people working in the kitchen of a restaurant. The complexity of dietary behavior can also be illustrated by the diversity of the objectives of nutritional interventions such as increasing the hygienic behavior in the catering industry; reducing the consumption of proteins and sodium by kidney patients to relieve the kidney(s) as much as possible; reducing the total energy intake to prevent or treat obesity; increasing the consumption of food products containing carbohydrates to improve achievements in endurance sports; increasing the knowledge about food preservation to prevent food poisoning, for example, resulting from microbial contamination; and reducing alcohol consumption to decrease the number of alcohol-related traffic accidents.

Dietary behavior is determined by many factors, such as the availability of food, the food policy of the government, social environment, advertising, and the experience and opinions people have regarding food safety. In general, three main groups of behavioral determinants can be distinguished: (1) attitude (what do people think of their behavior themselves?); (2) social influence (what is the role of the social environment?); and (3) possibilities (either internal or external to the person) for displaying a behavior. External factors affecting these behavioral determinants are age, education, sex, physiological variables, and habit. An attitude toward a specific behavior reflects whether a person's general feelings are favorable or unfavorable toward that behavior and is determined by the evaluation of all pros and cons of the behavior. To identify the specific pros and cons people may be asked to point out which consequences they believe the behavior is connected with (= beliefs). It is also important to know whether the consequence is considered an advantage or a disadvantage (= evaluations).

Social environment very much affects dietary behavior. There are two kinds of social influence: (1) direct influence (referring to the clear expectations of others as to how someone should behave), and (2) indirect influence (referring to modeling, imitating the behavior of others). The third group of influencing factors is the possibilities or impossibilities for displaying a behavior. Impossibilities for behavior can be external (e.g., unavailability of products, money, or time, and noncooperative members of the family) or internal (e.g., lack of information, skills, or perseverance) to the person.

DIETARY FIBER

See Fiber.

DIETARY GUIDELINES FOR AMERICANS

A list of nine key messages based on the preponderance of scientific evidence that are designed to help Americans make good decision regarding their lifestyle choices. Included are the following:

- Consume a variety of foods within and among the basic food groups while staying within energy needs.
- Control energy intake to manage body weight.
- Be physically active every day.
- Increase daily intake of fruits and vegetables, whole grains, and nonfat or low-fat milk and milk products.
- Choose fats wisely for good health.
- Choose carbohydrates wisely for good health.
- Choose and prepare foods with little salt.
- If you drink alcoholic beverages, do so in moderation.
- Keep food safe to eat.

These guidelines are updated every five years.

DIETARY HISTORY METHOD

See Interview Method.

DIETETIC TECHNICIAN, REGISTERED (DTR)

Individual who has completed a minimum of an associate degree in dietetics or a related area at a U.S. regionally accredited college or university, has completed a supervised clinical experience, and has passed a national examination.

DIETITIAN (RD)

Individual who has completed a minimum of a baccalaureate degree in dietetics or a related area in a U.S. accredited college or university, has completed a supervised clinical experience, and has passed a national examination. A dietitian is trained in the art of advising clients in the selections of foods appropriate to the age, nutrient needs, and health of the individual. A therapeutic dietitian works closely with a physician to ensure that the food choices are appropriate for the particular medical state the physician wishes to manage. These conditions may include specific nutrient differences, specific nutrient or food intolerances, or metabolic diseases requiring close management of the intake of specific food components, such as glucose, saturated fat, specific amino acids, and so on.

DIFFERENTIAL MISCLASSIFICATION

Errors in the necessary information (e.g., in exposure measurement) that are related to the state of disease. This type of misclassification has more serious consequences than the nondifferential or random misclassification. It can lead to either underestimation or overestimation of the effect.

DIFFUSION

A uniform distribution of solutes on both sides of a permeable membrane.

DIGESTION

The process of mechanical and chemical breakdown of food into absorbable units within the digestive tract.

DIGESTIVE TRACT

The section of the body beginning with the mouth and ending at the anus. Includes the mouth, esophagus, stomach, small intestine (duodenum, jejunum, ileum), cecum, large intestine, rectum, and anus.

DIGITALIS (DIGOXIN)

A drug that assists in the maintenance of a regular heartbeat. It is a cardiac glycoside.

DIGLYCERIDE (DIACYLGLYCEROL)

Two fatty acids esterified to glycerol.

5α-DIHYDROTESTOSTERONE

The active form of the male sex hormone, testosterone.

DIHYDROXY CHOLECALCIFEROL

The active form of vitamin D. Also called 1,25-dihydroxy cholecalciferol.

DILTIAZEM HYDROCHLORIDE

A calcium channel blocker that serves as an antianginal drug. Trade names: Apo-diltiaz, Cardizem, Dilacor, Diltia.

DIPEPTIDE

Two amino acids linked together by a peptide bond.

DIPHENOXYLATE HYDROCHLORIDE (WITH ATROPINE SULFATE)

An antidiarrheal drug. Trade names: Logen, Lomanate, Lomotil, Lonox.

DIPHENYLHYDRAMINE HYDROCHLORIDE

A ethanolamine derivative that serves as an antihistamine. It also is an antiemetic, an antivertigo agent, an antitussive, a sedative-hypnotic, and a dyskinetic. Trade names: Allerdryl, Benedryl, Hydramine, Nytol, Sominex.

DIPLOID

Having two equivalent sets of chromosomes.

DIRECT CALORIMETRY

The measurement of heat produced by a body or the combustion of food through the use of a calorimeter.

DISACCHARIDE

A carbohydrate containing two sugar (saccharide) units. Sucrose, mannose, and lactose are common disaccharides in the human diet.

DISSEMINATED INTRAVASCULAR COAGULATION (DIC)

Acquired clotting disorder occurring simultaneously with another medical condition in which clotting mechanisms become accelerated resulting in occlusion of the microcirculation. Common causes of DIC include obstetric complications, cancer, sepsis, and massive tissue damage.

DISTAL

Away from the center of the body.

DISTENTION

The condition of being expanded or extended beyond normal.

DISULFIDE BRIDGE

A covalent bond containing two sulfur molecules.

DIURESIS

Urine excretion in excess of normal.

DIURETICS

Pharmaceutic agents which increase urinary water loss.

DIURNAL VARIATION

Cyclical changes in one or more features of the body over a 24-hour period.

DIVERTICULITIS

Inflammation of a diverticulum, a small pocket in the wall of the intestine.

DIVERTICULOSIS

The presence of a number of diverticula in the intestine.

DNA

Deoxyribonucleic acid. The genetic material in the nucleus and mitochondria. DNA dictates all the genetically determined characteristics. Each of these characteristics is coded by the sequence of purine and pyrimidine bases that are connected together in a double-stranded helix. (See Protein Synthesis.)

DOPAMINE

A neurotransmitter synthesized from tyrosine in the adrenal medulla and the CNS.

DOUBLE-BLIND STUDY

An experiment designed such that neither the subject nor the investigator is aware of the treatment given to the subject.

DOWNSTREAM

Base sequences in either DNA or RNA that proceed further in the direction of expression.

DOXAZOSIN MESYLATE

A drug that is an α-blocker and serves as an antihypertensive medication. Trade name: Cardura.

DRUG-NUTRIENT INTERACTIONS

Drugs that interfere with the action of particular nutrients. In this circumstance, the drug becomes an antinutrient (see http://www.drug digest.org/dd/Home; http://www.drugs.com/drug_interactions.html; http://www.medicine.iupui.edu/flockhart/ for more information on interactions). Table 25 gives some examples of these interactions.

DUAL ENERGY RADIOGRAPHIC ABSORPTIOMETRY (DERA)

A procedure based on X-rays that measures bone mineralization. Also known as dual X-ray absorptiometry (DXA and DEXA).

DUAL PHOTON ABSORPTIOMETRY

Similar to DEXA but uses photons at two different energy levels to determine bone mineral content.

DUMPING SYNDROME

Characterized by the rapid rate of gastric emptying into the intestine after ingestion of food and frequently resulting in diarrhea, nausea, and weakness.

TABLE 25
Some Drugs That Affect Nutrient Intakes and Use

Drug	Effect
Phenethylamine and related compounds	Anorexia
Amphetamine	Anorexia
Ethanol	Inhibits intestinal absorption of folate, B_{12}; increases need for niacin, riboflavin, thiamin, and pyridoxine
Diphenylhydantoin (Dilantin)	Impairs use of folate
Oral contraceptives	Increases folate turnover
Azulfidine	Decreases folate absorption, B_{12}, and fat-soluble vitamins
Neomycin	Decreases lipid absorption
P-aminosalicylic acid	Promotes diarrhea and results in decreased absorption of almost all nutrients
Colchicine	Promotes diarrhea and results in decreased absorption of almost all nutrients
Biguanides (phenformin, metformin)	Decreases absorption of B_{12}
Bile salt sequestrants	Decreases fat and fat-soluble vitamin absorption

---

DUODENUM

The first 12 inches of the small intestine of the human.

DWARFISM

Abnormal (reduced) growth due to a deficiency in growth hormone production.

DYNAMIC STATE

A state of flux as happens in living cells. Components of the cell are constantly being synthesized and degraded such that there is little net gain except for those products of metabolism, which are storage products, such as glycogen and triacylglycerides.

DYNORPHIN

An appetite stimulant.

DYSGEUSIA

Abnormal taste perception.

DYSPHAGIA

Difficulty with swallowing.

DYSURIA

Painful or difficult urination.

E

EATING DISORDER

Eating behavior that leads to disease or disability, including any eating pattern that deviates from the cultural norm. The most common eating disorders include anorexia nervosa, bulimia nervosa, and compulsive overeating.

ECHOCARDIOGRAPHY

Diagnostic procedure that employs ultrasound to inspect the structures of the heart.

ECLAMPSIA

Coma and convulsions that may develop during pregnancy or immediately after parturition. Preceded by hypertension, edema, and proteinuria.

ECOLOGICAL STUDIES

Nonexperimental studies in which the unit of observation is not the individual but a group of people in a particular environment, such as workers in a factory or inhabitants of a city or a country. These studies can be useful if information on individuals is not available; exposure is then an overall measure for the population under investigation. The outcome variable under investigation in ecological studies is often mortality. A well-known phenomenon occurring in this type of study is the so-called ecological fallacy. On comparing countries, it may be found that the higher the average level of a risk factor A for a country, the higher the level of mortality due to disease B, while within each country (based on individual measurements of A and B) risk factor A is negatively associated with disease B.

EDEMA

Excess accumulation of water in the body, particularly in the periphery; also called dropsy or hydrops. A condition of disordered water balance. It usually occurs secondary to a primary disease. In this condition, water is accumulated in the tissues distal to the kidneys. Urine volume is very low and highly concentrated. As the fluids in the extracellular compartment increase, the functionality of the patient decreases. At first, the edema is noted in the extremities. Feet, ankles, legs, and hands become swollen, then, noticeably, there is an accumulation of fluid in the abdominal cavity and in the pericardial sac. This fluid accumulation makes it difficult for the patient to walk and, eventually, interferes with the vital functions of the internal organs such as the heart.

Depending on the primary disorder, the edema can be treated. If due to inadequate protein or thiamin intake, these nutrients can be supplied and the edema will subside as the patient's nutritional status improves. If, however, the edema is due to heart disease characterized by an impaired ability to pump the blood throughout the body, a loss in the pressure differential needed for peripheral fluid exchange and circulation through the renal tubules will occur. In this instance, the treatment is much more difficult since it depends on the successful treatment of the diseased heart. Edema can also result from a loss of vascular elasticity, which characterizes high blood pressure (hypertension).

Hypertension occurs when the vascular system is continually stimulated to constrict. In this disorder, the pressure of the blood is so high in the peripheral tissues that water cannot flow from the tissues to the blood in response to the usual pressure differential between the arteries, arterioles, capillaries, venules and veins, and the tissues they serve. However, if the blood pressure can be reduced through antivasoconstrictor medication, sodium intake restriction, and, if needed, weight reduction, then the edema will also be reduced.

EDEMATOUS DISORDERS

A group of diseases characterized by excessive water and sodium retention. Included are congestive heart failure, nephritic syndrome, and hepatic cirrhosis.

EDENTULOUS

Toothless.

EFLORNITHINE HYDROCHLORIDE

A drug that inhibits the enzyme, ornithine decarboxylase. It also inhibits hair growth. Trade name: Vaniqa.

EGG ALLERGY

Egg white is the most frequent cause of egg allergy. Egg white contains about 20 allergens, the most important being ovalbumin, ovotransferrin, and ovomucoid. The latter is heat resistant. Other egg allergens that have been isolated are lysozymes. There is evidence that some cross-reactivity exists between the allergens of the egg white and the egg yolk. Egg allergy is most frequently encountered in children (appearing in the first two years of life).

EICOSANOIDS

A group of compounds synthesized from arachidonic acid. The synthesis pathway is outlined in Figure 16, while the functions of the various compounds are listed in Table 26.

Eicosanoids are 20 carbon molecules having hormone-like activity. In their various forms, they are produced and released by many different mammalian cells rather than being produced by highly specialized cells as is the instance of insulin and the β cell in the islets of Langerhans. When each of these compounds is produced, their site of action is local. That is, whereas insulin may be transported from the pancreas to peripheral target cells, the eicosanoids are produced, released, and have as their targets the surrounding cells. For this reason, the eicosanoids are called local hormones. They have a variety of actions.

The eicosanoids fall into three general groups of compounds: (1) the prostaglandins (compounds of the PG series), (2) the thromboxanes (compounds of the TBX series), and (3) the leukotrienes (compounds of the LKT series). All of these compounds arise from a 20-carbon polyunsaturated fatty acid. This fatty acid is usually arachidonic acid (20 carbons; four double bonds at 5, 8, 11, and 14). However, in instances where the diet is rich in omega-3 (n-3) fatty acids, the precursor may be a 20-carbon-5 double-bond fatty acid, eicosapentaenoic acid (double bonds at 5, 8, 11, 14, and 17). Other eicosanoids can be synthesized from a 20-carbon fatty acid, dihomo-γ-linoleic acid, which has only three double bonds at carbons 8, 11, and 14. Each of these precursors yields a particular set of eicosanoids. They are called eicosanoids because they have 20 carbons; during their synthesis, they take up oxygen and are cyclized. Dihomo γ-linoleic acid is the precursor of prostaglandin E_1 (PGE$_1$), prostaglandin $E_1\alpha$ (PGE$_1\alpha$), and subsequent prostaglandins. Arachidonic acid is the

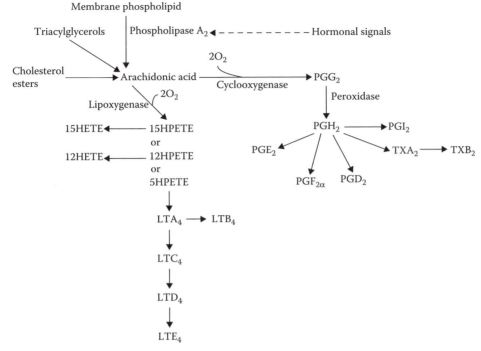

FIGURE 16   Eicosanoid synthesis from arachidonic acid.

TABLE 26
Functions of Eicosanoids

Eicosanoids	Function
PGG_2	Precursor of PGH_2.
PGH_2	Precursor of PGD_2, PGE_2, PGI_2, and $PGF_2\alpha$.
PGD_2	Promotes sleeping behavior. Precursor of PGF_2.
PGE_2	Enhances perception of pain when histamine or bradykinin is given.
	Induces signs of inflammation; promotes wakefulness.
	Precursor of $PGF_2\alpha$. Reduces gastric acid secretion.
	Vasoconstrictor in some tissues. Vasodilator in other tissues.
	Maintains the patency of the ductus arteriosis prior to birth.
$PGF_2\alpha$	Induces parturition. Bronchial constrictor. Vasoconstrictor especially in coronary vasculature. Increases sperm motility; stimulates steroidogenesis, corpus luteum; induces luteolysis.
PGI_2	Inhibits platelet aggregation.
PGE_1	Inhibits motility of nonpregnant uterus; increases motility of pregnant uterus. Bronchial dilator.
TXA_2	Stimulates platelet aggregation. Potent vasoconstrictor.
LTB_4	Potent chemotactic agent.

precursor of prostaglandins of the 2 series (PGE_2, $PGF_2\alpha$, etc.) and eicosapentaenoic acid is the precursor of prostaglandins of the 3 series (PGE_3, $PGF_3\alpha$, etc.). The cyclization of these 20 carbon fatty acids is accomplished by a complex of enzymes called the prostaglandin synthesis complex. The first step is the cyclooxygenase step, which involves the cyclization of C-9. The C-12 of the precursor to form the cyclic 9,11-endoperoxide 15-hydroperoxide (PGG_2) is shown in Figure 17. PGG_2

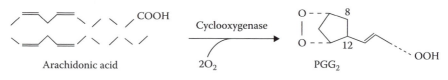

FIGURE 17   Cyclization of arachidonic acid to make PGG_2.

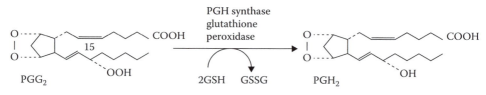

FIGURE 18   Oxygen removal to form PGH_2.

is then used to form prostaglandin H_2 (PGH_2) through the removal of one oxygen from the carbonyl group at carbon 15. This reaction is shown in Figure 18. Glutathione peroxidase and prostaglandin H synthase catalyze this reaction. Prostaglandin H synthase is a very unstable, short-lived enzyme with an mRNA that is one of the shortest-lived species so far found in mammalian cells. The expression of genes for this enzyme is under the control of polypeptide growth factors such as interleukin 1a and colony stimulating factor 1. Interferons α and β inhibit the expression and prostanoid production by the macrophages.

PGH_2 is then converted through the action of a variety of isomerases to PGD_2, PGE_2, prostacyclin I_2 (PGI_2), or prostaglandin $F_2\alpha$ ($PGF_2\alpha$). These are the primary precursors of the prostaglandins of the D, E, and F series and PGI or thromboxane. The conversion to subsequent prostaglandins is mediated by enzymes that are specific to a certain cell type and tissue. Not all of these subsequent compounds are formed in all tissues. Thus, PGE_2 and $PGF_2\alpha$ are produced in the kidney and spleen. Just prior to parturition, $PGF_2\alpha$ and PGE are produced in the uterus. PGI_2 is produced by endothelial cells lining the blood vessels. This prostaglandin inhibits platelet aggregation and thus is important to maintaining a blood flow free of clots. It is counteracted by thromboxane A_2, which is produced by the platelets when these cells contact a foreign surface. PGE_2, $PGF_2\alpha$, and PGI_2 are produced in the heart in about equal amounts. All of these prostaglandins have a very short half-life. No sooner are they released than they are inactivated.

The thromboxanes are highly active metabolites of the prostaglandins. They are formed when PGH_2 has its cyclopentane ring replaced by a six-membered oxane ring as shown in Figure 19. Imidazole is a potent inhibitor of thromboxane A synthase and is used to block thromboxane A_2 (TXA_2) production and platelet aggregation.

Thromboxane A_2 has a role in clot formation. The half-life of TXA_2 is less than 1 minute. Thromboxane B_2 (TXB_2) is its metabolic end product and has little biological activity. Measuring TXB_2 levels in blood and tissue can indicate the level of TXA_2 produced. PGD_2 and PGE_2 are involved in the regulation of sleep-wake cycles in a variety of species.

The cyclooxygenase reaction illustrated in Figure 19 can be inhibited by certain anti-inflammatory drugs such as aspirin, indomethacin, and phenylbutazone.

When the conversion of arachidonic acid to the prostaglandins is inhibited or when either of the other 20 carbon fatty acids are abundantly available, a different series of prostaglandins and leukotrienes are produced. Eicosapentaenoic acid is not as good a substrate for cyclooxygenase as is arachidonic acid. As a result, less of the arachidonic acid-related prostaglandins (even-numbered PGs and TBXs) are produced and more of the odd-numbered prostaglandins and leukotrienes are produced. Figure 16 shows the overall metabolic pathway for eicosanoid synthesis and degradation.

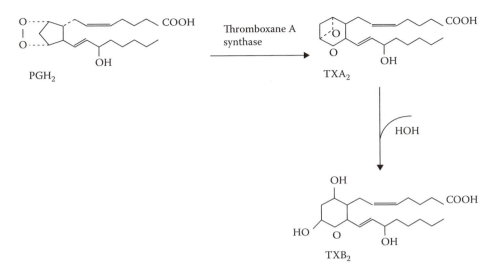

FIGURE 19   Formation of the thromboxanes.

Although the cyclooxygenase pathway is quite important in the production of prostaglandins, equally important is the lipoxygenase pathway. This pathway is catalyzed by a family of enzymes called the lipoxygenase enzymes. These enzymes differ from the cyclooxygenase enzymes in their catalytic site for oxygen addition to the unsaturated fatty acid. One lipoxygenase is active at the double bond at carbon 5 while a second is active at carbon 11 and a third is active at carbon 15. The products of these reactions are monohydroperoxy-eicosatetraenoic acids (HPETEs) and are numbered according to the location of the double bond to which the oxygen is added. 5HPETE is the major lipoxygenase product in basophils, polymorphonuclear leukocytes, macrophages, mast cells, and any organ undergoing an inflammatory response. 12HPETE is the major product in platelets, pancreatic endocrine cells, vascular smooth muscle, and glomerular cells. 15HPETE predominates in reticulocytes, eosinophils, T lymphocytes, and tracheal epithelial cells. The HPETEs are not in themselves active hormones; rather, they serve as precursors for the leukotrienes. The leukotrienes are the metabolic end products of the lipoxygenase reaction. These compounds contain at least three conjugated double bonds. The unstable 5HPETE is converted to either an analogous alcohol (hydroxy fatty acid) or is reduced by a peroxide or converted to leukotriene. The peroxidative reduction of 5'HPETE to stable 5-hydroxyeicosatetraenoic acid (5HETE) is similar to that of 12HPETE to 12HETE and of 15HPETE to 15HETE. In each instance, the carbon-carbon double bonds are unconjugated, and the geometry of the double bonds is trans, cis, and cis, respectively. In contrast to the active thromboxanes, which have very short half-lives, the leukotrienes can persist as long as four hours. These compounds comprise a group of substances known as the slow-acting anaphylaxis substances. They cause slowly evolving but protracted contractions of smooth muscles in the airways and gastrointestinal tract. Leukotriene C_4 is rapidly converted to LTD_4, which in turn is slowly converted to LTE_4. Enzymes in the plasma are responsible for these conversions. The products of the lipoxygenase pathway are potent mediators of the response to allergens, tissue damage (inflammation), hormone secretion, cell movement, cell growth, and calcium flux. The leukotrienes are more potent than histamine in stimulating the contraction of the bronchial nonvascular smooth muscles. In addition, LTD_4 increases the permeability of the microvasculature. The mono HETEs and LTB_4 stimulate the movement of eosinophils and neutrophils, making them the first line of defense in injury resulting in inflammation.

When dihomo-γ-linoleic acid or eicosapentaenoic acid serve as substrates for eicosanoid production, the products are either of the 1 series or 3 series. The products they form may be less active than those formed from arachidonic acid, and this decrease in activity can be of therapeutic value. Hence, ingestion of omega-3 fatty acids leads to the decreased production of prostaglandin E_2 and its metabolites; a decrease in the production of thromboxane A_2, a potent platelet aggregator and vasoconstrictor; and a decrease in leukotriene B_4, a potent inflammatory hormone and a powerful inducer of leukocyte hemotaxis and adherence. Counteracting these decreases are an increase in thromboxane A_3 (TXA_3), a weak platelet aggregator and vasoconstrictor; an increase in the production of PGI_3 without an increase in PGI_2, which stimulates vasodilation and inhibits platelet aggregation; and an increase in leukotriene B_5, which is a weak inducer of inflammation and a weak chemotxic agent.

EJECTION FRACTION

Percentage of the total diastolic volume of blood the heart ejects as it contracts.

ELASTIN

A protein found in connective tissue, ligaments, and vascular tissues. Rich in lysine and glycine. It is a very elastic protein.

ELECTROCARDIOGRAM (ECG OR EKG)

A record of the electrical activity of the heart that provides information about cardiac rhythm and function.

ELECTROLYTE

An electrically charged particle (anion or cation).

ELECTRON DONOR

In an electron acceptor/donor pair, the electron donor gives or donates electrons to the acceptor. An electron donor is a reducing agent.

ELECTRON TRANSPORT

See Oxidative Phosphorylation and Metabolic Maps, Appendix 2.

ELEMENTAL FORMULA

A liquid diet containing nutrients in a readily absorbed form.

ELIMINATION DIET

Dietary regimen where foods suspected to cause allergy or intolerance are eliminated from the diet for a period of at least two weeks. If symptoms are reduced or eliminated, foods are reintroduced one at a time and reactions are noted to confirm or rule out food involvement in allergy or intolerance.

ELISA

Enzyme-linked immunosorbent assay.

ELONGASE

An enzyme that adds acetyl units to a fatty acid previously synthesized by fatty acid synthetase.

ELONGATION FACTORS

Proteins that associate with ribosomes during the addition of amino acids to the polypeptide chain being formed.

EMBDEN–MEYERHOF PATHWAY

See Glycolysis. (See Metabolic Maps, Appendix 2.)

EMBOLISM

Obstruction of a blood vessel by a blood clot or a foreign body.

EMBRYO

The initial stage of development of the fertilized egg; usually the first 12 weeks in human pregnancy.

EMBRYOGENESIS

The process of maturation of the fertilized egg during the first 12 weeks of gestation in the human.

EMESIS

Vomiting.

EMETIC

A compound that stimulates vomiting. Example: ipecac.

EMULSIFIERS

Compounds that facilitate the dispersion of oil in water. Egg yolk serves as an emulsifier in the manufacture of mayonnaise.

EMULSION

A mixture of fat and water held together by an agent that has a lipophilic and a hydrophilic portion of its structure. Bile salts serve as emulsifying agents facilitating lipid digestion and absorption.

ENALAPRIL

An ACE inhibitor; serves as an antihypertensive drug. This is the generic name for this drug.

ENAMEL

The hard glistening substance covering the crown of the tooth.

ENCEPHALOPATHY

Disease of the encephalus. Dysfunction of the brain associated with advanced liver disease due to excess ammonia and accumulation of nitrogenous waste product and characterized by loss of consciousness.

ENDEMIC

Present in a community or population, as in diseases that are localized to a particular group of people.

ENDOCANNABINOIDS

Compounds involved in feeding behavior and body weight regulation. They are arachidonic acid derivatives that are synthesized when needed. They bind to CB_1 receptors and are rapidly degraded. The endocannabinoid system normally functions to increase food intake and energy storage. The system consists of two types of cannabinoid receptors, CB_1 and CB_2. CB_1 receptors are present in many central and peripheral sites involved in the control of energy homeostasis (e.g., brain, adipose tissue, gastrointestinal tract, liver, and muscle). CB_2 receptors are primarily expressed in the immune system and do not appear to play a major role in energy homeostasis or food intake. Both receptors are G-protein-coupled receptors whose primary function is to transduce specific extracellular stimuli into intracellular signals. In turn, these signals modulate glucose homeostasis, hepatic lipogenesis, and adipose tissue metabolism. In the adipose tissue, stimulation of CB_1 receptors has been shown to increase the lipoprotein lipase expression, down regulate adiponectin and reduce the expression of AMP kinase.

ENDOCARDITIS

Inflammation of the endocardium, heart valves, or cardiac prosthesis resulting from an infectious agent entering the bloodstream.

ENDOCRINE DISORDERS

Diseases of the endocrine glands that are characterized by either an overproduction or underproduction of the hormone that gland produces.

ENDOCRINE GLANDS

Specialized cells and tissues that release hormones into the bloodstream. These hormones have as their targets tissues some distance away from the tissue of origin.

ENDOCRINOLOGY

The study of the endocrine glands and their secretions.

ENDOCYTOSIS

The process of forming a vesicle within the secreting cell of material the cell will release upon appropriate signaling. The process is linked to the exocytotic process.

ENDOGENOUS

Growing from within the body.

ENDONUCLEASE

An enzyme the cleaves the internal bonds of DNA and RNA.

ENDOPLASMIC RETICULUM (ER)

See Cell Anatomy.

ENDORPHIN

A peptide produced in the brain that has sedative properties. β endorphin stimulates prolactin release.

ENDOSPERM

The portion of a seed in which the embryonic plant forms.

ENDOTHELIN

A 21–amino acid peptide that is a potent vasoconstrictor. It is produced by a wide variety of cell types in the gastrointestinal tract and cells in the vascular wall.

ENDOTOXIN

A bacterial toxin that is not freely released into the surrounding medium; may be a component of the bacterial cell wall; is heat stable; may cause symptoms of shock accompanied by diarrhea, fever, and leukocytosis.

END-STAGE RENAL DISEASE (ESRD)

See Chronic Renal Failure.

ENERGETICS

The physical laws of energy and thermodynamics that apply to all chemical reactions.

ENERGY BALANCE

When energy balance is zero, energy intake equals energy expenditure. When energy balance is positive, intake exceeds expenditure and weight is gained. When energy balance is negative, expenditure exceeds intake and weight is lost.

ENERGY INTAKE

The intake of energy needed to sustain the body and its associated activity. The U.S. recommendations for energy intake are shown in Table 27. The DRIs for energy can be accessed at http://www.nap.edu.

TABLE 27

Recommended Energy Intakes for Infants, Children, and Adults Based on Weight and Height (United States)

Category	Age	Weight (pounds)	Height (inches)	Recommended Energy Intake (kcal)
Infants	0–6 months	13	24	650
	6–12 months	20	28	850
Children	1–3 years	29	35	1300
	4–6	44	44	1800
	7–10	62	52	2000
Males	11–14	99	62	2500
	15–18	145	69	3000
	19–24	160	70	2900
	25–50	174	70	2900
	51+	170	68	2300
Females	11–14	101	62	2200
	15–18	120	64	2200
	19–24	128	65	2200
	25–50	138	64	2200
	51+	143	63	1900
Pregnant	First trimester			No change
	Second trimester			+300
	Third trimester			+300
Lactation	1–6 months			+500
	7–12 months			+500

Source: From National Research Council. 1989. *Food and Nutrition Board.* 10th ed. Washington, DC: National Academy Press. With permission. (See http://www.nap.edu for updates.)

ENERGY-PROTEIN MALNUTRITION

Protein-energy malnutrition (PEM or PCM). A condition in which the intake of macronutrients is inadequate. The needs for the essential nutrients and energy are determined by the age and health status of the individual. Rapid growth, infection, injury, and chronic debilitating disease can drive up the need for food and the nutrients it contains. It is difficult to segregate symptoms of protein deficiency from those due solely to energy deficit. The different symptoms are parts of a continuum called protein-energy malnutrition.

ENGINEERED FOODS

Foods designed by food scientists for specific purposes. These foods have specific properties and functions; they may have more fiber or less salt and/or less fat and/or unusual ingredients that are used as substitutes for usual ingredients.

ENHANCER ELEMENT

A cis-acting base sequence that binds one or more promoters. It can function in either orientation and in any location (upstream or downstream) relative to the promoter region.

ENKEPHALINS

Two forms: met-enkephalin and Leu-enkephalin; both are released by mesenteric neurons as a consequence of the processing of proopiomelanocortin. Each contains five amino acids. In the gut, they inhibit gut motility and mucosal secretions while stimulating sphincter tone. Enkephalins are also released by the CNS neurons, the hypothalamus, and 20 other areas outside the hypothalamus. Their function in the CNS is not altogether clear.

ENRICHED FOOD

Food product in which micronutrients such as iron or the B vitamins have been added.

ENRICHMENT

Process of restoring nutrients lost during processing to a food.

ENTERAL FEEDING

Feeding by way of a tube inserted through the nose to the stomach.

ENTERAL NUTRITION

Providing nutrition through a tube that enters the stomach or small intestine through the nasal passage or abdominal area. Used for patients who are unable to consume adequate nutrition by eating sufficient quantities of food.

ENTEROCHROMAFFIN CELLS

Cells present in the gastrointestinal tract that secrete hormones that in turn affect gastrointestinal function. Some of these hormones may also have effects on the regulation of food intake.

ENTEROCYTE

Absorptive cells lining the gastrointestinal tract.

ENTEROGLUCAGON

Also called glicentin; a 69-amino acid hormone related to pancreatic glucagon. It is synthesized by the mucosal L cells. May serve as a trophic factor for the intestinal mucosa.

ENTEROHEPATIC CIRCULATION

The path of bile salts and cholesterol from the liver to the gall bladder to the duodenum, returning to the liver via the portal circulation upon absorption from the ileum. Some vitamins and minerals also follow this pathway.

ENTEROSTATIN

A blood-borne factor that signals satiety.

ENTHALPY

The thermodynamic function of a system equivalent to the internal energy plus the product of pressure and volume.

ENTROPY

The randomness or disorder of a system.

ENZYMATIC OXIDATION

Enzyme-mediated oxidative degradation of a substance.

ENZYMES

Proteins that serve as catalysts of biological reactions.

EPIDEMIOLOGY

The study of the health status of a population.

EPIDERMIS

The top layer of the skin.

EPIGENETICS

Modifications in the expression of genes that do not involve a change in the base sequence of that gene. This occurs, for example, through the methylation of DNA.

EPINEPHRINE

A catecholamine synthesized from tyrosine in the adrenal medulla; a neurotransmitter.

EPITHELIAL CELLS

Cells on the body surface, skin cells; enterocytes are specialized epithelial cells.

EPITHELIUM

The layer of cells that provide the surface covering of the body; the nonvascular cell layer of skin, gastrointestinal tract, and respiratory tract.

EPLERENONE

An aldosterone receptor inhibitor useful as an antihypertensive drug. Trade name: Inspra.

EPOETIN ALFA

Same as erythropoietin. Trade names: Procrit, Epogen.

EPROSARTAN MESYLATE

Angiotensin II receptor antagonist; an antihypertensive agent. Trade name: Teveten.

ERGOCALCIFEROL

Vitamin D_2, a synthetic vitamin D derived from ergosterol; used as a food supplement to increase the food content of this vitamin.

ERGOGENIC, ERGONOMICS

A discipline relating human factors to the design and operation of machines or elements of the physical environment.

ERGOT ALKALOIDS

Mycotoxins that are 3,4-substituted indole alkaloids are produced by the mold *Claviceps purpurea*. There are two types of ergot alkaloids: type I, including ergotamine, ergotaminine, ergocristine, ergocristinine, ergostine, ergotamine, ergosine, α-ergocryptine, α-ergokryptinine, β-ergocryptine, β-ergokryptinine, and ergocornine; and type II, including ergine, arginine, ergometrine, ergometrinine, lysergic acid, isolysergic acid methylcarbinolamide, lysergic acid L-valine methyl ester, D-8,9-lysergic acid, ergosecaline, and ergosecalinine. Most ergot alkaloids are peptides of lysergic acid or isolysergic acid in cyclol form. Lysergic acid alkaloids are levorotatory and highly active pharmacologically. On the other hand, the isolysergic acid alkaloids are dextrorotatory and only weakly active. Thus, the biological activity of *Claviceps purpurea* can be ascribed only to the former type of alkaloids.

Ergot alkaloids as a group can result in toxic symptoms of both acute (tachycardia, hypertension, confusion, thirst, abdominal colic, vomiting, diarrhea, hypothermia of the skin) and chronic (disturbances in the gastrointestinal tract, angina pectoris, hypo- or hypertension, and the characteristic symptoms seen in ergotism) nature. Consumption of rye and other cereal grains contaminated by *Claviceps purpurea* causes ergotism. The mold can parasitize the female sex organs of the flowers of grasses, such as rye, wheat, and other grains. This phenomenon is characterized by a black or deep purple, hard, dense mass of cells, or sclerotium, which contains a plethora of compounds that are quite toxic. The sclerotium is capable of germination but may lie dormant in the ground during the winter. In the spring, with the alternation of cold (3°C–4°C) and relatively warm (≥14°C) temperatures, the sclerotium germinates. During the harvest the sclerotia may end up between the cereal grains. The consumption by humans of flour contaminated by the sclerotia of *Claviceps purpurea* results in epidemic ergotism. Two types of ergotism have been identified: (1) gangrenous ergotism (general lassitude; pains in the lumbar region, limbs, and calves; mild vomiting; swelling and inflammation of the feet and hands; alternating feeling of hot and cold; numbness; and gangrene), and (2) convulsive ergotism (sudden, painful, convulsive seizures beginning with the fingers or toes and spreading to the arms or legs; coma; drowsiness; giddiness; blindness; deafness; and swollen and edematous hands or feet).

ERUCIC ACID (CH3(CH2)7CH=CH(CH2)11COOH)

A toxic monounsaturated fatty acid, which is found in the plant family Cruciferae, notably in *Brassica*. The oils from rapeseed and mustard seed are particularly high in erucic acid (20%–55%). The toxic effects in animals include fat accumulation in the heart muscle, growth retardation, and liver damage. Because a large intake of erucic acid is necessary to induce myocardial damage in animals, the hazard of erucic acid toxicity in humans is probably minimal. A variety of rapeseed has been developed that produces an erucic acid-free oil. This plant is called canola and its oil is canola oil.

ERYTHROBLAST

An immature red blood cell characterized by the presence of a nucleus and large size. Usually found in the bone marrow.

ERYTHROCYTE

Red blood cells.

ERYTHROCYTHEMIA

Abnormal increase in the red blood cells in circulation.

ERYTHROMYCIN

An antibiotic that comes in many forms.

ERYTHROPOIESIS

The process for the synthesis of red blood cells.

ERYTHROPOIETIC PORPHYRIA

Presence of porphyrins in the urine due to excess red blood cell breakdown.

ERYTHROPOIETIN

Substance that stimulates red cell formation.

ESADDI

Estimated Safe and Adequate Daily Dietary Intakes. Refers to those nutrients for which there are indications of essentiality but for which the database is insufficient to make valid recommendations for intakes.

ESMOLOL HYDROCHLORIDE

A drug that serves as a beta blocker; an antiarrhythmic agent. Trade name: Brevibloc.

ESOPHAGEAL VARICES

Enlarged blood vessels in the collateral circulation of the esophagus.

ESSENTIAL AMINO ACIDS

Amino acids that cannot be synthesized in sufficient quantities in the body to meet the need for protein synthesis. (See Table 5; Amino Acids.)

ESSENTIAL FATTY ACID DEFICIENCY

Inadequate intake of linoleic and linolenic acids; characterized by dry, scaly skin; weight loss and/or inefficient use of food for weight gain; enlarged heart and kidneys; fatty liver; disturbed regulation of oxidative phosphorylation; impaired gonadal function; and poor reproduction.

ESSENTIAL FATTY ACIDS

Long-chain (18 carbons) unsaturated fatty acids needed by the body but which the body cannot synthesize. These include linoleic and linolenic acids for most species. Members of the cat family cannot synthesize arachidonic acid and therefore require this fatty acid in their diets in addition to linoleic and linolenic acids. Corn oil is a rich source of linoleic acid. Canola oil is a good source of linolenic acid.

ESSENTIAL NUTRIENTS

Nutrients needed by the body that must be provided in the diet. There are species and age differences in the nutrients needed. Some nutrients can be synthesized in the body, but the synthesis may be inadequate to meet the need of the consumer. The essential nutrients for humans include the amino acids, valine, leucine, isoleucine, threonine, phenylalanine, methionine, tryptophan, lysine, histidine, and arginine. Arginine can be synthesized but not in sufficient quantities in the growing child to meet the need for new tissue growth. Carbohydrate (glucose) can be synthesized. The fatty acids, linoleic, linolenic; the vitamins: retinol and its equivalents, vitamin D (can be synthesized if body is exposed to ultraviolet light), vitamin E, vitamin K, thiamin, riboflavin, niacin, vitamin B_6, pantothenic acid, folacin, vitamin B_{12} (cyanocobalamin), biotin, choline and ascorbic acid (can be synthesized by most species except primates, guinea pig, and fruit bat); the minerals: calcium, phosphorous, iron, copper, selenium, magnesium, zinc, manganese, chloride, sodium, potassium, molybdenum, and fluoride. The needs for some additional minerals are being studied. These are called the trace and ultratrace minerals, and the need for these is very difficult to establish.

ESTER

A compound containing an oxygen linkage; the product of the condensation of an acid and alcohol with the loss of a molecule of water.

ESTERIFIED CHOLESTEROL

Cholesterol to which a fatty acid is joined.

ESTROGENS

Steroid hormones produced by the ovary in a cyclic fashion and that are essential for female fertility as well as for the development of female characteristics (hair pattern, mammary cell development, etc.). Included in this group of female hormones are estradiol, 17β-estradiol, and estriol. They are also prepared commercially as conjugates. Trade names: Premarin, Cenestin. As an estrogen replacement it may be in a sulfate form with the trade name of Ogen or Ortho-Est.

ESTRUS

The portion or phase of the sexual cycle of female animals characterized by a willingness to accept the male.

ETANERCEPT

An antirheumatic drug. Trade name: Enbrel.

ETHANOL

The two-carbon alcohol (CH_3CHOH) resulting from the fermentation of glucose. It is found in alcoholic beverages: beer, wine, gin, whiskey, and so on. It is commonly referred to as alcohol although other carbon compounds having an –OH group are found in the food supply and produced during metabolism.

ETHANOL METABOLISM

See also Alcohol and Figure 4. Ethanol, once consumed, is absorbed by simple diffusion. The diffusion is affected by the amount of alcohol consumed, the regional blood flow, the surface area, and the presence of other foods. Absorption is fastest in the duodenum and jejunum; slower in the stomach, ileum, and colon; and slowest in the mouth and esophagus. The rate of absorption by the duodenum depends on gastric emptying time. Complete absorption may vary from two to six hours. The type of beverage can influence ethanol absorption. Ethanol in beer is absorbed slower than that found in whisky, which is slower than that in gin and red wine. Ethanol is water miscible and is rapidly distributed between the intracellular and extracellular compartments. The uptake of ethanol by the fat depots is minimal. Ethanol crosses the plasma membranes but, in so doing, changes them. When ethanol is in contact with a protein, it denatures it. Thus, large and frequent ethanol exposures result in damage to proteins both within and around the cells. The most damaged tissue is the liver since ethanol is carried directly to this tissue via the portal blood. While gut cells are also damaged, these cells have such a rapid turnover time (less than seven days) that damage due to intermittent ethanol consumption is not as long lasting as happens in the liver. Ethanol is metabolized to acetaldehyde. The acetaldehyde is converted to acetate, which can either be joined with a CoA or released to the circulation. If too much acetate is released, acidosis develops. Acetyl CoA can either be used for fatty acid synthesis or be shuttled into the mitochondria via carnitine to be oxidized as through the citric acid cycle. A fatty liver typifies the alcoholic. The fatty liver may progress to alcoholic hepatitis, cirrhosis, liver failure, and death. The fatty liver is due to accelerated hepatic fatty acid synthesis as well as due to an ethanol-induced impairment in hepatic lipid output. If the hepatocyte accumulates too much lipid, the cell will burst and die. Dead tissue within the liver is known as cirrhosis. When too much tissue dies, the liver may cease to function and the alcoholic dies.

ETHNOLOGY

The study of ethnic groups characterized by a common set of customs, beliefs, language, or cultural origin.

ETHOLOGY

A branch of knowledge dealing with human ethos, its evolution, and formation; the study of behavior.

ETIOLOGY

The study of the causes and development of a disease.

ETODOLAC

A nonsteroid anti-inflammatory, antiarthritic drug. Trade name: Lodine.

EUCARYOTES (EUKARYOTES)

Multicelled living beings. Cells are characterized by the presence of a membrane surrounding the nucleus.

EXCINUCLEASE

The excision nuclease enzyme that is involved in nucleotide exchange or repair of DNA.

EXOCRINE CELLS

Cells that produce secretions into the surrounding environment. Examples are mucous-producing cells of the respiratory tract and enzyme-producing cells of the intestinal tract.

EXOCYTOSIS

Process by which cells release compounds such as hormones.

EXOGENOUS NUTRIENTS

Nutrients in the diet.

EXON

The sequence of bases used to transcribe mRNA.

EXONUCLEASE

An enzyme that cleaves nucleotides from either the 3′ or 5′ ends of DNA or RNA.

EXOPHTHALMIC GOITER

Disease caused by excess thyroxine production. Also called Graves' disease, characterized by high metabolic rate; weight loss, particularly muscle and fat loss; bulging eyes; tremor; rapid heart rate; good appetite; and irritability.

EXPANDED FOOD AND NUTRITION EDUCATION PROGRAM (EFNEP)

Nutrition education program available in the United States to low-income mothers of young children. EFNEP is a program of the U.S. Department of Agriculture.

EXPERIMENTAL STUDIES

Studies in which the exposure conditions are chosen by the investigator. For ethical reasons, exposure restrictions exist. The most important one is that examining potentially toxic substances in humans is prohibited. This implies that potentially adverse effects of food components can only be investigated in animal studies. In experimental studies, two groups of subjects are compared with regard to the outcome variable—subjects exposed to the substance under investigation (treatment group) and subjects not exposed (control group). An essential condition of this type of study is that the exposure is randomly distributed over the subjects. Maintaining all conditions constant except for the exposure has to be achieved by randomization of the study subjects, as lifestyle and genetic background differ greatly from one person to another. If possible, the study should be double-blind. This means that the investigator as well as the study subjects do not know whether they are in the treatment group or the control group. In this way, the observations are not influenced by the investigator or the respondent.

EXPRESSION VECTOR

A cloning vector designed so that a coding sequence inserted at a particular site will be transcribed and translated into protein.

EXTERNAL VALIDITY

Determines whether the results can be generalized beyond the study population. Internal validity is a prerequisite for external validity. If an association is not validly assessed for the population under investigation, it cannot be generalized to other populations. For external validity, a judgment must be made as to the plausibility that the effect observed in the study population can be generalized.

EXTRACELLULAR

Outside of the cell, as in serum which surrounds the blood cells.

EXTRACELLULAR WATER

The fluid compartment that surrounds cells, tissues, and organs. It is distributed into several sub-compartments (plasma, interstitial, and lymph fluids; fluids around connective tissue, cartilage, and bone; and transcellular fluids), which are not clearly defined. About 45% of the total body water is found in the extracellular compartments.

EXTRAVASCULAR

Outside the vascular system as the fluids, which are between the cells in the tissues or between the capillaries and the cells they supply.

EXTRINSIC FACTOR

Vitamin B_{12}.

EXUDATE

Fluid that has left blood vessels and deposited in or on tissues.

EZETIMIBE

A selective cholesterol absorption inhibitor; an antihypercholesterolemic agent. Trade name: Zetia.

F

FACILITATED TRANSPORT

See also Absorption. Transport against a concentration gradient using a carrier. Facilitated transport does not require energy or sodium.

FAD, FMN (FLAVIN ADENINE DINUCLEOTIDE, FLAVIN MONONUCLEOTIDE)

Coenzymes that carry reducing equivalents (H^+) in reactions of intermediary metabolism. Riboflavin is an essential component of these nucleotides.

FAILURE TO THRIVE

Term usually referring to infants and children who fail to grow and develop in the normal way but in whom no definitive cause for this failure can be identified. The term can also be used to refer to the elderly who appear ill for no apparent cause.

FAMOTIDINE

H_2-recptor antagonist; antiulcerative. Trade names: Pepcid, Pepcid-AC, Pepcid RPO.

FANCONI'S SYNDROME

A genetic disease associated with abnormal metabolism of cystine. Characterized by abnormal renal function, glycosuria, phosphaturia, amino aciduria, and bicarbonate wasting.

FASTING BLOOD GLUCOSE

The level of glucose in the blood after 12–16 hours without food, usually between 80–120 mg/dL or 4–6 mmol/L. Levels below this range indicate hypoglycemia; levels above this range indicate hyperglycemia.

FAT

A mixture of triacylglycerols, phospholipids, sphingolipids, cholesterol, and other sterols. The material is solid at room temperature.

FAT-SOLUBLE VITAMINS

The vitamins that are soluble in fat solvents (alcohol, ether, chloroform, etc.). Includes retinol and its equivalents (vitamin A), vitamin D, vitamin E, and vitamin K.

FAT SUBSTITUTES

Synthetic compounds designed to provide the food characteristics of fat without the energy value. (See Simplesse, Olestra.)

FATTY ACID

A carboxylic acid with a long-chain hydrocarbon side group [$CH_3(CH_2)_nCOOH$]. The carbon chain can be saturated (no double bonds) or unsaturated (one or more double bonds). The existence of the double bond in the fatty acid changes the physical and chemical attributes of the fatty acid. Those with more than one double bond are more fluid than those without any double bonds. Those with multiple double bonds are more fluid than those with single double bonds. Short-chain fatty acids are more fluid than long-chain fatty acids. In general, fatty acids from vegetable sources are more fluid than those from animal sources. Those from marine animals and cold-water fish are more fluid than fatty acids from land animals.

Polyunsaturated fats or fatty acids have a variety of beneficial effects on metabolism. Three of the unsaturated fatty acids (linoleic, linolenic, and arachidonic acids) are considered essential to the normal functioning of cells and tissues. Mammals cannot produce linoleic or linolenic acids but can convert linoleic acid to arachidonic acid. Felines cannot do this, so members of this class of mammals require not only linoleic and linolenic acids but also arachidonic acid in their diets. Linoleic acid has 18 carbons and two double bonds, whereas α- and γ-linolenic acids have 18 carbons and three double bonds. α-Linolenic acid is a member of the ω3 family of fatty acids, while γ-linolenic acid is a member of the ω6 family. Arachidonic acid has 20 carbons and 4 double bonds. Linoleic acid is found in vegetable oils, while α-linolenic acid is found in soybean, canola and, to some small extent, the oils of cold-water fish. Industrial hydrogenation converts some of the double bonds to single ones. It can also result in changes in the configuration of some of the fatty acids. These structural changes involve the difference in the placement of the carbon chains and hydrogen atoms on each side of the double bond. In the normal or cis configuration, the carbon chains are on one side of the double bond while the hydrogen atoms are on the other side of the double bond. Under the conditions of hydrogenation, the fatty acid structure changes such that a trans configuration is formed. The hydrogen atoms are on opposite sides of the double bond and the carbon chains likewise are on opposite sides of the double bond. These fatty acids are called trans fatty acids. There are several different configurations of the same 18-carbon polyunsaturated fatty acid. In the systematic naming system for fatty acids, the placement and number of the double bonds is indicated. Thus, the 18-carbon fatty acid we commonly call α-linolenic acid has a systematic name of 9,12,15-octadecatrienoic acid. The numbers indicate the position of the double bonds counting carbons from the carboxyl end. Linoleic acid is 9,12-octadecadienoic acid (di means two double bonds), γ-linolenic acid is 6,9,12-octadecatrienoic acid (tri means three double bonds), and arachidonic acid is 5,8,11,14-eicosatetraenoic acid (tetra means four double bonds). There are options for the placement of the double bonds as well. The first double bond could occur between the ninth and tenth carbons in the chain (counting from the carboxyl end) or between the fifth and sixth carbons, with the other double bonds occurring between carbons numbered 12 and 13 and between 15 and 16.

FATTY ACID DESATURATION

See Metabolic Maps, Appendix 2. The conversion of saturated fatty acids to unsaturated fatty acids in the body. Desaturation occurs in the endoplasmic reticulum and in the microsomes. The enzymes that catalyze desaturation are the Δ9, Δ6, or Δ3 desaturases. They are sometimes called mixed function oxidases because two substrates (fatty acid and nicotinamide adenine dinucleotide phosphate [NADPH]) are oxidized simultaneously. Fatty acid desaturation can be followed by elongation and can be repeated such that a variety of mono- and polyunsaturated fatty acids are formed. The body converts the dietary saturated fatty acids (S) to unsaturated fatty acids (P) in order to maintain an optimal P:S ratio in the tissues. There is one desaturation reaction that cannot occur in mammals: the conversion of 18:1 to 18:2. Further, felines cannot elongate and desaturate 18:2 to 20:4, arachidonic acid. The activity of the desaturases can be increased through feeding high-saturated-fat and/or high-sugar diets. Both dietary maneuvers increase the need to synthesize unsaturated fatty acids. Desaturase activity is stimulated by insulin, triiodothyronine, and glucocorticoid. Desaturase activity is decreased when high polyunsaturated fats are fed.

FATTY ACID ELONGATION

See Metabolic Maps, Appendix 2. The lengthening of fatty acids by the addition of two carbon units (acetyl groups). Elongation occurs in either the endoplasmic reticulum or the mitochondria. The reaction differs depending on where it occurs. In the endoplasmic reticulum, the reaction sequence is similar to that described for the cytosolic fatty acid synthase complex. The source of the two-carbon unit is malonyl coenzyme A (CoA), and NADPH provides the reducing power. The intermediates are CoA esters and not the acyl carrier protein 4′-phosphopantetheine. The reaction sequence produces stearic acid (18:0) in all tissues that make fatty acids except the brain. In the brain, elongation can proceed further by producing fatty acids containing up to 24 carbons. In the mitochondria, elongation uses acetyl CoA rather than malonyl CoA as the source of the two-carbon unit. It uses either $NADH^+H^+$ or $NADPH^+H^+$ as the source of reducing equivalents and uses, as substrate, carbon chains of less than 16 carbons. Mitochondrial elongation is the reversal of fatty acid oxidation, which also occurs in this organelle.

FATTY ACID ESTERIFICATION

See Metabolic Maps, Appendix 2. The joining of a fatty acid to a carbon skeleton using oxygen. The resultant product is a monoglyceride, diglyceride, or triglyceride (triacylglyceride). Triacylglycerides are formed in a stepwise fashion. First, a fatty acid (usually a saturated fatty acid) is attached at carbon 1 of the glycerophosphate. The phosphate group at carbon 3 is electronegative and because it pulls electrons toward it, it leaves carbon 1 more reactive than carbon 2. The fatty acid (as acyl CoA) is transferred to carbon 1 through the action of a transferase. The attachment uses the carboxy end of the fatty acid chain and makes an ester linkage releasing the CoA. Now the molecule has electronegative forces at each end—the phosphate group on carbon 3 and the oxygen plus carbon chain at carbon 1. Now carbon 2 is vulnerable and reactive and another carbon chain can be attached. In this instance, the fatty acid is usually an unsaturated fatty acid. At this point, the 1,2 diacylglyceride-phosphate loses its phosphate group so that carbon 3 is now reactive. The 1,2 diacylglyceride can either be esterified with another fatty acid to make triacylglyceride or can be used to make the membrane phospholipids, phosphatidylcholine, phosphatidylethanolamine, phosphatidylinositol, cardiolipin, and phosphatidylserine.

FATTY ACID OXIDATION

See Metabolic Maps, Appendix 2. A process that occurs after the glycerides are hydrolyzed to glycerol and fatty acids. This oxidation is called β oxidation and occurs in the mitochondria. It is preceded by the transport of the fatty acid into the mitochondria via the acyl carnitine transport system. While most of the fatty acids that enter the β oxidation pathway are completely oxidized via the citric acid cycle and respiratory chain to CO_2 and HOH, some of the acetyl CoA is converted to the ketones, acetoacetate, and β hydroxybutyrate. The condensation of two molecules of acetyl CoA to acetoacetyl CoA occurs in the mitochondria via the enzyme β-ketothiolase. Acetoacetyl

CoA then condenses with another acetyl CoA to form HMG CoA. At last, the HMG CoA is cleaved into acetoacetic acid and acetyl CoA. The acetoacetic acid is reduced to β hydroxybutyrate, and this reduction is dependent on the ratio of NAD^+ to $NADH^+H^+$. The enzyme for this reduction, β hydroxybutyrate dehydrogenase, is tightly bound to the inner aspect of the mitochondrial membrane. Because of its high activity, the product (β hydroxybutyrate) and substrate (acetoacetate) are in equilibrium.

The oxidation of unsaturated fatty acids follows the same pathway as the saturated fatty acids until the double-bonded carbons are reached. At this point, a few additional steps must be taken that involve a few additional enzymes.

A fatty acid with a cis double bond is oxidized via β oxidation until it reaches the double bond. At this point, an isomerase enzyme, D_3 cis D_6 trans enoyl CoA isomerase, acts to convert the cis bond to a trans bond. The double bond is then opened and a hydroxyl group is inserted. In turn, this hydroxyl group is rotated to the L position and the remaining product can then reenter the β oxidation pathway. Other unsaturated fatty acids can be similarly oxidized. Each time the double bond is approached, the isomerization and hydroxyl group addition takes place until all of the fatty acid is oxidized.

While β oxidation is the main pathway for the oxidation of fatty acids, some fatty acids undergo α oxidation so as to provide the substrates for the synthesis of sphingolipids. These reactions occur in the endoplasmic reticulum and involve the mixed function oxidases. The reaction requires molecular oxygen, reduced NAD, and specific cytochromes. The reactions are energy-wasteful reactions because the endoplasmic reticulum does not have the citric acid cycle, nor does it have the respiratory chain, which takes the reducing equivalents released by the oxidative steps and combines them with oxygen to make water, releasing energy that is then trapped in the high-energy bonds of the ATP.

FATTY ACID SYNTHESIS

See Metabolic Maps, Appendix 2. Fatty acid synthesis occurs in the cytosol of the living cell using two carbon units (acetyl units) that are the result of glucose oxidation or amino acid degradation. Fatty acid synthesis begins with acetyl CoA. Acetyl CoA is converted to malonyl CoA with the addition of one carbon (from bicarbonate) in the presence of the enzyme acetyl CoA carboxylase. The reaction uses the energy from one molecule of ATP and biotin as a coenzyme. This reaction is the first committed step in the reaction sequence that results in the synthesis of a fatty acid. The activated carbon dioxide attached to the biotin-enzyme complex is transferred to the methyl end of the substrate. Although most fatty acids synthesized in mammalian cells have an even number of carbons, this first committed step yields a three-carbon product. This results in an asymmetric molecule that becomes vulnerable to attack (addition) at carbon 2 with the subsequent loss of the terminal carbon. The vulnerability is conferred by the fact that both the carboxyl group at one end and the CoA group at the other end are both powerful attractants of electrons from the hydrogen of the middle carbon. This leaves the carbon in a very reactive state, and a second acetyl group carried by a carrier protein with the help of phosphopantethine, which has a sulfur group connection, can be joined to it through the action of the enzyme malonyl transferase. Subsequently, the "extra" carbon is released via the β ketoacyl enzyme synthase, leaving a four-carbon chain still connected to an SH group at the carboxyl end. This SH group is the docking end for all the enzymes that comprise the fatty acid synthase complex. These enzymes catalyze the addition of two-carbon acetyl groups in sequence to the methyl end of the carbon chain until the final product, palmityl CoA, and then the 16-carbon palmitic acid is produced. Members of this fatty acid synthase complex include the aforementioned malonyl transferase and β ketoacyl synthase; β ketoacyl reductase, which catalyzes the addition of reducing equivalents carried by FMN; and an acyl transferase.

FATTY FOODS

Foods having a high percentage of their energy content as fat. See http://www.nal.usda.gov/fnic/foodcomp/Data/foods, 82 nutrients for the fat content of a wide variety of foods.

FAVISM

A condition that develops after consuming certain species (*Vicia faba*) of beans; characterized by fever, headache, abdominal pain, severe anemia, prostration, coma, and sometimes death.

FDA

Food and Drug Administration. A subunit of the U.S. Department of Health and Human Services.

FECAL ENERGY (FE)

The energy content of the feces. The FE is the weight of feces times the gross energy of a unit weight of feces. FE can be partitioned into energy of undigested food (FiE) and the energy of compounds of endogenous origin (FmE).

FECES

Excrement discharged from the anus containing undigested food, intestinal secretions, intestinal flora, and desquamated intestinal cells.

FELODIPINE

A calcium channel blocker; an antihypertensive agent. Trade names: Plendil, Renedil.

FENOFIBRATE

Fibric acid derivative that adsorbs cholesterol in the gastrointestinal tract; an anticholesterolemic-anti-triglyceridemic drug. Trade names: Lofibra, Tricor.

FERMENTATION

A processing technique affecting the oxidation of dietary carbohydrates, fats, and oils. Some types of fermentation are used for the production of substances that are undesirable in other products.

FERRITIN

An iron-binding protein that transports iron from the absorption site in the intestine to the site where it is used.

FERROPORTIN

A protein essential for iron efflux from liver, spleen, and duodenal cells. Its activity is regulated by hepcidin.

FERROUS GLUCONATE

An oral iron supplement. Trade names: Fergon, Simron. There are other iron supplements in ferrous sulfate form.

FETAL ALCOHOL SYNDROME

A condition in infants whose malformations can be traced to alcohol consumed by their mothers during pregnancy. Characterized by abnormal eye placement, abnormal nose and mouth development, and failure of the infant to grow and develop normally with full intellectual capacity. Various learning disabilities have been associated with this condition.

FETUS

An unborn child; stage of development of a human from embryo to birth, or from about 12 weeks post fertilization to full gestational age (approximately 40 weeks).

FEXOFENADINE

An H_1-receptor antagonist; an antihistamine. Trade name: Allegra.

FIBER

Dietary fiber refers to those carbohydrates that are indigestible and unabsorbed. The component glucose moieties are joined by β linkages rather than α linkages. They may also contain additional substituents, but their chief characteristic is that of nondigestibility by the α amylases of the gastrointestinal system. These nondigestible carbohydrates are plant products and fall into five major categories: (1) celluloses, (2) hemicelluloses, (3) lignins, (4) pectins, and (5) gums. The celluloses, hemicelluloses, and lignins provide bulk to the gastrointestinal contents due to their property of absorbing water. The increased bulkiness of the gut contents stimulates peristalsis and results in shorter passage time and more frequent defecation. In addition to its water-holding property, fibers of the lignin type adsorb cholesterol and noxious agents from the gut contents, aiding in their excretion through the feces. Pectins and gums also influence gastric emptying but in the opposite direction. These fiber types form gels that slow gastric emptying and the digestion and absorption of sugars, starches, and fats. Fruits are good sources of pectin, while cereal grains and the woody parts of vegetables are good sources of celluloses, hemicelluloses, and lignins. Dried beans and oats are good sources of gums. The intestinal flora can metabolize some of the undigested fiber, producing short-chain fatty acids that are then absorbed.

FIBRINOGEN

The precursor of fibrin that provides a network of fibers that forms the structural element in clot formation.

FIBROBLASTS

Progenitor cells that can differentiate into other more specific cells.

FIBROUS PLAQUE

Lipids collect on a fibrous network within or on the interior aspect of the arterial walls during the atherogenic process to form a projection into the lumen of the vessel and impede blood flow.

FINASTERIDE

A synthetic steroid derivative that inhibits androgen production. Trade names: Propecia, Proscar.

FINGERPRINTING

The use of restriction fragment length polymorphisms (LPs) or repeat sequences of DNA to establish a unique pattern of DNA for an individual.

FISH ALLERGY

Allergic reactions to fish. The codfish allergen is heat stable and resistant to proteolytic enzymes. In sensitive people, it elicits symptoms such as rhinitis, dyspnea, eczema, urticaria, nausea, and vomiting following ingestion of fish. Urticaria may occur after skin contact with fish. Shellfish can cause strong allergic reactions as well. Probably, fish families have a species-specific antigen as well as cross-reactive antigens. Antibodies and allergic reactions may be directed against a specific fish or multiple fish families.

FISH OILS

Marine oils, lipids extracted from cold-water fish and from sea mammals, are rich in omega-3 (N-3, ω-3) unsaturated fatty acids. These fatty acids affect (decrease) platelet aggregation because they stimulate the synthesis of thromboxane A_3. Thromboxane A_3 does not have the platelet-aggregating property of the other eicosanoids. In addition, eicosapentaenoic acid is used to make the anti-aggregating prostaglandin PGI_3. Animals fed $\omega3$-rich oils produce significantly more of the eicosanoids of the leukotrine B_5 (LTB_5) series. LTB_4 is an important inflammatory mediator whereas LTB_5 is not. Fish oil consumption results in an increased neutrophil LTB_5 production with a concomitant decrease in LTB_4 production. This diet-influenced change in LTB_4 and LTB_5 production seems to be related to a reduced incidence of autoimmune-inflammatory disorders such as asthma, psoriasis, and rheumatoid arthritis in populations consuming $\omega3$ fatty acids routinely. Tumorigenesis likewise can be influenced by the relative amounts of the various eicosanoids. Prostaglandin G of the 2-series acts as a tumor promoter. It downregulates macrophage tumoricidal activities and inhibits interleukin-2 production. Increased PGE_2 levels (from $\omega6$ fatty acids) have been associated with aggressive growth patterns of both basal and squamous cell skin carcinomas in humans. Products of the lipooxygenase pathway (stimulated by the ω-3 fatty acids) have the reverse effect.

FLATULENCE

Release from the anus of gases (methane, sulfur dioxide, etc.) produced in the large intestine through the action of intestinal flora on food residue. If the gas is not released, intestinal distention and discomfort result.

FLAVONOLS, FLAVONOIDS

A class of plant pigments that are widely present in human food. These pigments are polyhydroxy-2-phenylbenzo-γ-pyrone derivatives, occurring as aglycones, glycosides, and methyl ethers. They are divided into six main subgroups: (1) flavanone, 3-OH: flavanol; (2) flavone, 3-OH: flavonol; (3) anthocyanidin, 3-OH: catechin, 3-OH: condensed tannins; (4) isoflavanone; (5) chalcone; and (6) aurone. Flavonols are polyphenols. Included in this group are curcumin, limonin, and quercetin. These are strong antioxidants. Consumption of flavonols is inversely related to incidence of stroke. Their intake is also inversely related to serum C-reactive protein concentrations. The C-reactive protein is a marker of inflammation.

FLUDROCORTISONE ACETATE

An aldosterone-glucocorticoid replacement drug. Trade name: Florinef.

FLUID MOSAIC MODEL

A model of biological membranes in which integral membrane proteins float and diffuse laterally in a fluid–lipid bilayer.

FLUORIDATION

The addition of fluoride to water as a treatment of teeth to prevent decay.

FLUORIDE

An essential mineral. Present in low but varying concentrations in drinking water (1 mg/L), plants, and animals (fish: 50–100 mg per 100 g). It accumulates in human bone tissue and dental enamel. In appropriate amounts, fluoride serves to harden bones and teeth. If consumed in excessive amounts, fluoride is toxic. The normal daily intake is 1–2 mg. Daily ingestion of 20–80 mg of fluoride leads to fluorosis, a toxic state characterized by calcification of soft tissue with effects on function notably renal, muscle, and nerve function.

FLUOROSIS

A condition of excess fluoride intake chiefly characterized by a mottled appearance of the tooth enamel.

FLUOXETINE

An appetite suppressant.

FLUVASTATIN

An HMG-CoA inhibitor; serves to reduce the de novo synthesis of cholesterol by the liver. Trade name: Lescol.

FMN

Flavin mononucleotide. A nucleotide coenzyme containing riboflavin.

FOLACIN (FOLIC ACID)

An essential B vitamin that participates in one-carbon transfer. Folic acid (folate or folacin) is the generic term for pteroylmonoglutamic acid and its related biologically active compounds. A number of derivatives have vitamin activity. The basic structure of pteroylglutamic acid is shown in Figure 20. The derivatives include the addition of hydrogen at N5 and N10 and only one glutamate attached to para-aminobenzoic acid (Table 28). This derivative is called tetrahydrofolic acid (THF). Other derivatives can have a methyl group attached at N5, a methyl bridge between N5 and N10 or a methylene bridge at this position or an aldehyde group at either N5 or N10 or a HCNH group at N5. All of these derivatives have vitamin activity because vitamin activity is dependent on the presence of a pterin structure with variable hydrogenation or methyl addition at N5 or N10 and the presence of at least one glutamyl residue linked via peptide bonds to p-aminobenzoic acid. Methotrexate (4-amino-N10-methyl folic acid, an antineoplastic agent) and aminopterin (4-amino folic acid, a rodenticide) are folate antagonists and as such are useful pharmaceutical agents against cell growth. Folacin is an orange-yellow crystal with a melting point of 250°C. It is unstable to ultraviolet light, heat, oxygen, acid conditions, and divalent metal ions such as iron and copper.

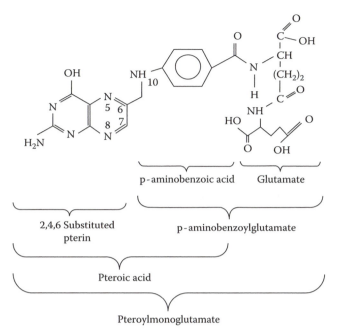

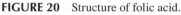

FIGURE 20   Structure of folic acid.

TABLE 28
Derivatives of Folic Acid

Derivative	N-5	N-10
Tetrahydrofolic acid	–H	–H
5-Methyfolic acid	–CH$_3$	–H
5,10-Methanylfolic acid	–CH=	–CH$_2$=
5,10-Methylenefolic acid	–CH$_2$=	–CH$_2$=
5-Formylfolic acid	–HCO	H
10- Formylfolic acid	H	–HCO

SOURCES

Folate is found in a wide variety of foods of both animal and plant origin. However, because it is so unstable, food sources may be insufficient to meet need. Good sources include meats, fruits, vegetables (especially asparagus), dry beans, peas and nuts, and whole grain cereal products. Many cereal products are now enriched with this vitamin to ensure an adequate intake by more than 95% of the U.S. population.

ABSORPTION, METABOLISM

Folate transport in the intestine is a carrier-mediated, pH-dependent process with maximum transport occurring after glutamation in the jejunum. There are specific folate-binding proteins that function in the absorption process. One is a low-affinity folate-binding protein found in the brush border membrane of the absorptive cell. There is another high-affinity folate-binding protein that is localized to the jejunal brush border cells. Affinity is optimized at pH 5.5–6.0. The high-affinity binding protein is similar to one found in the kidney. A number of drugs inhibit active folate transport. These include ethacrynic acid, sulfinpyrazone, phenylbutazone, sulfasalazine, and furosemide. All of these are amphipathic substances. That is, they are compounds with a polar-apolar character. Absorption is also inhibited by cyanide and 2,4-dinitrophenol, drugs that poison oxidative phosphorylation and thus reduce the ATP supply. ATP is necessary for the active transport process to work. Absorption can also occur by passive diffusion, but this is a secondary means for folate uptake. Very little folate appears in the feces.

After folate is absorbed, it circulates in the plasma as pteroylmonoglutamate. Folate that is not used by the cells is excreted in the urine as pteroylglutamic acid, 5-methyl-pteroylglumic acid, 10-formyl tetrahydrofolate, or acetamidobenzoylglumate. Uptake by cells is mediated by a highly specific folate-binding protein. This protein has been isolated from the membranes of a variety of cells, and a complementary DNA (cDNA) probe has been prepared. Folate appears to stimulate the transcription of the mRNA for this protein.

FUNCTION

Folate's main function is as a coenzyme in one-carbon transfer. However, before it can do this it must be activated. Activation consists of the reduction of folic acid to dihydrofolic acid and then to tetrahydrofolic acid as shown in Figure 21.

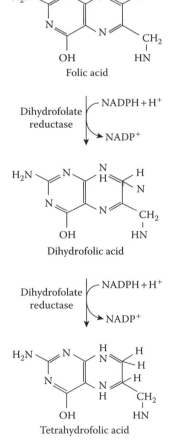

FIGURE 21 Activation of folic acid.

A number of folate derivatives have vitamin activity and these derivatives are interconvertible. Folate's chief function is in methyl group transfer and in this role vitamin B_{12} is also involved as shown in Figure 22. Folate serves as a coenzyme in other reactions as well. These are listed in Table 29.

The regulation of methyl group transfer is complex and involves a number of enzymes and substrates. While serine is a good source for the methyl group, methyl groups arise from other substrates as well. The major source of single methyl groups involves a cycle of reactions catalyzed by serine-hydroxymethyltransferase, 5,10-methylene-FH_4 reductase, and methionine synthetase. The last of these reactions is rate limiting for the cycle, whereas the second is inhibited by s-adenosylmethionine (SAM) as well as 5-methyl FH_4. As described in the section on vitamin

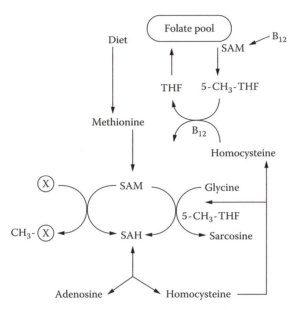

FIGURE 22   Involvement of folacin in methyl group transfer via S-adenosylmethionine (SAM).

TABLE 29
Metabolic Reactions in Which Folate Plays a Role as a Coenzyme

Enzyme	Role
Thymidylate synthetase	Transfers formaldehyde to C-5 of deoxyuridine monophosphate (dUMP) to form a deoxythymidine monophosphate (dTMP) in pyrimidine synthesis (see Figure 5).
Glycinamide ribonucleotide transformylase	Donates formate in purine synthesis (see Chapter 2).
5-Amino-4-imidazolecarboxamide transformylase	Donates formate in purine synthesis (see Chapter 2).
Serine hydroxymethyl transferase	Accepts formaldehyde in serine catabolism.
10-Formyl-FH_4 synthetase	Accepts formaldehyde from tryptophan catabolism.
10-Formyl-FH_4 dehydrogenase	Transfers formate for oxidation to CO_2 in histidine catabolism.
Methionine syntase	Donates methyl group to homocysteine to form methionine.
Formiminotransferase	Accepts formimino group from histidine.

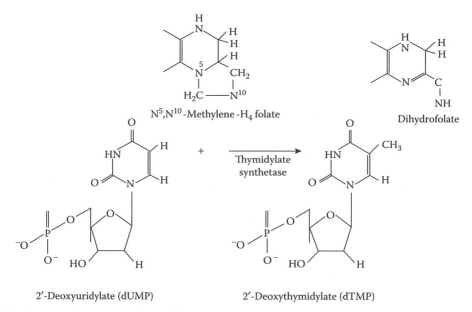

FIGURE 23   Methyl group transfer in DNA synthesis.

B_{12}, methionine synthesis depends on the transfer of labile methyl groups from 5-methyl folate to B_{12}, which, as methyl B_{12}, donates this methyl group to homocysteine resulting in methionine.

One-carbon transfer is particularly important in purine and pyrimidine synthesis. The mechanism of this transfer that involves folate (and also B_{12}) is illustrated in Figure 23, and it is immediately apparent why folate and vitamin B_{12} are so important to gene expression. While nuclear DNA, once made, merely reproduces itself within the cell cycle, new mRNA is made every minute as new proteins are needed by the cell. While some of the purine and pyrimidine bases can be salvaged and reused, this recycling is not 100% efficient. Messenger RNA has a *very* short half-life (seconds to hours) compared to the other nucleic acid species in the cell. Thus, newly synthesized purines and pyrimidines must be available. If not available, de novo protein synthesis and, of course, new cell formation will be adversely affected.

DEFICIENCY

While anemia, dermatitis, and impaired growth are the chief clinical symptoms of folate deficiency in humans, scientists are now beginning to recognize the importance of adequate folate intake in early embryonic development. Inadequate intake by the mother prior to and/or during the early stages of development can have teratogenic effects on the embryo. Embryonic development, particularly the neural tube, is impaired in folate deficiency. Choline deficiency also has this effect on neural development. As a result of inadequate maternal nutrition, infants with spina bifida and other neural tube defects are born. It is estimated that about 2500 infants per year are born with these defects. Available evidence indicates that women contemplating pregnancy should consume 400 mg of folate/day as a prophylactic measure. Inadequate folate intake can induce epigenetic change in the growing offspring that can be reversed by folacin supplementation.

Folacin is also important in the maintenance of stem cells and germ cells. Because folacin is important to DNA synthesis and chromosome maintenance, folacin intake is associated with telomere length. Reduced telomere length is associated with age-related deterioration in vascular and neural function. The 677C→T variants have a greater risk of having inadequate folacin status than those with a CC genotype. Further, those with a 19-base pair deletion polymorphism in the gene for dihydrofolate reductase are more likely to have decreased levels of red cell folate.

Low folate intake has been suggested as a factor in the development of colon cancer as well as bronchial squamous metaplasia (premalignant lesions) in smokers and cervical dysplasia (another premalignant lesion) in women. The association of folacin with the cell mutation that leads to cancer may be genetically determined as polymorphisms in four uracil-processing genes have been found to associate with mutagenic lesions. In deficient individuals, there is a decrease in thymidylate synthesis from deoxyuridylate that results in an imbalance of deoxyribonucleotide that in turn may lead to excessive uracil incorporation into DNA during replication. The presence of the methylenetetrahydrofolate (MTHFR) 677C→T variant increases folacin requirement. A 19-base pair deletion polymorphism in dihydrofolate reductase is associated with increased unmetabolized folic acid in plasma and decreased red blood cell folate. Low zinc intake compromises folate status by negatively affecting intestinal folate uptake. Other symptoms of deficiency are leukopenia (low white cell count), general weakness, depression, and polyneuropathy. The latter sign is probably related to the folate-B_{12} interaction. Low folate intake during the post weaning years increases genomic DNA methylation in experimental animals. Whether this occurs in humans is not known. However, methylation is one of the key reactions that dictate epigenetic change.

FOLLICULOSIS

Presence of lymph follicles in large numbers.

FOLLISTATIN

A peptide hormone that binds the hormones activin and inhibin through an interaction with their β-subunits. In doing so, this hormone exerts local control of activin function and thus reduces or blocks activin-stimulated follicle-stimulating hormone (FSH) secretion.

FOLLOW-UP STUDIES (COHORT STUDIES)

Population studies in which the subjects (also referred to as the cohort) are followed for some time (follow-up period). At the start of the study (also called the baseline), the cohort consists of people who are free of the disease under investigation and differ in exposure conditions. All persons are examined and information on variables of interest is collected. During the course of the study, the occurrence of disease is recorded. From this, the incidence of the disease in the study population can be calculated. Based on these data, inferences on the association between exposure and occurrence of disease can be drawn. An important advantage of a follow-up study is that exposure is measured before the disease has developed. The appropriate follow-up period depends on the associations that are studied. Because the majority of follow-up studies concern chronic diseases, the follow-up period is usually long. Consequently, results are only available after many years. Furthermore, for the assessment of associations between exposure and disease, it is necessary for the number of cases that manifest themselves during the follow-up period to be sufficiently large. This means that the cohort approach is not suitable for studying rare diseases.

Another advantage of follow-up studies is that a large number of both exposures and outcomes can be studied. At baseline, a large number of parameters are measured in all study subjects. For a cohort study on a chronic disease, for example, these parameters may include lifestyle factors such as diet, physical activity, and smoking habits, and biological variables such as blood pressure, serum cholesterol concentration, height, and weight. Recent developments in the design of cohort studies include storage of biological material such as serum and white or red blood cells. This can be very useful if during the follow-up period new hypotheses arise about the role of variables, which have not been measured at baseline. In this way, additional baseline information on the study subjects can still be obtained even after the study is complete.

There are two special types of cohort studies. For a study on a particular effect of an industrial chemical, a cohort can be selected from groups of industrial workers who have been exposed to the chemical. Such cohorts are referred to as special cohorts. The prevalence of adverse health effects in such a cohort can then be compared with that among workers in the same industry who have not been exposed to the chemical or with that in the general population. Because a cohort has to be followed for many years after exposure has been measured, a retrospective cohort study is sometimes carried out. This means that a cohort is selected that has been exposed in the past. The investigator then has to establish the appearance of adverse health effects for all individuals of that cohort at the time of the actual study.

FONTANEL

One of several membranous intervals at the angles of the cranial bones in the head of an infant.

FOOD ADDITIVES

See Additives.

FOOD ALLERGY

Immunological reaction to food or a food product. There are many foods that may cause allergic reactions, but in only a few have the allergens been isolated and identified. The most common foods are cow's milk, soy, fish, egg, nuts, peanut, and wheat. The clinical symptoms of allergic food reactions can be characterized as skin symptoms (itching, erythema, angioedema, urticaria, increase of eczema), respiratory symptoms (itching of eyes, nose, throat; tearing, redness of the eyes; sneezing, nasal obstruction; swelling of the throat; shortness of breath; cough), gastrointestinal symptoms (nausea, vomiting, abdominal cramps, diarrhea), systemic symptoms (hypotension, shock), and controversial symptoms (arthritis, migraine, glue ear, irritable bowel syndrome). Sometimes, the allergic reaction only develops if the food intake is followed by exercise. This is referred to as exercise-induced food allergy.

FOOD AND AGRICULTURAL ORGANIZATION (FAO)

An international organization dedicated to improving the health of third world nations through improvement of agricultural practices.

FOOD AVERSION

A psychogenic reaction to a food (product).

FOOD CONTAMINANTS

Substances that are included unintentionally in foods.

FOOD DIARY

A record kept by an individual of food and beverages consumed, their quantity, and method of preparation.

FOOD EXCHANGE LISTS

Lists of food developed by dietitians, which allow patients to exchange one food for another in planning their daily food intake. Lists of fruits, vegetables, meats, and so on, have been developed for the control of fat intake, sodium intake, total energy intake, or balancing the intake of carbohydrates, fats, and proteins as is needed to manage a diabetic condition. The American Dietetic Association Food Exchange System is widely used and can be obtained through correspondence with their headquarters (ADA, P.O. Box 97215, Chicago, IL 60678–7215).

FOOD FADS

Instances where certain foods are consumed frequently for reasons other than for providing needed nutrients.

FOOD FAT

See the fat content of common foods at http://www.nal.usda.gov/fnic/foodcomp/Data/food .82nutrients.

FOOD FREQUENCY METHOD

A method for recording and estimating food intake. Food frequency questionnaires ask about the usual intake frequency (and sometimes also the quantities) of a limited number of food products. Only products that contribute substantially to the intake of the nutrients of interest are selected. A disadvantage of this method is that no information on total food consumption is obtained. Since food consumption patterns differ widely from one population to another, a new food frequency list has to be designed and validated for each study.

FOOD GROUPS

Lists of foods having similar characteristics. Fruits, vegetables, meats, fish and seafood, milk and dairy products, breads and cereals, and fats and oils are the major food groups. The nutrient composition of these foods can be found online at http://www.nal.usda.gov/fnic/foodcomp/Data/foods,82nutrients.

FOOD GUIDE PYRAMID

Graphic representation of the U.S. Department of Agriculture's (USDA) dietary guidelines that displays complex carbohydrates at the base to emphasize their contribution to the daily diet and fats and sweets at the top.

FOOD INTAKE REGULATION

A system that controls the amount and kinds of foods consumed. It signals hunger and the initiation of eating, and signals satiety or the cessation of eating.

Most animals other than humans eat primarily to satisfy their nutritional needs; a human's motivation for eating (or not eating) frequently is to satisfy both nonnutritional and nutritional needs. A human being's food selection is based on a combination of forces arising from his or her culture, family, educational level, economic circumstances, individual needs and idiosyncrasies, and age. With advanced age, the responses to a number of food intake signals are muted.

In addition to the social, cultural, and economic influences on food intake, the selection of foods involves a complex interaction between these influences and the special senses: reactions of the eye (sight), ear (sound), nose (smell), mouth (taste), and the sensations of pain and touch. The appearance, texture, smell, and taste of food are inextricably bound to one's cultural heritage. The sensation of hunger, together with the food's appeal, determines whether and when food is consumed.

NEURONAL SIGNALS FOR HUNGER AND SATIETY

Internal cues regulate food intake through a number of signals and responses, which ultimately result in the initiation or cessation of feeding. These cues are in addition to the aforementioned ones, which involve the cerebrum. Both short- and long-term controls are exerted, which, over time, serve to regulate the food intake of normal individuals so that they neither gain nor lose weight. Food intake control rests, in part, with the integration of a variety of hormonal and nonhormonal signals that are generated both peripherally and centrally. The hypothalamus is thought to be the main integrator of these signals. Other discrete areas of the brain are also involved. The paraventricular nucleus located slightly in front of the dorsomedial nucleus is involved in glucose homeostasis and also senses body size. A number of hormones, diet ingredients, metabolites, and drugs have been shown to influence food intake and feeding behavior. Some of the more important ones are shown in Table 30. Hormones that can enhance food intake at one level can suppress it at another level. In addition, a number of peptides have been discovered that influence food intake. These are listed in Table 31.

Several of these hormones or peptides have specific actions with respect to the intake of specific food components. For example, increases in neuropeptide Y (NPY) result in increased carbohydrate intake while increases in the level of galanin and opioid peptides increase fat intake. Fat intake is suppressed when the blood level of enterostatin rises. Rising blood levels of glucagon suppresses protein intake. The consumption of a high-protein, low-fat, and low-carbohydrate diet increases ghrelin release that in turn results in a decrease in food intake. All of the aforementioned

TABLE 30
Factors That Affect Food Intake

Enhances	Suppresses
Insulin	Estrogen
Testosterone	Corticotropin-releasing hormone
Glucocorticoids	Substance P
Thyroxine	Glucagon
Low serotonin levels	Serotonin
Dynorphin	High-protein diets
β-Endorphin	High blood glucose
NPY	Growth-hormone-releasing hormone
Galanin	Enterostatin
Opioid peptides	Calcitonin
Somatostatin	Cholecystokinin (CCK)
Desacetyl-melanocyte-stimulating hormone	Amino acid imbalance
Histidine (precursor of histamine)	Pain
	Tryptophan (precursor of serotonin)
	High saturated fat intake
	TSH (thyroid-stimulating hormone)
	Thyrotropin-releasing factor

TABLE 31
Peptides (Cytokines) That Influence Feeding

Appetite-Stimulating Cytokines	Satiety Cytokines
Galanin	Cholecystokinin
NPY	Anorectin
Opioid peptides	Ghrelin
	Leptin
	Neurotensin
	TNF-α
	Bombesin
	Cyclo-his-pro

compounds are short-term signals that appear to regulate food selection as well as the amount of food consumed. Although most of these studies have been done in carefully prepared experimental animals (usually rats), there is sufficient indirect evidence to suggest that short-term food intake is similarly regulated in man. Indeed, mutations in the genes for the satiety peptides or for their receptors have resulted in obesity. Several animal models for genetic obesity have been shown to have these mutations. In humans, serotoninergic agents are being developed for use as treatments for obesity and eating disorders. These agents either block the binding of serotonin (5-hydroxy-tryptamine, 5-HT) to its receptor or upregulate the receptors' binding affinity. The 5-HT receptors are widespread throughout the cerebral cortex, the limbic system, the striatum, the brain stem, the choroid plexus, and almost every other region of the central nervous system. Serotonin in modest amounts stimulates feeding, while in large amounts it has the reverse effect. Drugs that block the serotonin receptors are useful in treating anorexia (decreased desire to eat), especially the anorexia that accompanies anxiety, depression, obsessive-compulsive disorders, panic disorders, migraine, and chemotherapy emesis. By blocking the receptors the serotonin has a longer residence time and can stimulate feeding. In contrast, drugs that potentiate the binding of serotonin to its receptor will result in a suppression of appetite and may be useful in treating the hyperphagia of Prader-Willi syndrome and that associated with other forms of genetic obesity.

Drugs, particularly those used in cancer chemotherapy, frequently have appetite suppression as a side effect. In part, this reduction in food intake may be due to disease and/or drug-induced changes in taste and aroma perception and, in part, due to the effects of the disease and/or drugs on the central nervous system, particularly the adrenergic and serotonergic receptors. Several drugs, chemically related to the catecholamines, are appetite suppressants. These drugs can be addictive and are controlled substances, so they are not particularly useful for appetite control.

Some steroids affect food intake. Adrenalectomized animals or humans with Addison's disease (glucocorticoid-deficient states) do not perceive normal hunger signals. If without food for extended periods of time, these individuals are difficult to undergo realimentation. However, once eating commences, a normal feeding pattern will be maintained. In excess, glucocorticoid stimulates feeding and patients with Cushing's disease (excess glucocorticoid production) or patients who are receiving long-term glucocorticoid treatment will report increased hunger and food intake. Patients with Cushing's disease are often characterized by large fat depots across the shoulders and in the abdomen. In addition, obese patients are frequently characterized by excess blood levels of both glucocorticoids and insulin. These hormones stimulate appetite and feeding.

Within the normal range of blood hormone levels, testosterone and estrogen, although also steroids, have opposite effects with respect to food intake. In experimental animals, day-to-day variations in food intake by females will follow the same pattern as their day-to-day variation in estrogen levels. When estrogen is high, food intake is suppressed and vice versa. Women who are anestrus due to ovariectomy or who are postmenopausal frequently lose their day-to-day estrogen-mediated food intake pattern. With this loss, they demonstrate a more even (and somewhat increased) food intake and subsequent body fat gain. This has been found in castrated female rats as well. The gain in body weight as fat is explained by the loss in food intake control exerted by the estrogens rather than by an estrogen-inhibiting effect on lipogenesis. Testosterone increases food intake marginally, but it also stimulates protein synthesis and spontaneous physical activity. As a result, body fat does not increase. As testosterone levels decline in males with age, protein synthesis declines and the body tends to sustain its fat synthetic activity. This results in a change in body composition with an increase in body fat stores. The age-related decline in testosterone production may not be accompanied by a decline in food intake.

Although food intake can vary from day to day in response to minor day-to-day variations in food supply, activity, and hormonal status, body weight is relatively constant. The mechanisms that control body weight are very complex, and the fine details of this regulation are far from clear. However, suffice it to say, major long-term deviations in either food intake or physiological state can affect body weight or energy balance. If food intake (energy intake) is curtailed for days to months, body weight will fall; similarly, if food intake is dramatically increased, body weight will increase.

FOOD INTAKE TABLES

Data from 9349 individuals were collected from the National Health and Nutrition Examination Survey (NHANES). These are two-day food intake records and have been divided into a variety of summary tables that provide information on nutrient intake, nutrients contributed by foods eaten away from home, and other such compilations. They can be accessed online at http://www.ars.usda.gov/Services/docs.htm?docid=18349. Other summary tables can be accessed by using the number 17041 instead of 18349.

FOOD INTOLERANCE

General term describing an abnormal physiological response to food or food additives that does not appear to be immunological in nature.

FOOD JAGS

Periods of time when one or more foods are consumed in large amounts or in amounts relatively greater than usual.

FOOD POISONING

See Food-Borne Illness.

FOOD-BORNE DISEASES

Diseases that develop as a result of consuming contaminated food. Food-borne diseases can be divided into food-borne infections or food-borne intoxications, depending on whether the pathogen itself or its toxic product (a microbial toxin or toxic metabolite, produced in the food or in the human body) is the causal agent. The most important bacterial food-borne pathogens causing infections include *Salmonella* (incubation time: 6–36 hours; duration of disease: 1–7 days), *Shigella* (incubation time: 6–12 hours; duration of disease: 2–3 days), *Escherichia coli* (incubation time: 12–72 hours; duration of disease: 1–7 days), *Yersinia enterocolitica* (incubation time: 24–36 hours; duration of disease: 3–5 days), *Campylobacter jejuni* (incubation time: 3–5 days; duration of disease: 5–7 days), *Vibrio parahemolyticus* (incubation time: 2–48 hours; duration of disease:

2–5 days), and *Aeromonashydrophila* (incubation time: 2–48 hours; duration of disease: 2–7 days). Examples of pathogens causing food-borne intoxications are *Staphylococcus aureus* (in food; incubation time: 2–6 hours; duration of disease: 1 day or less), *Clostridium botulinum* (in food; incubation time: 12–96 hours; duration of disease: 1–8 days), *Clostridium perfringens* (in intestine; incubation time: 8–22 hours; duration of disease: 1–2 days), and *Bacillus cereus* (emetic type—in food; incubation time: 1–5 hours; duration of disease: 1 day or less; diarrheal type—in intestine; incubation time: 8–16 hours; duration of disease: >1 day). Other microbial agents causing food-borne intoxications include toxins produced by fungi (mycotoxins) and algae, and toxic metabolites such as biogenic amines and ethyl carbamate produced by bacteria in yeasts. In general, five sources of bacteria are recognized as causing food-borne diseases: (1) fecal matter and/or urine of infected humans or animals; (2) nasal and throat discharges of sick individuals or asymptomatic carriers; (3) infections on body surfaces of food handlers (hands and arms); (4) infected soils, mud, surface waters, and dust; and (5) sea water, marine materials, and marine life. (See also Botulism; Ciguatera Poisoning; Contamination of Food; Ergot Alkaloids; Glycoalkaloids; Immunoactive Endotoxins; Lesion-Causing Bacterial Toxins; Membrane-Affecting Bacterial Toxins; Mycotoxins; *Salmonella*.)

FOOD-ORIENTED CHEMICALS

Chemicals with no nutritional value that are primarily associated with food. They include food additives (preservatives such as benzoic acid; antioxidants such as butylated hydroxyanisole [BHA]; sweeteners, such as sorbitol; food contaminants such as nitrate, lead, cadmium, polycyclic aromatic hydrocarbons), and natural toxins (aflatoxins).

FOOTPRINTING

A technique for identifying the site on DNA bound by proteins that protect certain bonds from attack by nucleases.

FOREMILK

The early milk of the lactating mother; also called the colostrum.

FORSKOLIN

A compound that activates adenylate cyclase and protein kinase C (PKC); enhances gene transcription of c-Fos, transforming growth factor β (TGF-$β_1$), and NPY.

FORTIFICATION

The addition of nutrients to food products as they are manufactured.

FOSINOPRIL SODIUM

An angiotensin-converting enzyme (ACE) inhibitor; antihypertensive agent. Trade name: Monpril.

FREE ENERGY

Energy not trapped or used further; usually dissipated as heat.

FREE RADICALS

Very reactive products of the autoxidation of unsaturated fatty acids. Some amino acids also may be radicalized. Free radicals are molecules with an unpaired electron.

FREEZE-DRYING

A processing technique that results in the dehydration of food at temperatures below freezing.

FRUCTOSE

A six-carbon sugar having a five-membered ring and a ketone group instead of an aldehyde group at its terminus.

FRUCTOSE INTOLERANCE

Inability to use dietary fructose; a rare genetic disease of fructose metabolism. Three hereditary diseases result from a mutation in one of three key enzymes of fructose metabolism: (1) fructokinase, (2) aldolase B, and (3) fructose 1,6-bisphosphatase. A mutation in the gene for fructokinase is characterized by elevated blood and urine levels of fructose. A second mutation has been identified in the gene for aldolase B. This is the enzyme that catalyzes the splitting of fructose 1-phosphate to glyceraldehyde phosphate and dihydroxyacetone phosphate. Aldolase B is located in the liver only. The mutation is such that the enzyme has a reduced affinity for its substrate, fructose 1-phosphate. The results of this reduced affinity include hypoglycemia due to an inhibition of glycogenolysis by fructose 1-phosphate. This hypoglycemia is not responsive to glucagon stimulation. In addition to the disturbance in glycogenolysis, patients with this disorder vomit after a fructose load; have elevated levels of urine and blood fructose; grow poorly with evidence of jaundice; and have hyperbilirubinemia (high levels of bilirubin in the blood), albuminuria (albumin in the urine), and amino aciduria (amino acids in the urine), and some patients may have damaged renal proximal convoluted tubules.

The third mutation involves only the liver enzyme fructose 1,6-bisphosphatase. The muscle enzyme is normal in activity. This enzyme is a key enzyme in the hepatic gluconeogenic pathway so, as one might expect, hypoglycemia is one of the characteristics of a mutation in this enzyme. Other characteristics include an enlarged liver, poor muscle tone, and increased blood lactate levels. All of these mutations are uncommon, and all are autosomal recessive traits. Heterozygotes are not detectable.

FRUCTOSE METABOLISM

See Metabolic Maps, Appendix 2. Fructose is converted to glucose after phosphorylation. Although two enzymes are available for the phosphorylation of fructose, one of these, fructokinase, is present only in the liver. Hexokinase can catalyze the phosphorylation of fructose. However, fructokinase is a much more active enzyme. Its activity is so high that, in fact, most of the dietary fructose, whether as the free sugar or a component of sucrose, is metabolized in the liver. This is in contrast to glucose, which is metabolized by all the cells in the body. As a result, fructose- or sucrose-rich diets fed to rats or mice will result in a fatty liver. This occurs because the dietary overload of fructose or sucrose exceeds the capacity of the liver to oxidize it, so the liver uses sugar metabolites as substrates for fatty acid and triacylglyceride synthesis. Until the hepatic lipid export system increases sufficiently to transport this lipid to the storage depots, the lipid accumulates, hence, the occurrence of fatty liver. Adaptation to a high-fructose intake can and does occur in normal individuals.

FSH

Follicle-stimulating hormone.

FTO

Gene related to fat mass and obesity; located near the gene for melanocortin 4 receptor.

FULL LIQUID DIET

Diet containing foods and beverages that are liquid at room temperature.

FUNCTIONAL FOODS

Foods that have functions beyond the ones conferred by the nutrients they contain. These foods may play a role in, for example, vision protection, cancer prevention, or some other aspect of life.

FUNCTIONAL GROUP

A portion of a molecule that participates in interactions with other substances. Examples are acyl, carboxy, carbonyl, ester, and sulfhydryl groups.

FURANOSE

A sugar with a five-membered ring.

FUROSEMIDE

A loop diuretic; antihypertensive agent. Trade names: Lasix, Novosemide, Apo-Furosemide.

G

GABA

Gamma amino butyric acid. A neurotransmitter formed through the decarboxylation of glutamic acid.

GABAPENTIN

An anticonvulsant. Trade name: Neurontin.

GALACTORRHEA

Persistent discharge of a milk-like fluid from the mammary gland not associated with parturition and lactation.

GALACTOSE

See Metabolic Maps, Appendix 2. A monosaccharide that, with glucose, forms the disaccharide, lactose, or milk sugar. Galactose is converted to glucose and eventually enters the glycolytic sequence as glucose-6-phosphate. Galactose is phosphorylated at carbon 1 in the first step of its conversion to glucose. It can be isomerized to glucose-1-phosphate or converted to uridinediphosphate glucose (UDP)-galactose by exchanging its phosphate group for a UDP group. This UDP-galactose can be joined with glucose to form lactose in the adult mammary tissue under the influence of the hormone prolactin. However, usually the UDP-galactose is converted to UDP-glucose and thence used to form glycogen.

GALACTOSEMIA

An inability to use galactose; a genetic disease of galactose metabolism. Characterized by abnormally high blood levels of galactose. Three autosomal recessive mutations in the genes for enzymes involved in galactose conversion to glucose have been described. Galactosemia results in each instance. Two of these mutations involve the gene for galactose-1-phosphate uridyltransferase. Two variants have been described. One is fairly innocuous in that the mutation occurs only in the enzymes found in the red cells. This variant is called the Duarte variant, and affected individuals have 50% less red cell galactose-1-phosphate uridyltransferase activity than normal individuals. These people have no other discernible characteristics.

The second variant is far more severe in its effects on the patient. The enzyme in the liver is abnormal and does not convert galactose-1-phosphate to UDP galactose. As a result, galactose-1-phosphate accumulates, and some is converted to the sugar alcohol galactitol via NADH aldose reductase action. Cataracts in the eye form in this disease accompanied by mental retardation and increased tissue levels of galactose-1-phosphate, galactitol, and galactonic acid. These last metabolites are excreted in the urine. Also, characteristics of this mutation in galactose-1-phosphate uridyltransferase are decreased blood glucose levels, decreased glycogenesis, decreased mutase activity, and decreased pyrophosphorylase activity. Since UDP-galactose is necessary for the formation of galactoyl lipids, chondroitin sulfate formation is decreased. A mutation in the gene for galactokinase also results in accumulations of galactose and galactitol and cataracts. The galactitol accumulation was found to be the causative agent in the formation of cataracts. Except for cataract formation due to galactitol accumulation, no other symptoms have been described for this form of galactosemia.

GALANIN

A 30-amino acid peptide found in the neurons of the gastrointestinal submucosa. It can inhibit the release of somatostatin, insulin, pancreatic polypeptide, and neurotensin. It serves as a stimulator of food intake.

GALLSTONES

Gallstones develop when the bile salts and cholesterol accumulate in the gallbladder. With time, the cholesterol precipitates out, providing a crystalline structure for the stone. Since the bile also contains a variety of minerals, these minerals form salts with the bile acids and are deposited within and around the cholesterol matrix. Eventually these stones irritate the lining of the gallbladder or may lodge themselves in the duct connecting the bladder to the duodenum. When this happens, the bladder becomes inflamed, the duct may be blocked, and the patient becomes unable to tolerate food. In some cases, treatment consists of reducing the irritation and inflammation through drugs, but often the patient has the gallbladder and its offending stones removed.

GALT

Gut associated lymphoid tissue; plays a role in the activity of the immune system.

GAMMA AMINO BUTYRIC ACID (GABA)

A metabolite produced when glutamic acid is decarboxylated. It is an inhibitory neurotransmitter that quiets excited neurons. Low levels of GABA are associated with convulsions.

GANGLIOSIDE

A cerebroside containing glucose and/or galactose and neuraminic acid (an amino uronic acid).

GASEOUS PRODUCTS OF DIGESTION (GE)

Combustible gases produced in the digestive tract by microbial fermentation of food. Methane is the chief combustible gas in the ruminant. Hydrogen, carbon monoxide, acetone, ethane, and hydrogen sulfide are produced in trace amounts.

GASTRIC ACID

Hydrochloric acid.

GASTRIN

A small peptide hormone produced by gastric cells. Gastrin stimulates the parietal cells to release hydrochloric acid.

GASTRITIS

Inflammation of the stomach.

GASTROENTERITIS

Inflammation of the stomach and intestines. Condition characterized by the return of gastric contents up the esophagus resulting in a "burning sensation" under the sternum.

GASTROINTESTINAL TRACT (GI TRACT)

Flexible muscular tube from the mouth, through the esophagus, stomach, small intestine, large intestine, and rectum to the anus.

GASTROINTESTINAL TRANSIT TIME

The time that elapses between food entry and fecal excretion of the residual nondigested food components.

GASTROJEJUNOSTOMY

Known as the Billroth II procedure, in which a connection between the stomach and the jejunum is surgically created.

GASTROPARESIS

A condition in which the movement of ingesta through the stomach is slower than normal.

GASTROPLASTY

Reduction of the stomach size via surgery.

GAUCHER'S DISEASE

A genetic disease due to a mutation in the gene for the synthesis of the enzyme glucocerebrosidase. This enzyme catalyzes the cleavage of the sphingolipid glucocerebroside. Characterized by accumulation of cerebrosides in the brain and other tissues.

GCN2

Transduction pathway in the liver for amino acid sensing.

GDP

Guanosine diphosphate. A dephosphorylated form of guanosine triphosphate (GTP) important in the activation of substances participating in the biosynthesis of proteins.

GEMFIBROZIL

A fibric acid derivative that serves to lower blood lipids. Trade name: Lopid.

GENE

Carrier of specific genetic code for a specific protein in the organism.

GENERALLY RECOGNIZED AS SAFE (GRAS)

See Additives.

GENETIC CODE

The sequence of purine and pyrimidine bases that are in a specific order and that dictate the amino acid sequence of all proteins synthesized by cells.

GENETIC DISEASES

Diseases due to mutations in the gene codes for specific proteins.

GENETICALLY MODIFIED FOODS

Food from species whose genetic code has been modified either through selective breeding or gene transfer. Genetic changes have been introduced to improve the quality of the food, to hasten its production, or to improve its physical characteristics.

GENOMICS

The study of the genetic code of plants and animals.

GENOTOXIC CARCINOGENS

Chemicals that attack DNA causing mutated cells to develop and reproduce in an uncontrolled manner.

GENOTYPE

The sequence of bases in DNA that provides inherited characteristics of an individual.

GEOPHAGIA

The eating of dirt; an abnormal appetite.

GERIATRICS

A medical subspecialty relating to the care and treatment of elderly people.

GERM

A pathogenic microorganism.

GERM PLASM

The heart of a plant seed from which a new plant grows.

GERONTOLOGY

The study of senescence or aging.

GESTATION

The period of growth initiated at conception and terminated by parturition (birth).

GESTATIONAL DIABETES

A carbohydrate intolerance, in variable severity, with onset first recognized during pregnancy. Detected during screening between 24 and 28 weeks gestation with a 50-g oral glucose test. If results at 1-hour postprandial are ≥140 mg/dL, the oral glucose tolerance test is used to confirm diagnosis.

GHRELIN

A satiety factor responsive to protein feeding and low-carbohydrate–low-fat feeding.

GIP

Gastric inhibitory peptide. A peptide hormone that inhibits gastric motility and acid secretion.

GLIMEPIRIDE

A sulfonylurea that acts as a hypoglycemic agent. Trade name: Amaryl.

GLIPIZIDE

A sulfonylurea that acts as a hypoglycemic agent. Trade name: Glucotrol. This compound is sometimes combined with metformin. Trade name: Metaglip.

GLOBIN

The polypeptide components of myoglobin and hemoglobin.

GLOBULIN

A protein that is globular in shape. There are several. Gamma globulin is a protein that carries antibodies to a variety of antigens, especially those related to communicable diseases. Hemoglobin is a globular protein in red blood cells that contains heme iron which, in turn, carries oxygen.

GLOMERULAR FILTRATION RATE

A test used as an indicator of renal function that reflects the ability of the kidney to filter and reabsorb fluids.

GLOMERULONEPHRITIS

A disease characterized by inflammation of the nephrons of the kidney. Glomerulonephritis occurs most often one to two weeks after a streptococcal throat or skin infection and generally affects children.

GLOSSITIS

A shiny red appearance of the tongue.

GLUCAGON

A polypeptide synthesized and released by α cells of the islets of Langerhans in the pancreas. Serves as an anti-insulin with respect to glucose homeostasis. Glucagon stimulates gluconeogenesis and glycogenolysis.

GLUCOGENIC AMINO ACIDS

Amino acids whose carbon skeletons can be used for glucose synthesis. These are listed in Table 32.

GLUCONEOGENESIS

The synthesis of glucose from noncarbohydrate precursors. See Metabolic Maps, Appendix 2.

Gluconeogenesis occurs primarily in the liver and kidney. Except under conditions of prolonged starvation, the kidneys do not contribute appreciable amounts of glucose to the circulation. Most tissues lack the full complement of enzymes needed to run this pathway. In particular, the rate-limiting enzyme phosphoenolpyruvate carboxykinase (PEPCK) is not found to be active in tissues other than liver and kidney. The other reactions use the same enzymes as glycolysis and do not have control properties with respect to gluconeogenesis. The rate-limiting enzymes are glucose-6-phosphatase, fructose-1,6 bisphosphatase, and PEPCK. Pyruvate kinase and pyruvate carboxylase are also of interest because their control is a coordinated one with respect to the regulation of PEPCK.

Oxaloacetate is essential to gluconeogenesis because it is the substrate for PEPCK, which catalyzes its conversion to phosphoenolpyruvate (PEP). This is an energy-dependent conversion, which overcomes the irreversible final glycolytic reaction catalyzed by pyruvate kinase. The activity of PEPCK is closely coupled with that of pyruvate carboxylase. Whereas the pyruvate kinase reaction produces one ATP, the formation of PEP uses two ATPs—one in the mitochondria for the pyruvate carboxylase reaction and one in the cytosol for the PEPCK reaction. PEPCK requires GTP provided via the nucleoside diphosphate kinase reaction that uses ATP. ATP transfers one high-energy bond to GDP to form ADP and GTP.

TABLE 32
Amino Acids That Contribute a Carbon Chain for the Synthesis of Glucose

Amino Acid	Enters As
Alanine	Pyruvate
Tryptophan → Alanine	Pyruvate
Hydroxyproline	Pyruvate
Serine	Pyruvate
Cysteine	Pyruvate
Threonine	Pyruvate
Glycine	Pyruvate
Tyrosine	Fumarate
Isoleucine	Succinyl CoA
Methionine	Succinyl CoA
Valine	Succinyl CoA
Histidine → Glutamate	α ketoglutarate
Proline → Glutamate	α ketoglutarate
Glutamine → Glutamate	α ketoglutarate
Arginine → Glutamate	α ketoglutarate

In starvation or uncontrolled diabetes, PEPCK activity is elevated as is gluconeogenesis. Starvation elicits a number of catabolic hormones that serve to mobilize tissue energy stores as well as precursors for glucose synthesis. Uncontrolled diabetes elicits similar hormonal responses. In both instances, the synthesis of the PEPCK enzyme is increased. Unlike other rate-limiting enzymes, PEPCK is not regulated allosterically or by phosphorylation–dephosphorylation mechanisms. Instead, it is regulated by changes in gene transcription of its single copy gene from a single promoter site. This regulation is unique because all of the known factors (hormones, vitamins, metabolites) act in the same place. They either turn on the synthesis of the mRNA for PEPCK, or they turn it off. What is also unique is the fact that liver and kidney cells translate this message into sufficient active enzyme protein that catalyzes the PEP formation. Other cells and tissues have the code for PEPCK in their nuclear DNA but do not usually synthesize the enzyme. Instead, these cell types synthesize the enzyme that catalyzes glycerol synthesis. In effect then, only the kidney and liver have active gluconeogenic processes.

The next few steps in gluconeogenesis are identical to those of glycolysis but are in the reverse direction. When the step for the dephosphorylation of fructose-1,6 bisphosphate occurs, there is another energy barrier, and instead of a bidirectional reaction catalyzed by a single enzyme, there are separate forward and reverse reactions. In the synthesis of glucose, this reaction is catalyzed by fructose-1,6-bisphosphatase and yields fructose-6-phosphate. No ATP is involved, but a molecule of water and an inorganic phosphate are produced. Rising levels of fructose-2,6-bisphosphatase allosterically inhibits gluconeogenesis while it stimulates glycolysis. AMP likewise inhibits gluconeogenesis at this step.

Lastly, the removal of the phosphate from glucose-6-phosphate via the enzyme complex glucose-6-phosphatase completes the pathway to yield free glucose. This is an irreversible reaction that does not involve ATP. The glucose-6-phosphate moves to the endoplasmic reticulum, where the phosphatase is located and glucose is released for use.

GLUCOSE

A six-carbon monosaccharide. The preferred metabolic fuel for most cell types, particularly those of the CNS.

GLUCOSE TOLERANCE TEST

The test performed on an individual who has fasted at least 12 hours and then is provided 75–100 g of glucose. Blood glucose levels are monitored at hourly intervals and compared to established norms to confirm the diagnosis of diabetes mellitus.

GLUCOSE TRANSPORTERS (GLUT 1, 2, 3, 4)

A group of special proteins that transport glucose into the cell. There are four glucose transporters, called GLUT 1, 2, 3, and 4. Some cell types have only one of these while others have more than one. The transporters differ slightly in their structure and function with respect to the function of the tissues that contain them. Table 33 lists the transporters and their location. The glucose transporter is referred to as a mobile transporter because when it is not in use, it is sequestered in an intracellular pool. When needed, it leaves its storage site, moves to the interior aspect of the plasma membrane, forms a loose bond with the membrane, picks up the glucose molecule, and moves it through the membrane into the cytosol whereupon the glucose can be phosphorylated and metabolized. Aberrations in the mobile glucose transporters affect glucose use.

GLUCOSINOLATES

See Type B Antinutritives.

TABLE 33
Location of the Mobile Glucose Transporters

Transporter	Location
GLUT 1	Ubiquitous but found mainly in brain, placenta, and cultured cells; is not particularly responsive to insulin regulation
GLUT 2	Liver, β cells of pancreas, kidney, intestine
GLUT 3	Ubiquitous in human tissue, CNS
GLUT 4	Adipose tissue, heart, skeletal muscle

GLUCOSURIA

Glucose in the urine.

GLUTAMIC ACID

A five-carbon amino acid with two carboxyl groups. Glutamate is the precursor of the neurotransmitter GABA.

GLUTAMINE

The amine of glutamic acid; the two carboxyl groups of glutamic acid are replaced by two amino groups. Plays a key role in transporting amino groups to the urea cycle.

GLUTATHIONE

A tripeptide with a free sulfhydryl group that, in a reduced state, helps maintain iron in its appropriate oxidized state (ferrous) in hemoglobin.

GLUTEN-SENSITIVE ENTEROPATHY

Characterized by the gastrointestinal intolerance to the proteins in wheat, rye, oats, and barley. Also known as nontropicalsprue, celiac disease, and idiopathic steatorrhea.

GLYBURIDE (GLIBENCLAMIDE)

A sulfonylurea that serves as a hypoglycemic agent. Trade names: Micronase, Diabeta, Euglucon, Glynase PresTab.

GLYCEMIC INDEX

An index that relates the specific food consumed to the elevation in blood glucose that the particular food elicits. Not all carbohydrate-containing foods elicit the same rise in blood glucose. The index has been used to design diet management plans for people with diabetes mellitus.

GLYCEROL

A three-carbon monosaccharide that, when phosphorylated, provides the backbone for the synthesis of triglycerides.

GLYCEROPHOSPHATE SHUTTLE

A shuttle for the transfer of reducing equivalents into the mitochondria from the cytosol. Shown in Figure 24, this shuttle is a rate-limiting step for glycolysis.

GLYCINE

A two-carbon nonessential amino acid.

GLYCOALKALOIDS

Minor components of potatoes and tomatoes that are toxic if consumed in large quantities. Steroidal alkaloids are mainly present as glycosides in the family of Solanaceae, including the potato and the tomato. The major glycoalkaloids in potatoes are solanine and chaconine, both glycosides of solanidine. Solanine and chaconine are potent irritants of the intestinal mucosa and cholinesterase inhibitors, the first being the most active. Poisoning with either substance can result in gastrointestinal symptoms of vomiting and diarrhea, and neurological symptoms such as irritability, confusion, delirium, and respiratory failure, which may ultimately result in death. Furthermore, poisoning is often accompanied by high fever. In general, the glycoalkaloid contents of potato tubers do not pose harmful effects in humans. Serious poisonings have been reported following the consumption of large amounts of potatoes with high glycoalkaloid contents ($\geq$200 mg/kg). Potatoes that have been exposed to light and those that are diseased by fungal infection or mechanically bruised may contain toxic levels of glycoalkaloids. The major glycoalkaloid in tomatoes is α-tomatidine, with tomatidenol as the aglycone. It is present in all parts of the plant. In the fruit, the concentration decreases during ripening. Poisonings in humans due to the consumption of tomatoes have not been reported.

GLYCOCHOLATE

Bile acid required for fat digestion and absorption.

GLYCOGEN

Glucose polymer formed in mammalian liver and muscle. A storage form of glucose. Glycogen, when stimulated to release its glucose by the catabolic hormones, glucagon, epinephrine, the glucocorticoids, and thyroxine, and/or by the absence of food in the digestive tract, provides glucose

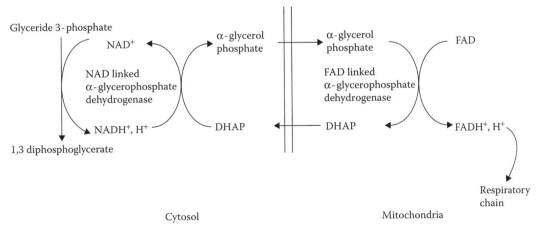

FIGURE 24 α-Glycerophosphate shuttle.

to the body. Because the glycogen molecule has molecules of water as part of its structure, it is a very large molecule and cumbersome to store in large amounts. An average 70-kg man has only an 18-hour fuel supply stored as glycogen, while the same individual might have up to a 2-month supply of fuel stored as fat. Muscle and liver glycogen stores have very different functions. Muscle glycogen is used to synthesize ATP for muscle contraction, whereas hepatic glycogen is the glucose reserve for the entire body, particularly the CNS. The amount of glycogen in the muscle is dependent upon the physical activity of the individual. After bouts of strenuous exercise, glycogen store will be depleted only to be rebuilt during the resting period following exercise. Hepatic glycogen stores are dependent on nutritional status. They are virtually absent in the 24-hour starved animal while being replenished within hours of ad libitum feeding. Clusters of glycogen molecules with an average molecular weight of 2×10^7 form quickly when an abundance of glucose is provided to the liver. The amount of glycogen in the liver is diet dependent. There is a 24-hour rhythmic change in hepatic glycogen that corresponds to the feeding pattern of the animal. In nocturnal animals such as the rat, the peak hepatic glycogen store will be found in the early morning hours, while the nadir will be found in the evening hours just before the nocturnal feeding begins. In humans accustomed to eating during the day, the reverse pattern will be observed.

GLYCOGEN STORAGE DISEASES

Genetic diseases that are characterized by excess glycogen stores. Rare autosomal recessive diseases due to mutations in the genes that encode different enzymes needed for glycogen metabolism.

GLYCOGEN SYNTHESIS

See Metabolic Maps, Appendix 2. Glycogen synthesis begins with glucose-1-phosphate formation from glucose-6-phosphate through the action of phosphoglucomutase. Glucose-1-phosphate then is converted to uridinediphosphate glucose (UDP-glucose), which can then be added to the glycogen already in storage (the glycogen primer). UDP-glucose can be added through a 1,6 linkage or a 1,4 linkage. Two high-energy bonds are used to incorporate each molecule of glucose into the glycogen. The straight chain glucose polymer comprises glucoses joined through the 1,4 linkage and is less compact than the branched chain glycogen, which has both 1,4 and 1,6 linkages. The addition of glucose to the primer glycogen with a 1,4 linkage is catalyzed by the glycogen synthase enzyme, while the 1,6 addition is catalyzed by the so-called glycogen branching enzyme, amylo $(1 \rightarrow 4, 1 \rightarrow 6)$ transglucosidase. Once the liver and muscle cell achieve their full storage capacity, these enzymes are product inhibited and glycogenesis is "turned off." Glycogen synthase is inactivated by a cAMP-dependent kinase and activated by a synthase phosphatase enzyme that is stimulated by changes in the ratio of ATP to ADP. Glycogen synthesis is stimulated by the hormone insulin and suppressed by the catabolic hormones. The process does not fully cease but operates at a very low level. Glycogen does not accumulate appreciably in cells other than liver and muscle, although all cells contain a small amount of glycogen. Note that a glycogen primer is required for glycogen synthesis to proceed. This primer is carefully guarded so that some is always available when glycogen is synthesized. This means that glycogenolysis never fully depletes the cell of its glycogen content.

GLYCOGENOLYSIS

See Metabolic Maps, Appendix 2. The process of releasing glucose from glycogen. Glycogenolysis is a carefully controlled series of reactions referred to as the glycogen cascade. It is called a cascade because of the stepwise changes in activation states of the enzymes involved. To release glucose for oxidation by the glycogenolytic pathway, the glycogen must be phosphorylated. This is accomplished by the enzyme glycogen phosphorylase. Glycogen phosphorylase exists in the cell in an inactive form (glycogen phosphorylase b) and is activated to its active form (glycogen phosphorylase a) by the enzyme phosphorylase b kinase. In turn, this kinase also exists in an inactive form, which is activated by the calcium-dependent enzyme, protein kinase, and active cAMP-dependent protein kinase. Each of these activations requires a molecule of ATP. Lastly, the cAMP-dependent protein kinase must have cAMP for its activation. This cAMP is generated from ATP by the enzyme adenylate cyclase, which, in itself, is inactive unless stimulated by a hormone such as epinephrine, thyroxine, or glucagon. As can be seen, this cascade of activation is energy dependent, with three molecules of ATP needed to get the process started. Once started, the glycolytic pathway will replenish the ATP needed initially as well as provide a further supply of ATP to provide needed energy. As mentioned earlier, the liver and muscle differ in the use of glycogen. This also affects how ATP is generated within the glycogen-containing cell and how much is generated by cells that do not store glycogen.

GLYCOLIPID

A complex lipid containing a carbohydrate moiety.

GLYCOLYSIS

See Metabolic Maps, Appendix 2. The glycolytic pathway for the anaerobic catabolism of glucose can be found in all cells in the body. This pathway begins with glucose, a six-carbon unit, and through a series of reactions produces two molecules of ATP and two molecules of pyruvate. The control of glycolysis is vested in several key steps. The first step is the activation of glucose through the formation of glucose-6-phosphate. In the liver and pancreatic β cell, this step is catalyzed by the enzyme glucokinase. A molecule of ATP is used and magnesium is required. Glucose-6-phosphate is a key metabolite. It can proceed down the glycolytic pathway or move through the hexose monophosphate shunt (see Hexose Monophosphate Shunt), or be used to produce glycogen. The amount of glucose-6-phosphate oxidized directly to pyruvate depends on the nutritional state of the animal, the type of cell, the genetics of the animal, and its hormonal state. Some cell types, the brain cell for example, do not produce glycogen. Some people do not have shunt activity in the red cells because the code for glucose-6-phosphate dehydrogenase has mutated such that the enzyme is not functional. Insulin-deficient animals likewise have little shunt activity due to the lack of insulin's effect on the synthesis of its enzymes. All these factors determine how much glucose-6-phosphate goes in which direction.

Two enzymes are used for the activation of glucose: glucokinase and hexokinase. In the liver, both enzymes are present. While hexokinase activity is product inhibited, glucokinase is not. The hexokinase in the nonhepatic tissues must be product inhibited to prevent the hexokinase from tying up all the inorganic phosphate (Pi) in the cells as glucose-6-phosphate. The Km for glucokinase is greater than that for hexokinase, so the former is the main enzyme for the conversion of glucose to glucose-6-phosphate in the liver. The other enzyme will phosphorylate not only glucose but also six other carbon sugars, such as fructose. However, the amount of fructose phosphorylated to fructose-6-phosphate is small in comparison to the phosphorylation of fructose at the carbon-1 position catalyzed by fructokinase.

Glucose-6-phosphate is isomerized to fructose-6-phosphate and then is phosphorylated once again to form fructose-1,6-bisphosphate. Another molecule of ATP is used, and again magnesium is an important cofactor. Both kinase reactions are rate-controlling reactions in that their activity determines the rate at which subsequent reactions proceed. The phosphofructokinase reaction is unique to the glycolytic sequence while the glucokinase or hexokinase step is not. Thus, one could argue that the formation of fructose-1,6-bisphosphate is the first committed step in glycolysis. Glycolysis is inhibited when phosphofructokinase is inhibited. This occurs when fatty acid levels in the cytosol rise and when the rates of lipolysis and fatty acid oxidation are high. Phosphofructokinase activity is increased when levels of fructose-6-phosphate rise or when cAMP levels rise. Stimulation also occurs when fructose-2,6-bisphosphate levels rise. In any event, glycolysis then proceeds with the splitting of fructose-1,6-bisphosphate into dihydroxyacetone phosphate (DHAP) and glyceraldehyde-3-phosphate. At this point, another rate-controlling step occurs that shuttles reducing equivalents into the mitochondria for use by the respiratory chain. This is the α-glycerophosphate shuttle (see Figure 24). This shuttle carries reducing equivalents from the cytosol to the mitochondria. DHAP picks up reducing equivalents when it is converted to α-glycerol phosphate. These reducing equivalents are produced when glyceraldehyde-3-phosphate is oxidized in the process of being phosphorylated to 1,3-diphosphate glycerate. The α-glycerophosphate enters the inner mitochondrial membrane whereupon it is converted back to DHAP, releasing its reducing equivalents to FAD that, in turn, transfers the reducing equivalents to the mitochondrial respiratory chain. The reason why this shuttle is rate limiting is due to the need to regenerate NAD^+. Without NAD^+, the glycolytic pathway ceases. $NADH^+$ is produced during glycolysis when reducing equivalents are accepted by NAD^+. $NADH^+$ itself cannot pass through the mitochondrial membrane, so substrate shuttles are necessary. Another means of producing NAD^+ is by converting pyruvate to lactate. This is a nonmitochondrial reaction catalyzed by lactate dehydrogenase. It occurs when an oxygen debt is developed as happens in exercising muscle. In these muscles, more oxygen is consumed than can be provided. Glycolysis is occurring at a rate faster than can be accommodated by the respiratory chain that joins the reducing equivalents transferred to it by the shuttles to molecular oxygen making water. If more reducing equivalents are generated than can be used to produce water, the excess equivalents are added to pyruvate to produce lactate. Thus, rising lactate levels are indicative of oxygen debt.

There are other shuttles that also serve to transfer reducing equivalents into the mitosol. These are the malate-aspartate shuttle and the malate-citrate shuttle. Neither of these are rate limiting with respect to glycolysis. The malate-aspartate shuttle has rate-controlling properties with respect to gluconeogenesis, while the malate-citrate shuttle is important in lipogenesis.

Once 1,3-bisphosphate glycerate is formed it is converted to 3-phosphoglycerate with the formation of one ATP. The 3-phosphoglycerate then goes to 2-phosphoglycerate and then to phosphoenolpyruvate (PEP). These are all bidirectional reactions that are also used in gluconeogenesis. The PEP is dephosphorylated to pyruvate with the formation of another ATP. Because of the great energy loss due to ATP formation at this step, this reaction is not reversible. Gluconeogenesis uses another enzyme, PEPCK, to reverse this step. Glycolysis uses pyruvate kinase to catalyze the reaction. At any rate, pyruvate can now be converted to acetyl CoA via pyruvate dehydrogenase or carboxylated to oxaloacetate via pyruvate carboxylase.

The glycolytic pathway is dependent upon both ATP for the initial steps of the pathway, the formation of glucose-6-phosphate and fructose-1,6-bisphosphate, and on the ratio of ATP to ADP and inorganic phosphate, Pi. In working muscle, the continuance of work and the continuance of glycolysis depend on the cycling of the adenine nucleotides and the export of lactate to the liver. ATP must be provided at the beginning of the pathway, and ADP as well as Pi must be provided in the later steps. If the tissue runs out of ATP, ADP, or Pi, or accumulates lactate and H^+, glycolysis will come to a halt and work cannot continue. This is what happens to the working skeletal muscle. Exhaustion sets in when glycolytic rate is downregulated by an accumulation of lactate.

GLYCOPROTEIN

A complex protein containing a carbohydrate moiety. Glycoproteins play a role in antigen recognition.

GLYCOSYLATED HEMOGLOBIN (A1C)

Molecules of glucose attached loosely to the hemoglobin molecule. Levels of A1C are indicators of glucose control. Values less than 5.7 indicate good glucose control; values in the range of 5.7–6.4 indicate an increased risk for the development of diabetes mellitus.

GMP

Guanosine monophosphate. A nucleotide containing guanine (a purine), ribose, and a high-energy phosphate group.

GOITER

An enlargement of the thyroid gland, usually due to an inadequate intake of iodine.

GOITROGEN

A compound that interferes with the normal secretion of thyroxine by the thyroid gland.

GONADOTROPINS

Hormones released by the pituitary gland that stimulate the gonads.

GOSSYPOL

A toxic yellow pigment found in cotton seeds.

GOUT

A condition in which uric acid excretion is impaired. The excess uric acid in the blood is deposited in tissues and joints, causing inflammation and discomfort.

G-PROTEIN

A protein that binds guanosine triphosphate or guanosinediphosphate. Located on the inner aspect of the plasma membrane.

G-PROTEIN-COUPLED RECEPTORS

Proteins located within plasma membranes and involved in downstream signaling. As an example, G-protein receptors are involved in the perception of taste by the taste buds in the mouth.

GRANISETRON HYDROCHLORIDE

A selective 5-hydroxytryptamine receptor antagonist; antiemetic, antinauseant. Trade name: Kytil.

GRAVES' DISEASE (HYPERTHYROIDISM)

A disease characterized by hyperplasia of the thyroid gland, excessive secretion of its hormones, and increased metabolic rate.

GRAVIDA

A pregnant woman.

GROWTH

A well-orchestrated series of processes that result in an increase in size of individual tissues, organs, and whole body.

GRP

Gastrin-releasing peptide. A neuroactive peptide originating in nerves of the gut and stimulating the release of gastrin from gastric cells.

GSH

Reduced glutathione.

GSSG

Oxidized glutathione. A tripeptide containing glutamic acid, cysteine, and glycine. Its sulfhydryl group can undergo reversible oxidation and reduction allowing the peptide to serve as a buffer. Its chief function is to serve as a reductant of toxic peroxides.

GTP

Guanosine triphosphate. A high-energy, phosphate-containing compound needed for protein synthesis.

GUAIFENESIN (GLYCERYL GUAIACOLATE)

A propanediol derivative that serves as an expectorant. Trade names: Anti-Tuss, Duratuss G, Glytuss, Halotussin L.A., Mucinex, Robitussin.

GUANINE

A purine base.

GUANOSINE

A nucleoside containing guanine and ribose.

GUSTATION

The sensation of taste

GUT HORMONES

Hormones produced by the endocrine cells of the gastrointestinal tract. Includes gastrin, cholecystokinin, bombesin, somatostatin, and others. At least 20 hormones have been identified. Most are small peptides.

GUT TRANSIT TIME (GUT PASSAGE TIME)

The time needed for food to pass from the mouth to the anus. Passage time correlates with the amount of fiber in the diet. High-fiber diets pass more rapidly than low-fiber diets. There is a large degree of individual variability in passage time. Passage time is increased with exercise as well as with food-borne illness and food ingredient intolerances. Passage time is decreased with high-fat diets. Constipation is characterized by long passage times.

GYNECOMASTIA

Inappropriate development of the mammary glands in males.

GYNOID OBESITY

Excess body fat deposited mainly on the hips and thighs.

H

HAGEMAN'S FACTOR

Precursor of kallikrein (serine protease) that participates in the production of bradykinin. The Hageman's factor also participates in the blood clotting process.

HAIRPIN

A double helical stretch of DNA formed by base pairing between neighboring strands.

HALF-LIFE

The time required for half of the amount of a given substance to disappear or be degraded.

HALOGENATED AROMATIC HYDROCARBONS

Organic cyclic compounds containing a fluoride, chloride, iodide, or bromide substituent. Thyroxin is an example.

HANES (NHANES I, II, III, OR HHANES)

Health and Nutrition Examination Survey sponsored by the U.S. Centers for Disease Control, a unit of the U.S. Public Health Service.

HARRIS-BENEDICT EQUATIONS

Equations used to estimate basal energy expenditure (see Table 14).

HASHIMOTO'S DISEASE

An autoimmune disease of the thyroid gland. The gland is enlarged with a firm goitrous appearance. The individual (usually female) is either euthyroid or hypothyroid with a mild myxedematous look. Thyroglobulin antibodies are of the IgG type, and complexes of the hormone and these antibodies are frequently deposited in the gland.

HDL

High-density lipoprotein. (See Lipoproteins.)

HEARTBURN

Burning sensation in the lower esophagus resulting from gastric acid reflux.

HEAT INCREMENT (HIE)

The increase in heat production associated with the consumption of food in a thermoneutral environment. It includes HdE, heat of product formation (HrE), heat of waste formation and excretion (HwE), and HfE.

HEAT OF ACTIVITY (HjE)

The heat produced by the activity of the skeletal muscular system in the course of performing actions such as standing, sitting, walking, running, and so on. Also called the activity increment.

HEAT OF COMBUSTION

The heat produced when a food substance is oxidized in a bomb calorimeter.

HEAT OF DIGESTION AND ABSORPTION (HDE)

The heat produced as a result of the action of digestive enzymes on the food within the digestive tract and the heat produced by the digestive tract in moving the digesta through the tract as well as moving the absorbed nutrients through the wall of the digestive tract.

HEAT OF FERMENTATION (HFE)

The heat produced in the digestive tract as a result of microbial action. This is an especially important heat component in ruminants.

HEAT OF PRODUCT FORMATION (HRE)

The heat produced in association with the metabolic processes of product formation from absorbed metabolites. In its simplest form, it is the heat produced by a biosynthetic pathway.

HEAT OF THERMAL REGULATION (HCE)

The additional heat needed to maintain body temperature when the environmental temperature drops below the zone of thermal neutrality. It is the additional heat produced as a result of an animal's efforts to maintain body temperature when the environmental temperature is either lower or higher than the zone of thermal neutrality. In either instance, excess energy is used.

HEAT OF WASTE FORMATION AND EXCRETION (HWE)

The additional heat production associated with the synthesis and excretion of waste products.

HEAT PRODUCTION

The heat produced by the body in the course of its metabolism.

HEAT SHOCK PROTEIN

A 90-kDa protein involved in gene transcription. Many unliganded forms of receptors form hetero-oligomers that include one or more receptors and a dimer of this heat shock protein. The purpose of this interaction may be to occlude DNA binding by the receptor when it is unbound by its usual ligand.

HEIGHT-WEIGHT INDICES

Various ratios or indices used to express weight in terms of height. Body mass index is one such expression and is used to indicate relative body fatness.

HELPER T CELLS

Component of the immune system that serves to direct antibody production by B cells in response to an antigen presented to the B cells by macrophages.

HEMATOCRIT

Volume of erythrocytes packed by centrifugation in a given volume of blood.

HEMATOPOIESIS

The production of blood cells. These include erythrocytes (hemoglobin-containing red blood cells) granulocytes, platelets, and mononuclear cells. Hematopoiesis is influenced by diet (adequate supplies of iron, copper, zinc, B vitamins), hormones and growth factors (erythropoietin, granulocyte macrophage stimulating factor, granulocyte colony-stimulating factor, and macrophage-stimulating factor), and cytokines (interleukins 1–13, stem cell factor, leukemia inhibitory factor, tumor necrosis factor, interferon). These factors direct and control the division and maturation of each of the different blood cell types.

HEME

The protein portion of hemoglobin that holds iron and is responsible for the carriage and release of oxygen by red blood cells.

HEME IRON

Iron held by heme.

HEMOCHROMATOSIS

A disease of iron metabolism in which iron accumulates in liver, under the skin, and in other tissues. Heart failure is a common consequence of this disorder.

HEMODIALYSIS

Process of removing toxic substances from blood with the aid of a synthetic semipermeable membrane.

HEMODILUTION

Dilution of the volume of red blood cells by an expansion of the extracellular water compartment.

HEMOGLOBIN

The iron-containing protein in the red blood cell responsible for carrying oxygen to the cells.

HEMOLYSIS

Rupture of the red blood cell.

HEMORRHAGIC DISEASE OF THE NEWBORN

Failure of the blood of the newborn to clot normally.

HEMORRHOIDS

Enlarged veins in the mucous membrane of the anus.

HEMOSIDERIN

An iron-containing compound that results from the breakdown of hemoglobin. It is a form of denatured ferritin.

HEPARIN

A mucopolysaccharide used in the prevention and treatment of thrombosis and embolism and as an anticoagulant.

HEPARIN SODIUM

An anticoagulant. Trade name: Hepalean.

HEPATITIS

Inflammation of the liver. Can be caused by pathogens or may be the result of exposure (either chronic or acute) to a toxin.

HEPATOCYTE

A liver cell.

HEPATOCYTE GROWTH FACTOR

A disulfide-linked protein that stimulates growth in a wide variety of tissues in addition to the liver.

HEPATOMEGALY

Enlargement of the liver.

HEPCIDIN

A hormone that is a key regulator of iron balance. During inflammation and/or infection, hepcidin-levels rise as do macrophage iron levels. Low levels of this hormone are associated with anemia, hypoxia, iron deficiency, and blood loss. Hepcidin acts by binding ferroportin on the plasma membranes, causing ferroportin to be internalized and degraded. Hepcidindeficiency seems to be the basis for hemochromatosis. Plasma hepcidin levels significantly predict interindividual iron absorption.

HERMAPHRODITE

A wide spectrum of problems that arises from incorrect gonadal differentiation. The true hermaphrodite is an individual who possesses both testicular and ovarian tissues.

HERS DISEASE

Genetic disease characterized by excess hepatic glycogen due to a mutation in the gene for hepatic phosphorylase.

HETERODIMERIZATION

The polymerization of two unlike compounds to DNA.

HETEROGEUSIA

Altered taste perception; may be due to specific drugs, toxins, or nutrient deficiencies. Zinc deficiency is an example.

HETEROZYGOTE

An individual having unlike copies of a gene coding for a given characteristic.

HEXOSE

A six carbon sugar.

HEXOSE MONOPHOSPHATE SHUNT

See Metabolic Maps, Appendix 2. An alternative pathway for the metabolism of glucose. The shunt provides an alternative pathway for the use of glucose-6-phosphate and generates phosphorylated ribose for use in nucleotide synthesis. It is estimated that approximately 10% of the glucose-6-phosphate generated from glucose is metabolized by the shunt.

The shunt contains two nicotinamide adenine dinucleotide phosphate (NADP)-linked dehydrogenases: glucose-6-phosphate dehydrogenase and 6 phosphogluconate dehydrogenase. These two enzymes are the rate-limiting steps in the reaction sequence. In the instance where there is an active lipogenic state, these reactions provide about 50% of the reducing equivalents needed by the lipogenic process. There is an excellent correlation between this dehydrogenase activity and lipogenesis. The microsomal P450 enzymes also use the reducing equivalents carried by $NADP^+$, as does the red blood cell in the maintenance of glutathione in the reduced state. The glutathione system in the red cell maintains the redox state and integrity of the cell membrane. If sufficient reducing equivalents are not produced by the shunt dehydrogenase reactions to reduce glutathione, the red cell membrane integrity is lost and hemolytic anemia results. This is important to the red blood cell function of carrying oxygen and exchanging it for carbon dioxide. There are a number of genetic mutations in the code for red cell glucose-6-phosphate dehydrogenase. The code is carried as a recessive trait on the X chromosome, and thus only males are affected. These mutations are usually silent. That is, the male, having a defective red cell glucose-6-phosphate dehydrogenase, does not know he has the problem unless his cells are tested or unless he is given a drug such as quinine or one of the sulfur antibiotics that increases the oxidation of $NADPH^+H^+$. When this happens, $NADPH^+H^+$ is depleted and is not available to reduce oxidized glutathione. In turn, the red cell ruptures. In almost all cases, the affected male has sufficient enzyme activity to meet the normal demands for $NADPH^+H^+$. It is only when stressed by drugs such as quinine that a problem develops.

In any event, glucose-6-phosphate proceeds to 6-phosphogluconolactone, a very unstable metabolite, which is, in turn, reduced to 6-phosphogluconate. The 6-phosphogluconate is decarboxylated and dehydrogenated to form ribulose 5-phosphate with an unstable intermediate (keto-6-phosphogluconate) forming between the 6-phosphogluconate and ribulose 5-phosphate. Ribulose 5-phosphate can be isomerized to ribose 5-phosphate or epimerized to xylulose 5-phosphate. Xylulose 5-phosphate and ribose 5-phosphate can reversibly form sedoheptulose 7-phosphate with release of glyceraldehyde 3-phosphate.

HIATAL HERNIA

Protrusion of the stomach through the esophageal opening into the chest cavity.

HIGH-DENSITY LIPOPROTEIN (HDL)

A protein-lipid complex responsible for the transport of lipids (triacylglycerides and cholesterol) in the blood from/to the liver to/from storage sites in the periphery. The complex is very dense and contains phospholipids as well as glycerides and sterols. Elevated HDL is associated with a reduction in risk for cardiovascular disease.

HIGH-ENERGY COMPOUND

A compound having high-energy phosphate bonds. When these bonds are broken, a large amount of energy is released.

HIGH-FIBER DIET

Diet characterized by significantly more fiber-containing foods than the norm; most high-fiber diets provide at least 20–35 g of mixed fiber daily.

HINDMILK

Milk produced by the mammary gland at or near the end of the lactation period.

HIRSUTISM

Heavy, abnormal growth of hair that may be either coarse and pigmented or fine, soft, and unpigmented. The condition in females is due to an inappropriate production of testosterone. Adrenal cortex tumors, androgen-producing tumors in the ovaries, hyperplasia of the androgen-producing cells (the stromal and thecal cells) of the ovaries, or polycystic ovary disease may be responsible for this hair growth.

HISTAMINE

A vasoactive amine, which is normally present in food products such as cheese, wine, cream, fish (especially sardine), sauerkraut, and sausages. Excessive intake of histamine can cause headache, abdominal cramps, tachycardia, urticaria, and in severe cases hypotension, bronchoconstriction, chills, and muscle pain. These symptoms appear within one hour after ingestion and may last for several hours. Histamine can also be produced by bacteria in the gut. It is metabolized very quickly by enzymes in the gut mucosa and liver.

HISTAMINE RELEASERS

Biologically active substances that can be involved in the pharmacological reactions of food intolerance. Known histamine releasers are lectins, present in certain legumes, fruits, and oat. Furthermore, foodstuffs like chocolate, strawberries, tomato, fish, eggs, pineapple, ethanol, and meat have been reported to cause histamine release. Symptoms following non-immunoglobulin E-mediated histamine release resemble allergic symptoms.

HISTIDINE

An amino acid that is essential for growth (see Table 5).

HISTIDINEMIA

A rare genetic disease characterized by an excess amount of histidine in the blood.

HISTONES

Conserved DNA-binding proteins that protect the DNA from free-radical attack.

HLA GENES

Genes that encode elements of the immune system, specifically those that dictate the formation of antibodies by white blood cells (leukocytes).

HMG CoA

3-hydroxy-3-methylglutaryl coenzyme A. A metabolic intermediate in cholesterol synthesis.

HMG CoA REDUCTASE

The rate-limiting enzyme in the synthesis of cholesterol. It is the target for statin drugs, which reduce the synthesis of cholesterol in the body.

HNIS

Human Nutrition Information Service of the U.S. Department of Agriculture.

HOLOENZYME

The complete active enzyme.

HOMEOSTASIS

A state of physiological equilibrium where anabolic and catabolic processes are in balance.

HOMOCYSTINURIA

A rare genetic disease characterized by a high level of homocystine in the urine due to an error in the gene for the vitamin B_6-dependent enzyme cystathionine synthetase.

HOMODIMERIZATION

The polymerization of two like compounds to DNA.

HOMOGENTISIC ACID

A metabolite in the pathway for the conversion of phenylalanine and tyrosine to fumarate and acetoacetate.

HOMOZYGOTE

An individual who has two identical genes coding for a given characteristic.

HORMONE

A substance synthesized and released by an endocrine cell, carried by the blood and having its site of action distal to its site of origin. There are some "local" hormones that are secreted and have as their site of action the same tissue. The eicosanoids are typical of this group of hormones.

HOSPICE CARE

Nonhospital comfort care offered to people with terminal diseases.

24-HOUR RECALL METHOD

See Interview Method.

HUMAN IMMUNODEFICIENCY VIRUS (HIV)

Virus that attacks the body's immune system; the virus is thought to cause acquired immunodeficiency syndrome (AIDS).

HUNGER

Physiologic drive to consume food.

HYBRIDIZATION

The specific reassociation of complementary strands of nucleic acids (DNA with DNA or RNA with RNA).

HYDRALAZINE HYDROCHLORIDE

A peripheral vasodilator that can serve as an antihypertensive agent. Trade names: Apresoline, Novo-Hylazin.

HYDROCHLOROTHIAZIDE (HCTZ)

A thiazide diuretic that can be used as an antihypertensive agent. Trade names: Apo-Hydro, Aquazide-H, Esidrix, hydroDIURIL, Oretic.

HYDROCORTISONE

An adrenal cortical hormone. Commercially available forms include liquids, tablets, and creams, and there are a number of compounds available. It has many uses in addition to being a hormone replacement: it can be an anti-inflammatory, it can be used to combat shock, and it can be used to soothe many types of dermatitis.

HYDROGENATED FATS

Fats whose double bonds have been converted to single bonds with the resultant change in physical state (oil or liquid state to a solid or semisolid state).

HYDROGENATION

The addition of hydrogen atoms to a compound; the conversion of unsaturated fatty acids to saturated fatty acids.

HYDROLASE

An enzyme that catalyzes the addition of water and thereby serves to split the compound into two fragments.

HYDROLYSIS

The process whereby a molecule is fragmented when water is added.

HYDROLYTIC RANCIDITY

A process resulting from the hydrolysis of glycerides to fatty acids and glycerol. It can be catalyzed by lipases (enzymes present in foods or originating from microorganisms), alkali, or acids. From a food safety point of view, hydrolytic rancidity has no important direct implication. Indirectly, however, it may be involved in combined actions. On the other hand, it can be considered desirable, for instance in strong-tasting cheeses. Hydrolytic rancidity can be minimized by cold storage, proper transportation, careful packaging, and sterilization.

HYDROPHILIC

A compound that will dissolve in water.

HYDROPHOBIC

A compound that will not dissolve in water but will dissolve in fat solvents such as alcohol, ether, or chloroform.

HYDROSTATIC PRESSURE

The pressure of fluids against their container.

HYDROSTATIC WEIGHING

A method for determining body fat where the body is weighed in air and then in water.

HYDROXYACID ANALOGUES

Used in the treatment of chronic renal failure; produced by the replacement of an amino group with a hydroxyl group to decrease the nitrogen load in the body.

HYDROXY-APATITE

The mineral complex that is deposited in the ground substance and provides hardness to bones and teeth.

HYDROXYLATION

The addition of a hydroxyl (−OH) group to a compound.

HYDROXYLYSINE

An amino acid in collagen. A special form of lysine that is made after the lysine is incorporated into the collagen protein.

HYDROXYPROLINE

A ring-structured nonessential amino acid.

HYPERALIMENTATION

Early term for parenteral nutrition; nutrition support provided when a hypertonic solution of nutrients is infused via the subclavian or umbilical vein.

HYPERAMMONEMIA

Excess (>40 mmol/L) levels of ammonia in blood.

HYPERANDROGENISM

Excess male hormone production and release into the blood stream.

HYPERBILIRUBINEMIA

Excess (>7 mmol/L) levels of bilirubin in blood.

HYPERCALCEMIA

Excess (>2.5 mmol/L) levels of calcium in blood.

HYPERCHOLESTEROLEMIA

Above normal levels of cholesterol in blood. Normal levels are <180 mg/dL or between 4 and 7 mmol/L.

HYPERCORTISOLISM (CUSHING'S DISEASE)

See Cushing's Syndrome.

HYPEREMESIS

Excessive vomiting.

HYPERGLYCEMIA

Levels of glucose >120 mg/dL (6 mmol/L) in blood for a fasting individual.

HYPERKALEMIA

Excessive levels of potassium (>5 mmol/L) in blood.

HYPERKINESIS (HYPERACTIVITY)

Excessive motor activity.

HYPERLIPEMIA (HYPERLIPIDEMIA)

Levels of lipids in excess of normal (5–6 g/L).

HYPERMAGNESEMIA

Excessive (>1.25 mmol/L) levels of magnesium in blood.

HYPERMETABOLISM

Above normal metabolic rate.

HYPERNATREMIA

Excessive (>145 mmol/L) levels of sodium in blood.

HYPERPARATHYROIDISM

Excess production of parathyroid hormone.

HYPERPHAGIA

Excessive food intake.

HYPERPLASIA

Increase in the number of cells.

HYPERPLASTIC ANEMIA

An increase in the size of the red blood cell with a reduction in its oxygen-carrying capacity. (See Anemia.)

HYPERPLASTIC OBESITY

Obesity characterized by an increase (above normal) in the size and number of adipocytes.

HYPERPROLACTINEMIA

Excess levels of prolactin in the blood. In males, this is usually due to a pituitary tumor. Such excess prolactin results in testis atrophy, a reduction in testosterone production, and a high incidence of impotence. Removal of the tumor reverses these characteristics.

HYPERSENSITIVITY

See Allergy.

HYPERTENSION

Blood pressure that exceeds 120/80 by 20%.

HYPERTHYROIDISM (GRAVES' DISEASE)

Excess thyroid hormone production.

HYPERTONIC SOLUTIONS

Solution with a greater osmolality than plasma; >290–300 mOsm/kg of water.

HYPERTROPHIC OBESITY

Obesity characterized by increase in adipocyte size.

HYPERTROPHY

Increased cell size.

HYPERURICEMIA

Excess (>0.29 mmol/L) level of uric acid in the blood; a key symptom of gout.

HYPERVITAMINOSIS

A toxic syndrome resulting from intake of vitamins in great excess of the required amounts.

HYPERVOLEMIA

Increased circulating blood volume.

HYPOCHLORHYDRIA

Decreased production of hydrochloric acid in the stomach.

HYPOCHROMIC MICROCYTIC ANEMIA

Red blood cells that are fewer in number and size and lack the normal amount of hemoglobin. (See Anemia.)

HYPODIPSIA

Decreased thirst.

HYPOGEUSIA

Abnormal taste perception; loss of taste perception.

HYPOGLYCEMIA

Lower than normal blood glucose level (<80 mg/dL blood or 4 mmol/L).

HYPOGLYCEMIC DRUGS

Drugs used in the management of type 2 diabetes mellitus. They fall into several different categories depending on their site of action. Some stimulate insulin release, some improve the responsiveness of the insulin receptors on the adipocytes and muscle, and some downregulate gluconeogenesis. Some drugs have more than one site of action. Metformin, a biguanide, (Glucophage) for example, potentiates the action of the insulin receptor thus decreasing insulin resistance. Metformin can assist in weight loss in the diabetic-obese person. Sulfonylurea (tolbutamide) stimulates insulin release, increases peripheral insulin sensitivity, and improves glucose signaling; however, unfortunately it also stimulates weight gain. Thiozolodine derivatives, that is, pioglitizone, increase insulin sensitivity, increase receptor activity, suppress gluconeogenesis, and improve glucose use. Benflourex decreases blood lipids and decreases insulin resistance.

HYPOGONADISM

Inadequate sperm production and/or androgen secretion. It may be a consequence of a hypothalamic disorder, pituitary failure, or testicular disease.

HYPOKALEMIA

Below normal blood levels of potassium (<2.5 mmol/L).

HYPONATREMIA

Below normal blood level of sodium (<136 mmol/L).

HYPOPROTEINEMIA

Below normal amounts of protein in the blood.

HYPOSMIA

Diminished sense of smell.

HYPOTHALAMUS

A part of the central nervous system that consists of a group of nuclei at the base of the brain in relation to the floor and walls of the third ventricle.

HYPOTHYROIDISM

Below normal activity of the thyroid gland resulting in low levels of active thyroid hormone in the blood.

HYPOTONIC SOLUTION

Solution with a lower osmolality than plasma: <290–300 mOsm/kg of water.

HYPOTONY

Decreased tone of the gastrointestinal tract that impedes transit time.

HYPOVITAMINOSIS

Below normal intakes of vitamins resulting in a deficient state.

HYPOVOLEMIA

Diminished circulating blood volume.

HYPOXIA

Subnormal content of oxygen in arterial blood.

I

IATROGENIC

An abnormal state in a patient induced by inappropriate or erroneous treatment.

IBUPROFEN

A nonsteroid anti-inflammatory, antipyretic, analgesic medication. Trade names: Advil, Motrin, Nuprin, Peda-profen. Dosages for both children and adults are sold.

IBS

See Irritable Bowel Syndrome.

IBW

Ideal body weight.

IDIOPATHIC DISEASE

A disease of no known cause.

IDIOPATHIC STEATORRHEA

See Gluten-Sensitive Enteropathy.

IDIOSYNCRATIC REACTION

An individual's intolerance of a certain food or additive. The underlying mechanism is unknown.

ILEOSTOMY

Procedure in which a part of the ileum is brought through the abdominal wall for defecation.

ILEUM

The last third of the small intestine.

ILIAC CREST

The crest or top of the ilium or the longest of the three bones comprising the pelvis. It is sometimes called the top of the hip bone.

ILEOCECAL VALVE

The valve at the junction between the large and small intestines.

IMMUNITY

The process whereby antibodies are developed to specific antigens.

IMMUNOACTIVE BACTERIAL ENDOTOXINS

Toxic substances produced by food-borne microorganisms.

IMMUNOGLOBULINS

Proteins that develop in response to antigens.

IMMUNOSUPPRESSION

Decreased ability to fight infection; decreased antibody response to antigens.

IMMUNOTHERAPY

Treatment with antibodies to enhance the response of the body to harmful substances. Treatment with very low doses of antigens to stimulate the body's production of antibodies to that antigen. The latter treatment is the basis for immunization against communicable diseases.

IMPEDENCE

The opposition to an alternating current composed of two elements: resistance and reactance.

IN UTERO

In the uterus.

INBORN ERRORS OF METABOLISM

Genetic diseases of metabolism caused by a mutation in specific genes for specific proteins, be they enzymes, carriers, membrane components, or intracellular materials.

INCIDENCE

The number of new events or cases of a disease in a population within a specified time period.

INDAPAMIDE

A thiazide-like diuretic that can serve as an antihypertensive agent. Trade names: Lozide, Lozol.

INDEPENDENT ACTION

Actions of substances at different sites of action, with no interaction between the components. Different mechanisms can underlie the same effect and this may mean that the effects of some components of a mixture consisting of a large number of substances are similar and are integrated into an overall effect (effect integration).

INDIGENOUS

Native to a particular geographic area.

INDIRECT CALORIMETRY

Determination of energy expenditure using the measurement of oxygen consumption.

INDISPENSIBLE NITROGEN

Nitrogenous compounds that must be sustained for good health.

INDOMETHACIN

A nonsteroid anti-inflammatory drug that is also an antipyretic and an analgesic. Trade names: Apo-Indomethicin, Indchron ER, Indocid SR, Indocin, Indocin SR, Novo-Methacin.

INFARCT

Death of local tissue fed by an obstructed artery or occluded vein.

INFECTIOUS DISEASE

Any disease caused by the invasion and multiplication of an invading pathogen.

INFLAMMATORY BOWEL DISEASE

See Crohn's Disease.

INFORMATION BIAS

Errors in the necessary information, leading to errors in the classification of subjects. The misclassification can be characterized as random (or nondifferential) or differential.

INHIBIN

A female hormone whose level rises as luteinizing hormone (LH) and follicle-stimulating hormone (FSH) levels fall. It rises in concert with progesterone. Its function in the estrus cycle is unclear.

INITIATION FACTORS

Proteins that associate with the small subunit of the ribosome specifically at the stage of the initiation of protein synthesis.

INORGANIC

Compounds that are not carbon compounds but are minerals and mineral salts.

INOSITOL

A carbohydrate that is an essential ingredient of the inositol phosphate second messenger system. Inositol is a six-carbon sugar that is related to D-glucose. Its structure is shown in Figure 25.

It occurs in nature in nine possible isomeric forms. However, only one, myoinositol, is biologically important as a nutrient. Myoinositol is a water-soluble, cyclic, six-carbon compound (cis-1,2,3,5 trans-4,6-cyclohexane-hexanol). Inositol is widely distributed in foods of both plant and animal origin. In plants and animals, it exists as part of the phosphatidylinositol (PI) of the cell membranes or as free inositol. Phytic acid, a component of many grain products, can be converted to myoinositol with the removal of the phosphate groups (see Figure 26).

Phytate or phytic acid can bind calcium, magnesium, and other divalent ions within the intestinal compartment, making them unavailable for absorption by mucosal cells. Once the phytate is dephosphorylated through the action of phytase the inositol residue remains. The divalent ions are released and the free inositol is absorbed. Both free inositol and cell membrane PI are found in foods of animal origin.

ABSORPTION AND METABOLISM

Dietary PI is acted on by the luminal enzyme phospholipase, and converted to lysophosphatidylinositol. This compound can then be further hydrolyzed to produce glycerophosphorylinositol and then free inositol or acted upon by an acyltransferase in the intestinal cell, which converts it back to PI. This is then transported out of the gut absorptive cell as a component of lipoproteins.

Free inositol in the lumen is transported into the luminal cells via an active, energy-dependent, sodium-dependent transport process quite similar to that which transports glucose. Although similar, it is not identical to the glucose transport process. Free inositol is then transported in the blood at a concentration of about 30 μm/dL.

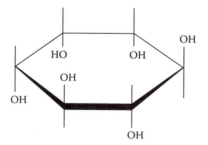

FIGURE 25 Myoinositol structure.

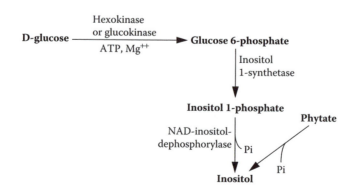

FIGURE 26 De novo synthesis of free inositol from either glucose or phytate.

Inositol can be synthesized from glucose by a variety of mammalian cells. Synthesis in the testes, brain, kidney, and liver has been reported. Humans can synthesize up to 4 g/day in the kidneys alone. Synthesis from glucose proceeds from glucose to glucose 6-phosphate to inositol 1-phosphate to inositol. The enzymes are glucokinase or hexokinase followed by inositol 1-synthetase and then NAD-inositol-dephosphorylase.

FUNCTION

Inositol functions as a constituent of the membrane phospholipid PI. Free inositol is added to diacylglycerol (DAG) via a CDP reaction producing PI and CMP. The enzyme catalyzing this reaction is CDP diacylglycerol:inositol phosphatidyltransferase, sometimes called PI synthetase. This synthesis takes place in the microsomes and the enzyme has a Km of 4.6 mM for inositol (see Figure 27). Phosphatidylinositol can also be synthesized via an exchange reaction where free inositol can exchange for either choline or ethanolamine in either phosphatidylcholine or phosphatidylethanolamine. The Km for the Mn^{++} dependent reaction is 0.024 mM. Once formed, the PI migrates from the microsomes, where it is formed to any one of the membranes within and around the cell. It comprises approximately 10% of the phospholipids in the cellular membranes. Recently, its function as a part of a unique cellular second messenger system (different from the cyclic adenosine monophosphate [cAMP] system) has been explored. This system, called the PIP system or PIP cycle, (where PIP stands for PI phosphate), has been reported to function in insulin release by the pancreatic insulin-producing β cells, in the regulation of protein kinase C, in the mobilization of

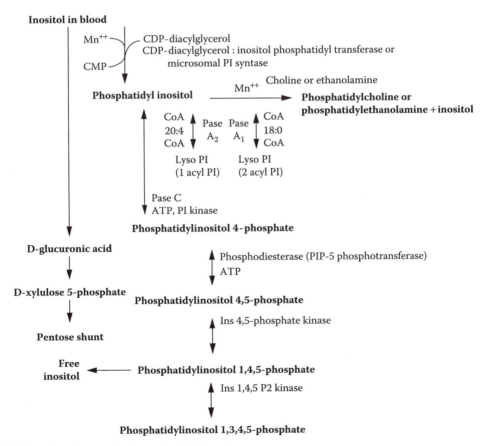

FIGURE 27   Inositol metabolism and the PIP cycle.

intracellular calcium, and in the regulation of Na$^+$K$^+$ATPase activity, and may have a role in blood clotting, blood pressure regulation, and renal function.

Once formed, PI serves as a substrate for one of several enzymes. Phospholipase A$_1$ acts on PI to produce lyso PI (2 acyl PI). Phospholipase A$_2$ acts to produce a 1 acyl PI. Both A$_1$ and A$_2$ act to remove one of the fatty acids from the phospholipids; A$_1$ removes the fatty acid (usually stearic acid, 18:0) from the glycerol carbon 1 while A$_2$ removes the fatty acid (usually arachidonic acid, 20:4) from the glycerol carbon 2. When phospholipase A$_2$ is activated, arachidonic acid is released and this fatty acid serves as the substrate for prostaglandin synthesis. Prostaglandins are another group of hormone-like substances that are important in the regulation of blood pressure and blood clotting. A third enzyme also has PI as its substrate. This enzyme is ATP PI kinase (phospholipase C) and initiates the PIP cycle (see in Figure 27). Phospholipase C action is mediated by the guanine nucleotide–binding protein called the G protein. Phospholipase C cleaves the phosphorylated inositol from the glycerol backbone, producing DAG and PI 4,5-phosphate (PIP$_2$). The DAG serves to activate protein kinase C, an important regulatory enzyme discovered in 1979. Neutral DAG remains within the membrane while the liberated inositol 4,5-bisphosphate migrates into the cytoplasm and, in the process, is again phosphorylated to form inositol 1,4,5-phosphate (PIP$_3$). This compound causes a release of calcium ion from nonmitochondrial vesicular, intracellular stores. The triphosphate inositol binds to a receptor protein associated with these stores to effect this release. The Ca^{++} release from the endoplasmic reticulum is elicited via an opening of a gated channel. Cyclic AMP–dependent phosphorylation of the receptor protein seems to be involved. The magnesium ion is also involved. Inositol 1,4,5-phosphate can then either be dephosphorylated to release free inositol or phosphorylated once again to form inositol 1,3,4,5-phosphate (PIP$_4$) via the enzyme D-myoinositol 1,4,5-triphosphate 3-kinase. This kinase is stimulated by a Ca^{++} in the presence of calmodulin and protein kinase C, and thus the level of the inositol 1,4,5-phosphate is carefully regulated. Inositol 1,3,4,5-phosphate also is an active metabolic regulator in that it modulates calcium ion concentration through either the reuptake of Ca^{++} into the intracellular stores or through control of the Ca^{++} transfer process between inositol 1,4,5-phosphate sensitive and insensitive pools. The kinase enzyme might be the target for the enzyme protein tyrosine kinase. All of the aforementioned phosphorylations of inositol are reversible, and the amounts of each of the phosphorylated intermediates produced depend on the hormonal status of the individual as well as on the availability of inositol for PI synthesis. Insulin, various growth factors, PGF$_{2\alpha}$ (one of the prostaglandins) have all been shown to stimulate the PI cycle. In normal humans, inositol needs are presumed to be met by endogenous synthesis.

INOSITOL PHOSPHATE

A phospholipid in the plasma membrane that releases phosphoinositol when stimulated by phospholipase C.

INOSITOL PHOSPHATE CYCLE

See Inositol.

INSENSIBLE WATER LOSS

Water lost through the skin and through the lungs that is not noticed by the individual.

INSERT

An additional length of base pairs in DNA that is introduced artificially.

INSULIN

The hormone synthesized and released by the β cells of the islet of Langerhans in response to rising levels of blood glucose.

INSULIN PUMP

A small instrument that senses changes in blood glucose and delivers insulin subcutaneously so as to maintain an optimal insulin-glucose relationship.

INSULIN RECEPTOR

Protein that is embedded in the plasma membrane of the insulin-sensitive cell. When insulin is bound to its receptor, a cascade of signals is generated that includes the movement of glucose transporters to the plasma membrane and the subsequent metabolism of the incoming glucose. Mutations in the genes for the receptor phenotype as diabetes mellitus.

INSULIN RECEPTOR SUBSTRATE 1

A cytosolic compound that associates with proteins containing SH2 domains; that is, tyrosine phosphatase when insulin binds to its receptor on the cell membrane.

INSULIN RELEASE

Insulin release by the β cells of the pancreas involves a number of interrelated metabolic reactions in both the cytosol and the mitochondria. The islet must sense that blood glucose levels are rising. This is a critical step in insulin release. The glucose-phosphorylating enzyme, glucokinase, serves this function. GLUT 2 transports glucose through the plasma membrane making this glucose available to glucokinase. The glucose is then processed through glycolysis. Once glucose is made available to glucokinase, this enzyme migrates to the mitochondrial membrane pore protein. The ATP produced by the mitochondrial OXPHOS system is needed by glucokinase as well as by the sodium-potassium pump. Insulin secretion also involves some ion shifts. The Na^+K^+ pump becomes active as does the K^+ channel, allowing these ions to move in and out of the cell. The calcium ion moves in. This ion serves two functions: (1) it stimulates OXPHOS, and (2) in sulin exocytosis.

INSULITIS

Inflammation of the insulin-producing β cells of the pancreas.

INTAKE ENERGY (IE)

The gross energy of the food consumed.

INTERCELLULAR COMPARTMENT

The water that surrounds cells and is contained in the intracellular space. Plasma is part of this compartment and surrounds the red blood cells in the blood.

INTERMEDIATE-DENSITY LIPOPROTEIN

Lipoprotein resulting from removal of triglycerides from very-low-density lipoproteins and chylomicrons.

INTERNAL VALIDITY

The validity of the inferences drawn for the population under investigation. In general, internal validity can be influenced by three types of bias: (1) selection bias, (2) information bias, and (3) confounding bias. However, the distinction between these three is not always strict.

INTERSTITIAL FLUID (ISF)

Fluid located between cells and in some body cavities such as joints, pleura, and the gastrointestinal tract. The fluid provides a medium for passage of nutrients to and from cells.

INTERSTITIAL SPACES

Space between tissues.

INTERVENTION STUDIES

See Experimental Studies.

INTERVIEW METHOD

A method for estimating food intake. Two frequently used interview methods are the 24-hour recall method and the dietary history method. In the 24-hour recall method, a complete description of the total food intake during the 24 hours preceding the interview is requested. As with the 2-day record method, a single 24-hour recall does not give a good estimate of food consumption by individuals because of the large day-to-day variation in food intake. With the dietary history method, respondents are asked about their usual food intake during a specific period of time, usually the 2–4 weeks preceding the interview. This method gives a better indication of the usual dietary intake by individuals. Since a dietary history interview takes about 1–2 hours, this method cannot be applied in studies in which many thousands of people participate.

INTESTINAL BYPASS

A surgical procedure wherein part or all of the small intestine is removed and the remaining fragments connected. The gastrointestinal tract is thus reduced in length.

INTRACELLULAR COMPARTMENT

Body water compartment consisting of fluids within the cells.

INTRAVASCULAR

Within the vascular tree. An intravascular (IV) injection is one where a substance is injected into a vein.

INTRAVENOUS THERAPY

Provision of fluids and/or nutrients or drugs into a vein.

INTRINSIC FACTOR

A protein secreted by the gastric cells and which is needed for the absorption of vitamin B_{12}.

INTRON

The sequences of bases in a gene that are transcribed but removed during RNA editing.

INVERT SUGAR

A mixture of glucose and fructose that results from the hydrolysis of sucrose.

INVERTASE (SUCRASE)

Enzyme that catalyzes the hydrolysis of sucrose to glucose and fructose.

INVERTED REPEATS

Two copies of the same sequence of DNA repeated in opposite orientations on the same molecule; adjacent inverted repeats constitute a palindrome.

IODIDE

The ion of iodine, an essential nutrient required primarily for the synthesis of thyroxin. The deficiency disorder is called goiter and is characterized by thyroid gland enlargement.

ION

An element with either a positive or negative charge.

IPECAC SYRUP

An alkaloid emetic.

IPRATROPIUM BROMIDE

An anticholinergic bronchodilator. Trade name: Atrovent.

IRBESARTAN

An angiotensin II receptor antagonist that serves as an antihypertensive agent. Trade name: Avapro.

IRON

An essential mineral nutrient (see http://www.nap.edu for the recommended daily intake) that serves as a component of hemoglobin, myoglobin, and the cytochromes. Iron is essential for the synthesis of red blood cell hemoglobin and is also important for embryonic neuron development and memory function. Iron functions in the urea cycle, lipogenesis, and cholesterogenesis. Anemia is a sign of inadequate intake of iron. Low iron intakes are associated with a greater risk of hypertension as well. Hemochromatosis results from excess iron intake. Excess iron intake affects feed efficiency (weight gained/unit food consumed) of farm animals. Iron intake affects the expression of genes for hepcidin, ferroportin, divalent mineral transporter 1, and transferrin receptor. High iron intake down regulates the expression of these genes. Age also affects the expression of these genes. As an individual ages expression is reduced. Iron absorption efficiency is poor, with an estimated 12% of intake being absorbed. Iron is transported from the enterocytes to its site of use by the protein, transferrin. The iron is stored chelated to ferritin. Hemosiderin also stores iron. Hemosiderin is a form of denatured ferritin. Iron is excreted in the feces.

Hepcidin regulates iron absorption efficiency. Levels of hepcidin and ferritin are closely correlated. Hepcidin interacts with the iron efflux transporter, ferroportin.

IRON ABSORPTION

A very inefficient process. Iron is transferred from the intestinal mucosa to transferrin. Transferrin then transports this iron to the rest of the body. Individuals who have had a gastric bypass operation are characterized by reduced iron absorption and their iron status can be compromised. Hepcidin is a good predictor of dietary iron bioavailability.

IRON DEFICIENCY

Inadequate intake of iron; characterized by anemia.

IRRADIATION OF FOOD

Preservation technique based on the irradiation of food with X-rays.

IRS-1

Insulin receptor substrate-1, a 131-kDa intracellular protein essential for most of insulin's intracellular actions. It possesses 21 potential tyrosine phosphorylation sites. After multiple phosphorylations, it binds the PIP3 kinase that in turn activates the PIP signal pathway. Through this phosporylation, it alters the activities of a number of glucose-metabolizing enzymes as well as key metabolic processes. Insulin has an influence via this substrate on protein and fat metabolism as well as glucose metabolism.

ISCHEMIA

Impaired blood flow causing oxygen and nutrient deprivation resulting in pain and, if severe, in the death of some or all parts of the tissue.

ISLET AMYLOID PROTEIN

A neuropeptide-like protein produced by the β cell of the pancreas. Its function is not known.

ISLET OF LANGERHANS

The particular segments of the pancreas having an endocrine function. These islets consist of several cell types, one of which is the β cell that produces the hormone insulin. Another is the α cell that produces glucagon, and a third, the D cell, produces somatostatin.

ISOLEUCINE

An essential amino acid; it can prevent the accumulation of tissue triglycerides in diet-induced obese mice. It can also upregulate the expression of peroxisome proliferator-activated receptor (PPAR)α and uncoupling protein (UCP) in these mice.

ISOPRENOIDS

Members of the steroid class of compounds. Isoprenoids include carotenes and ubiquinone.

ISOPROTERENOL

A drug that comes in many forms. It is an adrenergic broncodilator and a cardiac stimulant. Trade names: Isoproterenol, Isuprel, Vapo-Iso, Isoprel, Norisodrine, Medhaler-iso.

ISRADIPINE

A calcium-channel blocker that serves as an antihypertensive agent. Trade name: DynaCirc.

ISOELECTRIC POINT

The pH of a protein in solution at which there are equal numbers of positive- and negative-charged groups.

ISOENERGETIC (ISOCALORIC)

State where the energy consumed is equal to the energy expended.

ISOLEUCINE

An essential amino acid (see Table 5).

ISOPRENE

A five-carbon unit used in the synthesis of sterols.

ISOTONIC SOLUTION

Solution with an osmolality similar to plasma; 290–300 mOsm/kg of water.

ISOTOPIC DILUTION TECHNIQUE

A technique using very small amounts of isotopically labeled substrate to measure the volume and amount of a large pool of that substrate. The technique is based on the Fick principle, where the volume and concentration of the infused labeled substrate is known. It is infused, and at a set time later a known volume is withdrawn and the concentration determined. This allows the computation of the volume of distribution of the substrate in the larger volume of the body. The equation for this computation is

$$C_1/V_2 = V_2/C_2$$

IU (INTERNATIONAL UNIT)

An amount defined by the International Conference for Unification of Formulae.

J

JAUNDICE

A disease characterized by a yellow color of the skin, which arises when bilirubin accumulates in the subcutaneous layer of cells and in the blood; can be a symptom of hepatitis.

JEJUNOSTOMY

Surgical opening in the jejunum.

JEJUNUM

The middle third of the small intestine.

JELLY

A colloidal suspension of fruit juice. The suspension is created by the hydration of pectin.

JOULE

A unit of work or energy in the metric system. The amount of work done by a force of 1 N acting over a distance of 1 m.

K

KALLIKREINS

A group of serine proteases that act on blood proteins to produce bradykinin, a potent vasodilator.

KALLMAN'S SYNDROME

A disorder where patients have anosmia (loss of the sense of smell) and hypogonadism.

KELP

Seaweed.

KERATIN

A scleroprotein found primarily in fingernails, hair, horns, and so on; contains a large amount of sulfur.

KERNICTERUS

Jaundice of a newborn with degenerative lesions in parts of the brain.

KESHAN DISEASE

Selenium deficiency disease resulting in cardiomyopathy.

KETO ACID

Used in the treatment of chronic renal failure; produced by the replacement of an amino group with a keto group to decrease the nitrogen load in the body.

KETOGENIC AMINO ACIDS

Amino acids that, when catabolized, yield ketones. These include leucine, phenylalanine, tyrosine, lysine, threonine, and tryptophan.

KETONEMIA

A condition characterized by excessive levels of ketones in the blood. Rising levels of blood ketones increase the need for buffering power since they tend to lower pH. Ketonemia is a characteristic feature of uncontrolled type 1 diabetes.

KETONURIA

A condition characterized by excessive levels of ketones in the urine. In diabetes mellitus, fatty acid oxidation is incomplete. As a result, acetone, β-hydroxybutyrate, and acetoacetate, products of incomplete fatty acid oxidation, accumulate. These are the ketone bodies.

KETOPROFIN

A nonsteroid anti-inflammatory; this drug is a nonopioid analgesic and an antipyretic. Trade names: Orudis, Orudis KT, Onuvail.

KETOROLAC TROMETHAMINE

A nonsteroid anti-inflammatory analgesic drug. Trade name: Torodol.

KIBBLED

Coarsely ground meal or grain.

KIDNEY FAILURE

See Chronic Renal Failure.

KIDNEY STONES

Precipitates of calcium phosphate or oxalate. These stones vary in size from the size of coarse gravel to that of a pea. Also called calculi; the condition is called urolithiasis or nephrolithiasis.

KILOCALORIE (KCAL)

The amount of energy required to raise the temperature of 1 kg water 1°C. 1 kcal = 4.189 kJ.

KINETIC ENERGY

Mechanical energy.

KJELDAHL METHOD

Chemical method for determining the nitrogen content of foods and animal tissues. The quantity of nitrogen is multiplied by 6.25 to obtain the approximate protein content of the sample (6.25 is an average conversion factor). Specific foods and specific tissues may have different conversion factors.

KLINFELTER'S SYNDROME

Seminiferous tubule dysgenesis; the most common cause of male hypogonadism. The condition results from an extra X chromosome to give an XXY genotype. The phenotypes of this genotype are small testes, gynocomastia (partial breast development), azoospemia (poor or no sperm production), and elevated levels of gonadotropins.

K_M

Michaelis constant for enzyme reactions. The affinity of the enzyme for its substrate determines Km. If the affinity is high, the reaction will proceed very quickly. If two enzymes work on the same substrate, the one with the greater affinity will be more active and have a higher Km.

KREBS CYCLE

See Citric Acid Cycle and Metabolic Maps, Appendix 2. Located in the mitochondria. This is a central cyclic pathway where a two-carbon acetyl group is joined to a four-carbon oxaloacetate to form citrate. As the cycle turns, two molecules of CO_2 carbon dioxides are produced, as are four reducing equivalents.

KWASHIORKOR

An African word that refers to the development of protein-deficiency disorder in the young post-weaned child. The child is usually between 1 and 3 years old; cultural food practices or taboos may limit the kinds and amounts of protein given to the child. Concurrent infections, parasites, seasonal food shortages, and poor distribution of food amongst the family members may also contribute to the development of protein deficiency. Growth failure is the single most outstanding feature of protein malnutrition. The child's height and weight for his or her age will be less than that of his or her well-nourished peer. Tissue wastage is present but may not be apparent if edema is present. The edema begins with the feet and legs and gradually presents itself in the hands, face, and body. If edema is advanced, the child may not appear underweight but many appear "plump." The edema is thought to result from insufficient ADH production and a deficient supply of serum and tissue proteins needed to maintain water balance. The protein-deficient child is usually apathetic, has little interest in his or her surroundings, and is listless and dull. This child is usually "fussy" and irritable when moved. Mental retardation may or may not result. Hair changes are frequently observed. Texture, color, and strength are affected. Black, curly hair may become thin, lusterless, and brown or reddish brown in color. Lesions of the skin are not always present, but if present, they give the appearance of old, flaky paint. Depigmentation or darkly pigmented areas may develop with a tendency for these areas to appear in places of body friction such as the backs of legs, groins, and elbows. Diarrhea is almost always present. The diarrhea may be a result of the inability of the body to synthesize the needed digestive enzymes so that the food that is consumed can be utilized, and/or it may be the result of concurrent infections and parasites. Anemia due to an inability to synthesize hemoglobin as well as red blood cells is invariably present. Hepatomegaly (enlarged liver) is usually observed.

L

LABETALOL HYDROCHLORIDE

An α and β blocker; an antihypertensive agent. Trade names: Normodyne, Trandate.

LABILE

Easily degraded; unstable.

LACTALBUMIN

One of the whey proteins in milk.

LACTATE

One of the end products of glycolysis.

LACTATE DEHYDROGENASE

Enzyme that catalyzes the removal of reducing equivalents from lactate to produce pyruvate.

LACTATION

Milk production and release by the mammary gland. The process is under the control of the hormone prolactin and can be diminished in poorly nourished mothers. Lactation increases the mother's need for most nutrients.

LACTIC ACIDOSIS

Condition where lactate levels are elevated above normal; occurs in the muscles of exercising people, in uncontrolled diabetes mellitus, and also in patients with mitochondrial disease due to one or more mutations in the mitochondrial genome. Lactic acidosis can also develop in patients who have taken prescription drugs that the kidney cannot clear rapidly enough or whose liver is not functioning normally.

LACTOFLAVIN

An outdated name for riboflavin (vitamin B_2).

LACTOSE

A disaccharide present in milk; when hydrolyzed by lactase, glucose and galactose result.

LACTOSE INTOLERANCE

Inability to digest lactose due to decreased (or absence of) lactase activity. In the absence of lactase, lactose is not hydrolyzed (digested) and acts as an osmotic agent stimulating peristalsis with the clinical symptoms of flatulence, bloating, cramps, and diarrhea. Current evidence indicates that lactose intolerance is more common than lactose tolerance. Notable exceptions to these observations are Caucasians of Scandinavian or Northern European background. Less than 5% of these populations has lactose intolerance, and they traditionally consume diets containing large amounts of milk and milk products.

Lactose intolerance is age related. The prevalence of lactose intolerance is greater in adult populations than in populations of children, suggesting that if there is a genetic tendency toward lactase deficiency, this tendency may be modified by such environmental factors as milk availability, sanitation, adequacy of diet with respect to essential nutrients, and the presence of parasites. That lactose intolerance does not appear until after weaning and is related to milk drinking or avoidance suggests that high milk consumption may be a stimulus for prolonging lactase activity in the mucosal brush border during the postweaning period. Genetic studies of lactose-intolerant families suggest that true lactase deficiency is an autosomal recessive trait. Therapy for lactose-intolerant individuals consists simply of restricting lactose intakes. Some individuals tolerate fermented products such as yogurt and cheese fairly well, while varying amounts of milk or ice cream induce the typical symptoms of diarrhea and flatulence.

LACTULOSE

A laxative. Trade names: Ceplulac, Chronulac, Constulose, Duphalac, Enulose, Kristolose, Lactulax.

LAETRILE

A compound having questionable nutritional value. It is extracted from apricot pits and contains cyanide (a poison). Other names of the compound include amygdalin and vitamin B_{17}. Amygdalin is a β-cyanogenicglucoside. Neither the U.S. Food and Drug Administration (FDA) nor its Canadian equivalent recognize this substance as a vitamin.

LARD

Pig fat.

LDL

See Low-Density Lipoprotein.

LDL RECEPTOR

A protein on the surface of the cell that has a particular affinity for LDL. When aberrant, lipids transported to the adipose tissue are not transported into the cell and stored. This results in an increase in LDL in the blood. An increase in LDL is associated with an increased risk of cardiovascular disease (CVD).

LEAD

A mineral that is toxic to the neuromuscular system.

LEAN BODY MASS

That fraction of the body exclusive of stored fat. This fraction is considered to be the active metabolic fraction.

LECITHIN

The trivial name for the phospholipid phosphatidyl choline.

LECTINS

See Type A Antinutritives.

LEEK

A member of the onion family.

LEGUMES

A large family of plants that have nodules on their roots containing nitrogen-fixing bacteria. Peas and beans are legumes. Some legumes contain substances that interfere with vitamins or have other antinutrient effects. These are listed in Table 34.

TABLE 34
Antinutritional and/or Toxic Factors That May Be Present in Certain Legumes

Type of Factor(s)	Effect of Factor(s)	Legumes Containing the Factor(s)
Antivitamin A	Lipoxidase oxidizes and destroys carotene (provitamin A).	Soybeans.
Antivitamin B_{12}	Increases requirement for vitamin B_{12}.	Soybeans.
Antivitamin D	Causes rickets unless extra vitamin D is provided.	Soybeans.
Antivitamin E	Damages the liver and muscles.	Alfalfa, common beans (*Phaseolus vulgaris*), peas (*Pisum sativum*).
Cyanide-releasing glucosides	Releases hydrocyanic acid. The poison may also be released by an enzyme in *Escherichia coli*, a normal inhabitant of the human intestine.	All legumes contain small amounts of these factors. However, certain varieties of lima beans (*Phaseolus lunatus*) may contain much larger amounts.
Favism factor	Causes the breakdown of red blood cells in certain susceptible individuals.	Fava beans (*Vicia faba*).
Gas-generating	Certain indigestible carbohydrates are acted upon by gas-producing bacteria in the lower intestine.	Many species of mature dry legumes but not peanuts; the immature seeds contain much lower amounts.
Goitrogens	Interfere with thyroid hormone.	Peanuts and soybeans.
Trypsin inhibitors	The inhibitor(s) binds with the enzyme trypsin.	All legumes contain trypsin inhibitors. These inhibitors are destroyed by heat.
Lathyrogenic neurotoxin	Consumption of large quantities for severe neurologic disorders.	Lathyrus pea (*Lathyrus sativus*) grown in India. Common vetch (*Vicia sativa*) may also be lathyrogenic.
Metal binders	Bind copper, iron, manganese, and zinc.	Soybeans, peas (Pisum sativum).
Hemagglutinins	The agents cause the red blood cells to clump together.	Occurs in all legumes to some extent.

Source: Adapted from Ensminger et al. 1994. *Foods and Nutrition Encyclopedia.* 2nd ed., 1284–5. Boca Raton, FL: CRC Press.

LEPTIN

A cytokine produced by the adipocyte. Leptin signals the brain that the fat store is full and that satiety has been attained. Mutation of either the leptin gene or the gene for its receptor has been associated with the development of obesity.

LESCH NYHAN SYNDROME

A rare genetic disease affecting only males that is due to a mutation in the gene for hypoxanthine-guanine phosphoribosyl transferase, an enzyme that is essential in making guanosine from the purine guanine. The disorder is characterized by mental retardation, self-mutilation, and renal failure.

LESION-CAUSING BACTERIAL TOXINS

See also Food-Borne Illness. Bacteria that produce toxins that in turn cause lesions. *Bacillus cereus* are gram-positive, rod-shaped, spore-forming, aerobic bacteria, which produce enterotoxins (type I and II) as well as several enzymes of pathogenic relevance (e.g., hemolysin and lecithinase).

Type I (diarrheal type) is a proteinous enterotoxin (molecular weight 50,000), which is formed in the intestine. This enterotoxin is heat-sensitive and can be degraded by trypsin. Type II (emetic type) is an enterotoxin (molecular weight ≤5000), which is formed in the food during the logarithmic phase of bacterial growth. Type II is stable at pH 10 and heat-resistant.

It has been reported that *Bacillus cereus* counts ranging from 36,000 to 950 million cells/g of food result in enteritis. Type I enterotoxin occurs most frequently and is mildly toxic. After an incubation period of 8–16 hours, 50%–80% of consumers develop abdominal cramps and diarrhea, which may last for 24 hours. Type II enterotoxin is less common. After a short incubation period of 1–5 hours, violent vomiting occurs. Symptoms may last for 8–10 hours. The sudden onset of symptoms, short duration of illness, characteristic lack of fever, requirement for large numbers of organisms to produce response, and variability of fecal isolation of the organism are all suggestive of the noninfective nature of the disease and indicate that cereus food-borne illness is an intoxication.

The six factors affecting the growth and survival of *Bacillus cereus* are as follows:

1. Temperature (growth of *Bacillus cereus*: 7°C–50°C [optimum: 30°C–35°C]; germination of spores: –1°C–59°C [optimum: 30°C])
2. Acidity (growth of *Bacillus cereus*: pH 4.9–9.3)
3. Type of substrates and nutritional factors (growth of *Bacillus cereus*: affected by the amino acid composition of the medium, especially by arginine, cysteine, glutamic acid, histidine, isoleucine, leucine, methionine, phenylalanine, serine, threonine, and valine; enterotoxin production is further enhanced by adding glycine, lysine, aspartic acid, and tyrosine)
4. Presence of other microorganisms (*Streptococcus lactis* produces an antibiotic, nisin, that suppresses growth of *Bacillus cereus* in milk at low temperatures [≤5°C] of storage. The antibiotic has no effect at 15°C or higher, whereas the spores of *Bacillus cereus* appear to be resistant to nisin.)
5. Sodium chloride (NaCl tolerance: 5%)
6. Time (generation time: 27 minutes)

Sources contributing to *Bacillus cereus* contamination are soil and dust; principal food types involved include custards, cereal products, puddings, sauces, and meatloaf. There is no evidence that human factors are involved in the contamination. Type I enterotoxin is mainly associated with sauces, pastries, and so on, and type II enterotoxin with cooked or fried rice. The main prevention measure is adequate and immediate cooling after cooking. This should be carried out in shallow layers, enabling fast heat transfer; storage should be at ≤10°C.

LESIONS

A wound or injury; an abnormality of a cell or tissue that is indicative of disease.

LETHARGY

Lack of energy; drowsiness.

LEUCINE

An essential amino acid (see Table 5).

LEUCOVORIN CALCIUM (CITROVORUM FACTOR)

Formyl derivative (active reduced form of folic acid); a vitamin important in red cell formation.

LEUKEMIA

A cancer in which white blood cell production is uncontrolled.

LEUKOCYTES

White blood cells.

LEUKOTRIENES

Eicosanoids synthesized from arachidonic acid. (See Eicosanoids.)

LEVETIRACETAM

An anticonvulsant; antiepileptic. Trade name: Keppra.

LEVODOPA

A drug used to manage Parkinson's disease. Trade names: Dopar, Larodopa.

LEVOFLOXIN

An antibiotic. Trade name: Levaquin.

LEVOTHYROXINE SODIUM

Compund used in thyroid hormone replacement. Trade names: Eltroxin, Levo-T, Levothyroid, Levoxine, Levoxyl, Novothyrox, Synthoid, Thyro-tabs, Unithyroid.

LEVULOSE

Fructose.

LH

Luteinizing hormone: released by the pituitary and serves to stimulate estrogen and progesterone production in females and testosterone in males.

LHA

Lateral hypothalamus.

LIBRARY

A collection of cloned fragments of DNA. Libraries may be either genomic DNA (in which both introns and exons are included) or cDNA (in which only the exons are expressed in a particular cell or tissue).

LIDOCAINE HYDROCHLORIDE

Local anesthetic, amide derivative, ventricular antiarrhythmic. Trade names: LidoPen, Auto-injector, Xylocaine.

LIFE EXPECTANCY

The number of years a human can expect to live; can vary depending on nutritional status, genetics, environment, and physical activity.

LIGATION

The enzyme-catalyzed reaction that results in the joining of two substrates.

LIGNIN

A complex indigestible fiber that provides structure to very mature vegetables.

LIMITING AMINO ACIDS

Amino acids are required for normal protein maintenance, but if they are supplied in subnormal amounts they are referred to as limiting.

LINGUAL LIPASE

A lipase found in the saliva that initiates the digestion of triacylglycerides. (See Lipid Digestion.)

LINOLEIC ACID

An essential fatty acid of the n-6 or ω6 family of fatty acids.

LINOLENIC ACID

Two forms: (1) α-linolenic, and (2) γ-linolenic. Linolenic acid is an essential fatty acid. α-Linolenic is a member of the n-3 or ω3 family of fatty acids, while γ-linolenic is a member of the n-6 or ω6 family of fatty acids.

LIPASE

An enzyme responsible for the hydrolysis of the ester bond that links a fatty acid to its glycerol backbone.

LIPCORTIN

See Lipocortin.

LIPID ABSORPTION

See Absorption.

LIPID DIGESTION

The digestion of food lipids consists of a series of enzyme-catalyzed steps resulting in absorbable components. Food lipids (fats and oils) are digested initially in the mouth and then in the stomach and intestine. The digestion of lipid is begun in the mouth with the mastication of food and its mixing with the acid-stable lingual lipase. The mixing action separates the lipid particles, exposing more surface area for enzyme action and providing the opportunity for emulsion formation. These changes in physical state are essential steps that precede absorption. In the stomach, the proteins of lipid-protein complexes are denatured by gastric hydrochloric acid and attacked by the proteases (pepsin, parapepsin I, and parapepsin II) of the gastric juice with the resultant release of lipid. Little degradation of fat occurs in the stomach except that catalyzed by lingual lipase. Lingual lipase originates from glands in the back of the mouth and under the tongue. This lipase is active in the acidic environment of the stomach. However, because of the tendency of lipid to coalesce and form a separate phase, this lipase has limited opportunity to attack triacylglycerols. Those that are attacked release a single fatty acid, usually a short- or medium-chain one. The remaining diacylglycerol is subsequently hydrolyzed in the duodenum. In adults consuming a mixed diet, lingual lipase is relatively unimportant. However, in infants having an immature duodenal lipase, lingual lipase is quite important. In addition, this lipase has its greatest activity on the triacylglycerols commonly present in whole milk. Milk fat has more short- and medium-chain fatty acids than fats from other food sources.

Although the action of lingual lipase is slow relative to that of lipases found in the duodenum, its action to release diacylglycerol and short- and medium-chain fatty acids serves another function—these fatty acids serve as surfactants. Surfactants spontaneously adsorb to the water-lipid interface, conferring a hydrophilic surface to lipid droplets and thereby providing a stable interface with the aqueous environment. The dietary surfactants are the free fatty acids, lecithin, and the phospholipids. The action of acid-stable lingual lipase provides more fatty acids to supplement the dietary supply. All together these surfactants plus the churning action of the stomach produce an emulsion that is then expelled into the duodenum as chyme.

Once the chyme enters the duodenum, its entry stimulates the release into the blood stream of the gut hormone cholecystokinin. Cholecystokinin stimulates the gallbladder to contract and release bile. Bile salts serve as emulsifying agents and serve to further disperse the lipid droplets at the lipid-aqueous interface, facilitating the hydrolysis of the glycerides by the pancreatic lipases. The bile salts impart a negative charge to the lipids, which in turn attracts the pancreatic enzyme colipase.

Pancreozymin stimulates the exocrine pancreas to release pancreatic juice, which contains three lipases (lipase, lipid esterase, and colipase); the three lipases act at the water-lipid interface of the emulsion particles. One lipase acts on the fatty acids esterified at positions 1 and 3 of the glycerol backbone, leaving a fatty acid esterified at carbon 2. This 2-monoacylglyceride can isomerize, and the remaining fatty acid can move to carbon 1 or 3. The pancreatic juice contains another less specific lipase (called a lipid esterase), which cleaves the fatty acid from cholesterol esters, monoglycerides, or esters such as vitamin A ester. Its action requires the presence of bile salts. The lipase that is specific for the ester linkage at carbons 1 and 3 does not have a requirement for the bile salts and, in fact, is inhibited by them. The inhibition of pancreatic lipase by the bile salts is relieved by the third pancreatic enzyme, colipase. Colipase is a small protein (molecular weight of 12,000 Da) that binds to both the water-lipid interface and the lipase thereby anchoring and activating the lipase. The products of the lipase-catalyzed reaction, a reaction that favors the release of fatty acids having 10 or more carbons, are these fatty acids and monoacylglyceride. The products of the lipid esterase-catalyzed reaction are cholesterol, vitamins, fatty acids, and glycerol. Phospholipids present in food are attacked by phospholipases specific to each of the phospholipids. The pancreatic juice contains these lipases as prephospholipases, which are activated by the enzyme trypsin.

As mentioned earlier, the release of bile from the gallbladder is essential to the digestion of dietary fat. Bile contains the bile acids, cholic acid, and chenodeoxycholic acid. These are biological detergents or emulsifying agents. At physiological pH, these acids are present as anions so they are frequently referred to as bile salts. At pH values above the physiological range, they form aggregates with the fats at concentrations above 2–5 mM. These aggregates are called micelles. The micelles are much smaller in size than the emulsified lipid droplets. Micelle sizes vary depending on the ratio of lipids to bile acids but typically range from 40 to 600 Å.

Micelles are structured such that the hydrophobic portions (triglycerols, cholesterol esters, etc.) are towards the center of the structure, while the hydrophilic portions (phospholipids, short-chain fatty acids, bile salts) surround this center. The micelles contain many different lipids. Mixed micelles have a disc-like shape whereby the lipids form a bilayer and the bile acids occupy edge positions rendering the edge of the disc hydrophilic. During the process of lipase and esterase digestion of the lipids in the chyme, the water-insoluble lipids are rendered soluble and transferred from the lipid emulsion of the chyme to the micelle. In turn, these micelles transfer the products of digestion (free fatty acids, glycerol, cholesterol, etc.) from the intestinal lumen to the surface of the epithelial cells where absorption takes place. The micellar fluid layer next to this cell surface is homogenous, yet the products of lipid digestion are presented to the cell surface and, by passive diffusion, these products are transported into the absorptive cell. Thus, the degree to which dietary lipid is absorbed once digested depends largely on the amount of lipid to be absorbed relative to the amount of bile acid available to make the micelle. This, in turn, is dependent on the rate of bile acid synthesis by the liver and bile release by the gallbladder. The primary bile acids, cholic acid, and chenodeoxycholic acids, are produced from cholesterol by the liver. They are secreted into the intestine and the intestinal flora convert these acids to their conjugated forms by dehydroxylating carbon 7. Further metabolism occurs at the far end of the intestinal tract where lithocholate is sulfated. While the dehydroxylated acids can be reabsorbed and sent back to the liver via the portal blood, the sulfated lithocholate is not. It appears in the feces. The bile acids are recirculated via the entero-hepatic system such that very little is lost. It has been estimated that the bile acid lost in the feces (~0.8 g/day) equals that newly synthesized by the liver such that the total pool remains between 3–5 g. The amount secreted per day is on the order of 16–70 g. Since the pool size is only 3–5 g, this means that these acids are recirculated as much as 14 times a day. The function of the bile acids is thus quite similar to that of enzymes. Neither are "used up" by the processes they participate in and facilitate. In the instance of fat absorption, the bile acids facilitate the formation of micelles, which in turn facilitate the uptake of the dietary fatty acids, monoglycerides, sterols, phospholipids, and other fat-soluble nutrients by the enterocyte of the small intestine. Not only do these bile acids recirculate so too does cholesterol.

LIPIDS

See also Fats, Fatty Acids, Phospholipids, and Cholesterol. The lipids are a group of compounds that are insoluble in water and soluble in such solvents as diethyl ether, carbon tetrachloride, alcohol, chloroform, and benzene. They are present in various amounts in all living cells. Nerve cells and adipose cells are rich in lipid content; muscle cells and epithelial cells have less.

In addition to being a very important source of energy, lipids serve a variety of other functions. They perform a basic role in the structure and function of biological membranes. In the body, they are the precursors of a variety of hormones and important cellular signals. They help to regulate the uptake and excretion of nutrients by the cell. Each cell has a characteristic lipid content. Lipids are energetically more dense than carbohydrate, having an average energy value of 37.7 kJ/g. Some lipids are saponifiable; others are not. Saponifiable lipids, when treated with alkali, undergo hydrolysis at the ester linkage resulting in the formation of an alcohol and a soap. Triacylglycerol (triglyceride), for example, when treated with sodium hydroxide is hydrolyzed yielding a mixture of soaps and free glycerol. Traditionally, lipids have been classified into three groups, each with subgroups:

1. Simple lipids: esters of fatty acids with various alcohols
   (a) Fats—esters of fatty acids with glycerol (acylglycerols)
   (b) Waxes—esters of fatty acids with long-chain alcohols
   (c) Cholesterol and cholesterol esters
2. Compound lipids: esters of fatty acids that contain chemical groups in addition to fatty acids and alcohol
   (a) Phospholipids—esters of fatty acids, alcohol, a phosphoric acid residue, and usually an amino alcohol, sugar or other substituent
   (b) Glycolipids—esters of fatty acids that contain carbohydrates and nitrogen (but not phosphoric acid) in addition to fatty acids and alcohol
   (c) Lipoproteins—loose combinations of lipids and proteins
3. Derived lipids: substances derived from the above groups by hydrolysis; they are the results of saponification

LIPOCORTIN

Also called annexin; serves to inhibit the enzyme phospholipase A_2.

LIPOFUSCIN

Granules of pigments found in aging tissues; highly insoluble lipid-protein complexes held together by multiple cross-linkages.

LIPOGENESIS

The synthesis of fatty acids, triacylglycerols, cholesterol, and phospholipids. (See Fatty Acid Synthesis, Cholesterol Synthesis, Phospholipid Synthesis, and Metabolic Maps, Appendix 2.)

LIPOIC ACID

A critical coenzyme in the oxidative decarboxylation of pyruvate and α-ketoglutarate. It participates in the pyruvate dehydrogenase complex where lipoic acid is linked to the ε-amino group of a lysine residue from the enzyme dihydrolipoyl transacetylase. As the lipoamide undergoes reversible acylation/deacylation, it transfers acyl groups to CoA and results in reversible ring opening/closing in the oxidation of the α-keto acid. Lipoic acid can be synthesized endogenously to meet need and is not a vitamin.

LIPOLYSIS

The hydrolysis of triacylglycerides and subsequent oxidation of fatty acids. (See Fatty Acid Oxidation and Metabolic Maps, Appendix 2.)

LIPOMA

An adipose tissue tumor; a nonmalignant neoplasm composed of mature fat cells.

LIPOPROTEIN LIPASE (LPL)

Enzyme that catalyzes the initial step of hydrolyzing the fatty acids from the glycerol backbone.

LIPOPROTEINS

Lipoproteins are multicomponent complexes of lipids and protein that form distinct molecular aggregates with approximate stoichiometry between each of the components. They contain polar and neutral lipids, cholesterol, or cholesterol esters in addition to protein. The protein and lipid are held together by noncovalent forces. The protein component (apolipoprotein) is located on the outer surface of the micellar lipid structure, where it serves a hydrophilic function. Lipids, which are primarily hydrophobic molecules, are not easily transported through an aqueous environment such as blood. However, when they combine with proteins, the resulting compound becomes hydrophilic and can be transported in the blood to tissue, which can use or store these lipids. Membrane lipoproteins, like glycoproteins, are essential components of membrane transport systems and as such are important in the overall regulation of cellular activity.

Lipoproteins are conjugated amphipathic proteins containing lipid and protein moieties having a density of 1.006–1.063. Lipoproteins carry not only the absorbed food lipids but also the lipids synthesized or mobilized from organs and fat depots. Nine different lipid-carrying proteins have been identified and each plays a specific role in the lipid transport process. In addition, there are several minor proteins that may be involved in some aspects of lipid cycling and uptake. The proteins involved in lipid transport are listed in Table 35. Mutations in the genes, which encode these proteins, can lead to aberrant lipid transport and the individual may have either abnormally high or low blood lipid values. The hepatic and intestinal apolipoproteins can be distinguished using electrophoresis, a technique of separating proteins based on their electrophoretic mobility.

The intestinal cell has three apolipoproteins called A-1, A-IV, and B-48. The apolipoprotein B-48 is unique to the enterocyte and is essential for chylomicron release by the intestinal cell. Apo A-1 is synthesized in the liver. Apo B-48 is actually an edited version of the hepatic apo B-100. It is the result of an apo-B mRNA editing process that converts codon 2153 to a translational stop codon. Apo B-48 is thus an edited form of apo B-100, and this editing is unique to the intestinal cell. Failure to appropriately edit the apo B gene in the intestinal cell will result in a disorder called familial hypobetalipoproteinemia. In this disorder, there will be a total or partial (depending on the genetic mutation) absence of lipoproteins in the blood. Hypobetalipoproteinemia can also develop should there be base substitutions in the gene for the apo B protein. In addition to very low blood lipids, patients with this disorder also have fat malabsorption (steatorrhea). The feces contain an abnormally large amount of fat and have a characteristic peculiar odor. In this disorder, not only is the triacylglyceride absorption affected, so too are the fat-soluble vitamins. Without the ability to absorb these energy-rich food components and vital fat-soluble vitamins, the patient does not thrive and survive. Fortunately, this genetic mutation is not very common. It is inherited as an autosomal recessive trait.

TABLE 35
Proteins Involved in Lipid Transport

Protein	Function
Apo A-II	Transport protein in HDL.
Apo B-48	Transport protein for chylomicrons; synthesized in the enterocyte in humans.
High density lipoprotein binding protein (HDLBP)	Binds HDL and functions in the removal of excess cellular cholesterol.
Apo D	Transport protein similar to retinol-binding protein.
Apo (a)	Abnormal transport protein for LDL.
Apo A-I	Transport protein for chylomicrons and HDL; synthesized in the liver, and its synthesis is induced by retinoic acid.
Apo C-III	Transport protein for VLDL.
Apo A-IV	Transport protein for chylomicrons.
CETP	Participates in the transport of cholesterol from peripheral tissue to liver; reduces HDL size.
LCAT	Synthesized in the liver and is secreted into the plasma where it resides on the HDL. Participates in the reverse transport of cholesterol from peripheral tissues to the liver; esterifies the HDL cholesterol.
Apo E	Mediates high affinity binding of LDLs to LDL receptor and the putative chylomicron receptor. Required for clearance of chylomicron remnant. Synthesized primarily in the liver.
Apo C-I	Transport protein for VLDL.
Apo C-II	Chylomicron transport protein–required cofactor for LPL activity.
Apo B-100	Synthesized in the liver and is secreted into the circulation as part of the VLDL. Also serves as the ligand for the LDL receptor–mediated hepatic endocytosis.
LPL	Catalyzes the hydrolysis of plasma triglycerides into free fatty acids.
Hepatic lipase	Catalyzes the hydrolysis of triglycerides and phospholipids of LDL and HDL. It is bound to the surfaces of both hepatic and nonhepatic tissues.

The particles of absorbed lipid and transport proteins are called chylomicrons. They are present in the blood of feeding animals but are usually absent in starving animals. As the chylomicrons circulate, they acquire an additional protein, apo C-II. This additional protein is an essential cofactor for the recognition and hydrolysis of the chylomicron by the capillary endothelial enzyme, lipoprotein lipase (LPL). The LPL hydrolyzes most of the core triglycerides in the chylomicron, leaving a remnant that is rich in cholesterol and cholesterol esters. During the LPL-catalyzed hydrolytic process, the excess surface compounds, that is, the phospholipids and apolipoproteins B, A-I, and A-IV, are transferred to high-density lipoproteins (HDLs). In exchange, apo-E is transferred from the HDL to the cholesterol ester-rich chylomicron remnant. These remnants are then cleared from the blood by the liver. On the hepatocyte is a lipoprotein receptor that recognizes apo-E, and this receptor plays an important role in remnant clearance.

The circulation of chylomicrons is a relatively stable way of ensuring the movement, in an aqueous medium (blood), of hydrophobic molecules such as cholesterol and triacylglycerols from their point of origin, the intestine, to their point of use or storage. There are several unique proteins that facilitate this movement. These lipid-transporting proteins determine which cells of the body receive which lipids. At the target cell, the particles lose their lipid through hydrolysis facilitated by an interstitial LPL, which is found in the capillary beds of muscle, fat cells, and other tissues using lipid as a fuel. The LPL is synthesized by these target cells, but it is anchored on the outside of the cells by a polysaccharide chain on the endothelial wall of the surrounding capillaries. Should this LPL be missing or genetically aberrant (type I lipemia or chylomicronemia) so that the chylomicrons cannot be hydrolyzed, the chylomicrons accumulate and the individual would have a lipemia characterized by elevated levels of triacylglyceride and cholesterol containing chylomicrons. Also characteristic of this condition is the presence of an enlarged liver and spleen, considerable abdominal discomfort, and the presence of subcutaneous xanthomas (clusters of hard saturated fatty acid and cholesterol-rich nodules). Like familial hypolipoproteinemia, this condition is rare. Of interest is the observation that despite the very high blood lipid levels of these people, few die of coronary vessel disease. Their shortened lifespan is due to an inappropriate lipid deposition in all of the vital organs, which, in turn, has a negative effect on organ function and life span.

ENDOGENOUS LIPID TRANSPORT

Fatty acids, triglycerides, cholesterol, cholesterol esters, and phospholipids are synthesized in the body and are transported from sites of synthesis to sites of use and storage. While the transport of these lipids is, in many instances, similar to that of dietary lipids, there are differences in processing and in some of the proteins involved. Endogenous fat transport involves the production and secretion of very-low-density lipoproteins (VLDLs) by the liver. These lipid-protein complexes are rich in TG but also contain cholesterol. The polypeptides that transport these lipids comprise approximately 10% of the weight of the VLDL. They include the polypeptides apo-B, B-100, apo-C-I, apo-C-II, apo C-III, and apo-E. Several of these polypeptides are also involved in exogenous lipid transport. Once the VLDLs are released by the hepatocyte, they are hydrolyzed by the interstitial LPL and intermediate-density lipoproteins (IDLs) are formed. These are cleared from circulation as they are recognized and bound to hepatic IDL receptors. The hepatic receptors recognize the apo-E that is part of the IDL. Any of the IDL that escapes hydrolysis at this step is available for hydrolysis by hepatic LPL. This hydrolysis leaves a cholesterol-rich particle of low density (LDL). The LDL has apo B-100 as its polypeptide carrier, and both hepatic and extrahepatic cells have receptors that recognize this polypeptide. Normally, about 70% of LDL is cleared by LDL receptors and most of this is cleared by the liver. From the foregoing, it is apparent that considerable lipid recycling occurs in the liver. The VLDLs originate in the liver and the liver is the primary site for LDL disposal. However, other organs and tissues also participate in disposal but their participation is minor compared to that of the liver.

GENETIC BASIS FOR LIPOPROTEINEMIA

There are a number of proteins involved in the uptake, synthesis, and disposal of lipids. The genes for the transport proteins, apo A-I, apo A-II, apo A-IV, apo (a), apo B, apo D, apo C-I, apo C-II, apo C-III, apo D, and apo E, have been identified as having mutations that result in lipid transport abnormalities. In addition to these transport proteins, there are reports of abnormalities in other aspects of lipid transport. These include the receptors that are involved in lipoprotein processing, the peripheral LPL and the hepatic LPL, and the rate-limiting enzymes of lipid synthesis and use. Many of these proteins have been isolated and studied in detail. Several of their cognate genes have been identified and mapped. Listed in Table 36 are the chromosomal locations of these genes. With this many genes involved in the uptake, synthesis, transport, and degradation of the circulating lipids, it is not surprising to find mutations that phenotype as either lipemia or fat malabsorption. Not all of these diseases of lipid transport are associated with atherosclerosis. Also shown in Table 36 are some of the genetic defects and estimates of their frequency.

TABLE 36
Location of Genes Involved in Lipoprotein Metabolism

Gene	Chromosome Location	Characteristics of Mutation	Frequency of Mutation
Apo A-II	1	Transport protein in HDL	?
Apo B 48	2 p 23–24	Hypobetalipoproteinemia	1:1,000,000
HDLBP	2 q 37		?
Apo D	3	Transport protein similar to retinol-binding protein	?
Apo (a)	6	Abnormal transport protein for LDL	?
LPL	8 p 22	Defective chylomicron clearance	1:1,000,000
Apo A-I	11	Defective HDL production (Tangier's disease)	1:1,000,000
Apo C-III	11		?
Apo A-IV	11		?
Hepatic LPL (HTGL)	15 q 21	Defective IDL clearance	?
CETP	16 q 22.1		?
LCAT	16 q 22.1	Familial lecithin:cholesterol transferase deficiency; two types	Rare
LDL receptor	19	Familial hypercholesterolemia	1:500
Apo B-100	2	Familial defective apo B-100	1:500–1:1000
Apo E	19	Type III hyperlipoproteinemia	1:5000
Apo C-I	19	Transport protein for VLDL	?
Apo C-II	19	Defective chylomicron clearance	1:1,000,000

Defects in exogenous fat transport are manifested in several ways. Defective chylomicron formation due to mutations in either the apo-B gene or its editing leads to and is characterized by fat malabsorption. This includes the malabsorption of fat-soluble vitamins as well. Twenty different mutations have been identified in the gene for the apo-B protein. These mutations are inherited via an autosomal recessive mode and are characterized not only by fat malabsorption but also by acanthocytes, retinitis pigmentosa, and muscular neuropathies. To a large extent, these symptoms can be attributed to a relative deficiency of fat-soluble vitamins due to malabsorption. While a defect in the apo-B gene can account for defective fat absorption, there may be another mutation (in the microsomal triglyceride transfer protein) that also might result in fat malabsorption. This transfer protein is essential for apo-B translocation and subsequent synthesis of chylomicrons. Defects in this transfer protein would impair apo-B availability and chylomicron formation. In these defects, very low levels of chylomicrons are found in the blood. Persons with this disorder are rare (one in a million). In this circumstance, the severity of the disease is related to the size of the mutated gene product and whether it can associate with the lipids it must carry. The size of the truncated apo-B can vary from apo B-9 (41 residues) to apo B-89 (4487 residues). Except in the case of the apo B-25, the result of a deletion of the entire exon 21, all the truncated forms reported to date are C-T transitions or base deletions. These deletions can involve misaligned pairing deletion mechanisms. Frameshift mutation can be compensated by a reading frame restoration of the apo-B gene.

Familial hyperchylomicronemia is characterized by elevations in chylomicrons having both tri-glycerides and cholesterol. Hyperchylomicronemia was found to be due to mutations in the genes that encode the enzyme LPL needed for the hydrolysis of chylomicrons. This enzyme is a glyco-protein having an apparent monomeric molecular weight of about 60,000 Da on sodium dodecyl sulfate (SDS) gel electrophoresis and 48,300 Da by sedimentation-equilibrium ultracentrifugation. The enzyme is linked to the endothelial cells of the capillary system. The LPL is quite similar to hepatic triglyceride lipase, an enzyme found in the hepatic sinusoids. The main difference between the two lipases is that the interstitial lipase has a requirement for the lipid-carrying protein apo C-II for full activity, whereas hepatic LPL does not. Mutations in the gene for apo C-II can result in aberrant lipase activity because apo C-II serves as a cofactor in the LPL-catalyzed reaction. Hepatic triglyceride lipase has no such requirement. Aberrations in the hepatic triglyceride lipase result in an accumulation of VLDLs rather than accumulations of chylomicrons. Mutations in the genes for LPL and apo C-II are very rare, occurring at a frequency of one in a million. The gene for LPL has been mapped to chromosome 8, while that for apo C-II has been mapped to chromosome 19 and the hepatic LPL to chromosome 15. Other features of these disorders include an inflammation of the exocrine pancreas and eruptive xanthomas. Chylomicronemia does not appear to be atherogenic. The mutations in the LPL gene appear to be insertions or deletions or due to aberrant splicing, while those in the apo C-II gene seem to be due to splice site mutations or small deletions. Twenty-two mutations in the apo C-II gene have been reported. With respect to the aberrant splicing of the LPL gene in three unrelated humans, it has been reported that a C→A mutation in position 3 of the acceptor splice site of intron 6, exists that causes the aberrant splicing. The major transcript showed a deletion of exons 6 through 9. Trace amounts of both a normally spliced LPL mRNA and a second aberrant transcript devoid of exon 7 were found. In one patient, a 3^I splice mutation on one allele was reported, while on the other allele was found a missense mutation resulting in Gly 188→Glu substitution. All three subjects were classed as hyperchylomicronemic due to LPL deficiency.

The absence of LPL activity in certain tissues or in certain individuals can be attributed to mutations in the LPL promoter region. Studies of tissue-specific expression of LPL showed that cis-acting elements located within the -1824- bp of the 5^I flanking region was required for the expression of LPL. These include nuclear factors recognizing both the CCAAT box and the octamer sequence immediately flanking the transcriptional start site. Those tissues that have no LPL activity lack this promoter region. Since humans and mice have identical CCAAT and octamer sequences, one could suppose that humans having an intact LPL gene of normal sequence but lacking LPL activity might have a deficient or mutated promoter region; proof that this might occur is presently lacking.

Mutations in the gene for hepatic LPL result in elevated blood levels of triglycerides and choles-terol, and these elevations are related to an increased risk for atherosclerosis. Hepatic LPL must be secreted by the hepatocyte into the sinusoids to function as a catalyst for the hydrolysis of core TG and surface phospholipids of chylomicron remnants, HDL, and IDL. Through its activity, it aug-ments the uptake of HDL cholesterol by the liver (reverse cholesterol transport) and is involved in the reduction of HDL size from HDL_2 to HDL_3. Hepatic LPL aids in the clearance of chylomicron remnants by exposing the apo-E epitopes for enzymatic action. Missense mutations in the hepatic LPL gene include substitutions of serine for phenylalanine at amino acid position 267, threonine for methionine at position 383, and asparagine for serine at position 291. These mutations result in poorly secreted enzyme, and thus the phenotypic expression of the mutation is low hepatic lipase activity. The frequency of the Asn 291 Ser mutation in a population having premature CVD has been reported as 5.2%.

Defects in chylomicron remnant clearance are much more common than any of the aforemen-tioned mutations. Defective clearance due to mutations in the apo-E gene results in a lipemia known as type III hyperlipoproteinemia. It is associated with premature atherosclerosis, and patients with these defects have high serum triglyceride levels as well as high serum cholesterol levels. Xanthomas are found in nearly three-fourths of the population with these defects. The lipemia is responsive to energy restriction using diets that have 40% of energy from carbohydrate, 40% from fat, and 20% from protein. Weight loss is efficacious for most people with this defect. The apo-E gene codes for the protein on the surface of the chylomicron remnant that is the ligand for receptor-mediated clearance of this particle. A number of mutations in the apo-E gene have been reported, and the phenotypes of these mutations are grouped into three general groups labeled E_2, E_3, and E_4. Those of the E_2 group fail to bind the particles to the cell surface receptor for the chylomicron remnant. Those of the E_3 and E_4 groups have generally low remnant clearance rates. The apo-E allele and phenotype frequency varies. The E_2 frequency is about 8%, the E_3 about 77%, and the E_4 about 15% of the total population with an apo-E mutation. Apo-E gene mutations occur in about 1% of the population. Since apo-E is involved in both endogenous and exogenous lipid transport and clearance, a faulty apo-E gene is devastating. Mature human apo-E is a 299 amino acid polypeptide. Apo-E, as well as other apolipoproteins, contains 11 or 22 amino acid repeated sequences as one of its key features. These appear to encode largely amphipathic helices, which are needed for lipid binding. There is a high degree of conservation among species of nucleotide sequences in the gene fragment that encodes the amino acid repeats. The gene for apo-E has been mapped to chromosome 19 as have the genes for apo C-I, apo C-II, and LDL. There appears to be a tight linkage among these genes, which coordinates their expression. Among the common mutations are amino acid substitutions at positions 112 and 158 while less frequent substitutions occur at other positions in the polypeptide chain. Several of these involve the exchange of neutral amino acids for acidic amino acids with the net result of alterations in polypeptide charge and subsequent inadequate binding to the appropriate cell surface receptors. In a rare form of the disorder, the mutation is such that no useful apo-E is formed. Transgenic mice have been constructed with an apo-E mutation that mimics apo-E deficiency. These mice, like humans, develop hypercholesterolemia and increased susceptibility to atherosclerosis. When these mice were fed low-fat (5%) or high-fat (16%) diets, a differential serum cholesterol pattern was observed: those fed the high-fat diet had significantly higher levels of cholesterol, VLDL, and LDL than those fed a low-fat or stock diet. The transgenic mice, even when fed the stock diet, had significantly higher levels of cholesterol, VLDL, and LDL than the normal control mice. There was a gender difference as well. Male transgenic mice were less diet responsive in terms of their cholesterol levels than female transgenic mice. There is some sequence homology between humans and mice in the apo-E DNA, and one could infer that these responses to dietary fat intake in mice could be observed in humans as well.

While the aforementioned transgenic approach used the gene knockout paradigm (an extreme in the variants of apo-E mutants), it nonetheless suggests that variation in the apo-E genes could determine the responsiveness of humans with apo-E defects to dietary manipulation. Indeed, such nutrient–gene interactions have been reported. The dietary fat clearance in normal subjects appears to be regulated by the genetic variance in apo-E sequence and this in turn is related to fat intake. Not only is triacylglycerol clearance affected, so too is cholesterol clearance. One study reported that the apo-E genotype declares the response to cholesterol intake with respect to blood cholesterol levels and that this genotype influences cholesterol synthesis. Those subjects who responded poorly to an oral cholesterol challenge vis-à-vis blood cholesterol clearance had higher rates of cholesterol synthesis than those who could rapidly clear their blood of cholesterol after an oral challenge. One of the more interesting variants of the apo-E is called the Milano variant. In this variant, blood lipid levels are elevated but these elevations are not associated with an increased risk of atherosclerosis.

Cholesterol traffic is also controlled by the LDL receptor and the transport protein apo B-100. Mutations in the gene for the LDL receptor or in the gene for apo B-100, the ligand for the LDL receptor, result in high serum levels of cholesterol. The former results in the disorder called familial hypercholesterolemia and occurs with a frequency of about 1 in 500. Familial hypercholesterolemia is associated with early death from atherosclerosis in humans and related primates. Dietary fat saturation affects transcription of LDL receptor mRNA in that feeding a diet containing saturated fat results in decreased LDL receptor mRNA compared to feeding an unsaturated-fat diet. These results suggest that unsaturated fatty acids may interact with proteins that in turn serve as either cis- or trans-acting elements for this gene in much the same way as polyunsaturated fatty acids affect fatty acid synthetase gene expression.

Familial defective apo B-100 hypercholesterolemia is due to a mutation in the coding sequence of the apo-B gene at bp 3500 that changes the base sequence such that glutamine is substituted for arginine. This is in the LDL receptor-binding region of the apo-B protein and results in a binding affinity less than 4% of normal. Polymorphic variation in the genes for both the LDL receptor and the apo B-100 have been reported for mice, and this variation has provided the opportunity to identify the genetic and molecular constraints of lipoprotein gene expression. Both apo-B and apo-E serve as ligands for the LDL receptor. In contrast to apo-E, apo-B has little homology with the other apolipoproteins. Apo-B in mice is quite variable, and this variation imparts or confers a diet-responsive characteristic in inbred mouse strains vis-à-vis polypeptide sequence and activity. That is, some mouse strains have reduced levels of plasma apo-B when fed a high-fat diet compared to controls fed a stock diet, while other mouse strains are unresponsive to diet vis-à-vis their plasma apo B-100 levels. Such polymorphism also exists in humans. Apo-B has been mapped to chromosome 2 and produces two gene products: (1) apo B-100, and (2) apo B-48. In the intestine, the apo-B primary transcript is co- or post-transcriptionally modified. This modification converts codon 2153 from a glutamine (CAA) to an in-frame, premature termination codon (UAA), thereby causing translation to terminate after amino acid 2152. This mRNA editing thus explains the difference in size of these two proteins. If more of the apo-B gene is deleted, hypocholesterolemia is observed. This is because apo B-48 is required for the transport of the chylomicrons from the intestine. If lacking, chylomicron formation is impaired and low serum cholesterol levels are observed. Both familial defective apo B-100 and familial hypercholesterolemia are characterized by high levels of LDL. Both are associated with CVD, but only the familial hypercholesterolemia is characterized by tendon xanthomas. Both are inherited as autosomal dominant disorders. Collectively, these mutations have a cumulative frequency of 1 in 250. However, because polymorphism in the apo-B gene can and does occur, there is the possibility that collectively the frequency is much greater than, or perhaps as high as, 1 in 5. If this is the case, then the population variation in plasma cholesterol levels could be explained on the basis of these genetic differences alone apart from those mutations that are associated with the rest of the genes, which encode components of the lipid transport system.

Genetically determined abnormalities in LDL metabolism may also be due to mutation in the large glycoprotein, apo (a). Apo (a) is a highly variable, disulfide protein bonded to apo B-100. It is thought to resemble plasminogen. In fact, the genes that encode Lp(a) and plasminogen are very close to each other on the long arm of chromosome 6. In general, LDLs containing apo (a) do not bind well to the LPL receptor and people having significant amounts of apo (a) have a two- to three-fold increase in CVD risk. Many individuals have little or no apo (a), and it has been suggested that those who have it are abnormal with respect to LPL activity.

Several mutations in the genes that encode endogenous lipid transport have been reported. The reverse cholesterol transport pathway is part of this endogenous lipid transport system. It involves the movement of cholesterol from peripheral tissues to the liver. The peripheral tissues cannot oxidize cholesterol and so must send it to the liver, where it is prepared for excretion via cholesterol 7 α-hydroxylase, as bile acids. This pathway uses the HDL to shuttle the cholesterol in this direction. HDL consists primarily of apo A-1 and cholesterol, which is esterified by the enzyme lecithin:cholesterol acyl transferase (LCAT). Mutations in the LCAT gene have been reported and they result in one of two diseases: (1) familial LCAT deficiency, or (2) fish eye disease. Thirteen different mutations have been identified, and in one mutation a single T→A transversion in codon 252 in exon 6, converting met (ATG) to Lys (AAG), was observed. Three unrelated families were found to have this mutation; however, the severity of their disease varied. In these families, no other mutation in LCAT was observed. Of the remaining 12 LCAT mutations, 10 were point mutations, 3 were frameshifts, and 1 consisted of a three base insertion, which maintained its reading frame. For fish eye disease, three mutations have been reported. This disorder is less serious than familial LCAT deficiency and is characterized by dyslipoproteinemia and corneal opacity. LCAT activity is 15% of normal and there is a reduced level of HDL in the plasma. In contrast, familial LCAT deficiency is characterized by a variety of symptoms including lipoprotein abnormalities, renal failure, premature atherosclerosis, reduced levels of plasma cholesterol esters, and high plasma levels of cholesterol and lecithin.

The LCAT enzyme requires apo A-I as a cofactor. If there is a mutation in the gene for apo A-I, defective HDL production results. This is a rare mutation and its frequency is estimated as one in a million. Individuals with this defect have premature CVD, corneal clouding, and very low HDL levels. Plasma apo A-I has a variety of charge isoforms with similar antigenicity and amino acid composition. Humans, baboons, African green monkeys, and cynomolgus monkeys have been studied, and there are species differences in hepatic and intestinal apo A-I production. In all instances the differences in apo A-I were reported between intestine and liver. In the liver, there was a twofold higher level of apo A-I mRNA than in the intestine, and the abundance of this mRNA was species specific. The apo A-I gene is regulated at the level of transcription, and a portion of the species-specific difference in apo A-I gene expression is due to a sequence divergence in the 5' regulatory region, including the exon/intron 1 of the apo A-I gene. The capacity to produce HDLs is both genetically controlled and tissue specific and probably explains why some genotypes respond normally to a high-fat diet by producing more HDL while other genotypes become hypercholesterolemic under the same conditions. Attempts to create a transgenic mouse expressing a human apo A-I gene have not been fully successful, but they have provided additional information about the relationship of apo A-I to HDL size. The human apo A-I gene was inserted into mice, and in these mice both the mouse and the human genes were expressed. This dual expression suggests a species difference in the control of this expression. In other words, the control points differed and this resulted in a broader spectrum of HDL particles.

Defective HDL metabolism due to a mutation in the apo A-I gene results in a rare autosomal dominant disorder described in a small group of villagers in Italy. Affected individuals have reduced levels of HDL cholesterol and apo A-I levels but have no increased risk of CVD. The disorder, named apo A-I Milano, is due to a point mutation in the apo A-I gene, changing codon 173 so that cysteine is used instead of arginine. Normal apo A-I has no cysteine, so this change has effects (because of the sulfide group in the cysteine) on the apo A-I structure.

Defective lipoprotein processing has already been discussed with respect to LDP, LCAT, and apo C-II deficiencies. A deficient CETP has been reported due to a mutation of the gene for this protein located on chromosome 16. A mutation in this gene has been used to explain the atherogenicity of high-fat diets in primates, but to date no evidence of such a mutation in humans has been put forward.

NUTRIENT-GENE INTERACTIONS IN LIPID TRANSPORT

The aforementioned observations of diet and genetic factors suggest that CVD could develop as a result of a nutrient-gene interaction. There are a number of genes involved in the regulation of blood lipid levels. Further, the diet influence involves not only the amount of fat consumed but also the type of fat and the amount and type of carbohydrate consumed. For example, the editing of the apo-B gene is enhanced by dietary carbohydrate. A number of genes have carbohydrate response elements and it is possible that this gene has this element in its promoter region. A carbohydrate response element has been identified in the apo-E gene. Carbohydrate influences mRNA stability and RNA processing of this gene. Similarly, the gene that encodes the seven enzyme complexes of mammalian fatty acid synthetase has a fatty acid response unit in its promoter. The expression of this gene is downregulated by dietary polyunsaturated fatty acids. The lipid transport genes might also have a lipid response element.

Dietary lipids even in the absence of direct effects on transcription and translation do influence the phenotypic expression of specific genotypes either because of overconsumption or because they have effects on certain hormones, that is, insulin, the steroid hormones, or the catabolic hormones that regulate or influence lipid synthesis, oxidation, and storage. The level of cholesterol in the blood depends on the diet consumed and how much cholesterol is being synthesized. The cholesterol content of the gut LDL of a person on a low-cholesterol diet might run as low as 7%–10% of the total lipid in the lipoprotein, while the hepatic LPL of this same individual might be as high as 58% of total lipid. People consuming a low cholesterol–low saturated fat diet may reduce the contribution of the diet to the blood cholesterol while increasing the hepatic de novo cholesterol synthesis. Persons having an LPL receptor deficiency are characterized by high serum cholesterol levels and, in some cases, by high serum triacylglyceride levels. The reason these blood lipids are elevated is because the individuals cannot utilize the lipids carried by the LPL due to errors in the receptor molecule. Further, because these circulating lipids do not enter into the adipose and hepatic cells in normal amounts, the synthesis of triacylglycerides and cholesterol is not appropriately downregulated. Hence, this individual has elevated serum lipids not only because the LPL lipid is not appropriately cleared from the blood but also because of high rates of endogenous lipid synthesis. Individuals with this disorder have lipid deposits in unusual places, such as immediately under the skin, around the eyes, on the tendons, and in the vascular tree. It is this last feature that probably accounts for the shortened life span of these people with the cause of death being CVD. As can be seen from the metabolic characteristics of this disorder, low-cholesterol diets are probably useless in reducing serum cholesterol levels since de novo synthesis of cholesterol from nonlipid precursors can and does occur. Treatment with lipid adsorbents (high-fiber diets, the drug cholestyramine) will help reduce the cholesterol (but not triacylglycerides) coming from the intestine, and there are drugs that can safely lower de novo cholesterol synthesis as well as increase intracellular lipid oxidation. All of these therapies may help reduce the serum lipid levels, but even doing this only treats the symptoms and not the genetic disorder. For that, gene therapy is needed to correct the genetic disorder that is the basic underlying cause of the symptoms.

Heart disease in its various forms is also associated with elevated levels of VLDL. A specific genetic error has not been identified; however, the disorders have been subdivided into three general categories. In one, type III lipemia, patients are characterized by elevated serum cholesterol, phospholipid, and triacylglyceride levels; elevated VLDL levels (and sometimes LDL levels); fatty deposits on the tendons and in areas on the arms just under the skin; vascular atheromas; and ischemic heart disease. This type of lipemia is inherited as an autosomal dominant trait in 1 person in 5000. Another lipemia (type IV) having a normal cholesterol level but an elevated triacylglyceride level and elevated VLDL levels is also associated with ischemic heart disease and premature atherosclerosis. It is frequently seen in obese patients with type 2 diabetes. People with diabetes mellitus have five times the risk of normal people for developing premature atherosclerosis and its associated coronary events. Cardiovascular disease, followed by renal disease, is the leading cause of death for people with diabetes mellitus.

Those people with type 1, insulin-dependent diabetes mellitus are more likely to develop a lipemia (type V lipemia) that is slightly different from the aforementioned type 2 diabetes mellitus–related lipemia. While the incidence of both is 2 in 1000, those with the latter problem inherit their trait in an autosomal recessive manner while those with diabetes-related lipemia inherit their trait as an autosomal dominant trait. Elevated chylomicron and VLDL levels and reduced dietary fat tolerance characterize this type of lipemia. Patients with this disorder are usually of normal body weight.

LIQUID DIET

A wide variety of diets fit this category. Clear liquids include broths, clear juices, tea, and gelatin; full liquids include such items as ice cream, pureed soups, and so on. Formulated products are available that provide all the needed nutrients for individuals who cannot chew or digest foods in the normal state. These are appropriate for long-term use by such patients.

LISINOPRIL

Angiotensin-converting enzyme (ACE) inhibitor; antihypertensive. Trade names: Prinivil, Zestril.

LITHIASIS

The process of stone formation in the gallbladder, bile duct, kidney, ureters, or urinary bladder.

LITHIUM

A mineral used to treat mania; interferes with the activity of the Na^+K^+-dependent ATPase on the plasma membranes of nerve cells.

LITHIUM CARBONATE; LITHIUM CITRATE

Alkali metal antimanic; antipsychotic. Trade names: Carbolith, Eskalith CR, Lithobid, Lithonate, Lithotabs, Cibalith-S.

LITHOTRIPSY

Procedure of shattering calculi via a high-frequency sound in the kidney, urinary tract, and gallbladder.

LIVER DISEASE

A generic term that covers a variety of pathologic states of the liver.

LIVER FAILURE

A state in which the liver ceases to function.

LNAA

Large neutral amino acids; branched-chain and aromatic amino acids.

LOCUS

The position of a chromosome occupied by a gene or its allele.

LONGEVITY

Life span.

LOPERAMIDE

A piperidine derivative that works as an antidiarrheal. Trade names: Imodium A-D, KaopectateII Caplets.

LOSARTAN POTASSIUM

Angiotensin II receptor antagonist, antihypertensive. Trade name: Cozaar.

LOVASTATIN (MEVINOLIN)

HMG-CoA reductase inhibitor that reduces blood cholesterol levels. Trade names: Altocor, Mevacor.

LOW BIRTH WEIGHT INFANT

An infant whose weight at the end of gestation is less than expected based on the mother's size and the duration of pregnancy. Typically, these infants weigh less than 2500 g.

LOW-DENSITY LIPOPROTEIN (LDL)

A lipid protein complex consisting of a carrier protein, triglycerides, and cholesterol. Elevated LDL levels are associated with an increased risk of coronary vessel disease. (See Lipoproteins.)

LOW-FAT DIET

Therapeutic diet characterized by significantly fewer fat-containing foods than the usual diet; most low-fat diets contain 10%–20% of total energy from fat daily.

LOW-FIBER DIET

Therapeutic diet characterized by significantly fewer fiber-containing foods than the usual diet; most low-fiber diets contain less than 10–20 g of mixed fiber daily.

LOW GLYCEMIC INDEX DIET

A diet providing foods that elicit low glucose-raising potential. May have use in the management of type 2 diabetes mellitus.

LOW-RESIDUE DIET

Diet characterized by significantly fewer residue-producing foods than the usual diet; most low-residue diets also include foods low in fiber. In addition to restrictions found on the low-fiber diet, the low-residue diet typically restricts milk and milk products to one or two servings daily.

LOW-SODIUM DIET

Diet characterized by significantly less sodium-containing foods than the usual diet; low-sodium diets range from a "no added salt diet" with approximately 4000 mg/day (174 mEq) to a severe restriction at 500 mg/day (22 mEq).

LUMEN

Interior aspect of a vessel.

LUPUS ERYTHEMATOSUS

An autoimmune disease that affects the skin, joints, blood vessels, heart, kidneys, lungs, and brain.

LUXUS CONSUMPTION

Consumption of food beyond basic needs.

LYCOPENE

A carotene-like compound that has no vitamin activity.

LYMPH

Fluid present in the vessels of the lymphatic system; newly absorbed lipid is carried via the lymphatic system from the small intestine to the jugular, where the thoracic duct joins this vein.

LYSINE

An essential amino acid (see Table 5). When consumed with glucose, there is a threefold rise in insulin and glucagon release with a subsequent fall in blood glucose.

LYSOSOMES

Intracellular structures that contain digestive enzymes that attack material taken into the cells.

M

M (μ)

Greek letter prefix, which indicates 10^{-6} fraction of a liter or gram.

MACROBIOTIC (ZEN) DIET

A diet that is based on brown rice and can be deficient in a number of essential nutrients.

MACROCYTE

Immature red blood cell.

MACROCYTIC ANEMIA

An anemia characterized by large immature red cells. (See Anemia, Table 9.)

MACRONUTRIENTS

Major sources of energy and building materials for the organism. Macronutrients include lipids, carbohydrates, proteins, and water. (See Carbohydrates, Lipids, Protein, Water.)

MACROPHAGES

Cells of the immune system that are the first line of defense against pathogens. These cells are large mononuclear phagocytes that work by engulfing the foreign substance and neutralizing it.

MACROSOMIA

Enlarged cells; also used to describe a very large infant born to a mother with gestational diabetes.

MACULAR DEGENERATION

Degenerative changes in the central part (the macula) of the retina. This change is irreversible and is the leading cause of visual impairment in the United States today.

MAGNESIUM

An essential mineral that serves as a cofactor in phosphatase- and kinase-catalyzed reactions; these are the reactions that result in the hydrolysis of ATP to ADP and Pi. One of the most important of these reactions is the activation of amino acids for protein synthesis through the action of the enzyme aminoacyl-t-RNA synthetase. Another involves the attachment of mRNA to the ribosome. A third is the phosphorylation of glucose to form glucose-6-phosphate.

MAGNESIUM CHLORIDE, MAGNESIUM SULFATE

Mineral supplement. Trade name: Slow-Mag.

MAGNESIUM CITRATE (CITRATE OF MAGNESIUM)

Magnesium salt; antacid; antiulcerative; laxative. Trade names: Citroma, Citro-Mag, Citro-Nesia, Evac-Q-Mag.

MAGNESIUM HYDROXIDE (MILK OF MAGNESIA)

Magnesium salt, laxative. Trade names: Milk of Magnesia, Phillips Chewable, Phillips' Milk of Magnesia.

MAGNESIUM L-LACTATE DIHYDRATE

Mineral supplement, slow release. Trade name: Mag-Tab SR.

MAGNESIUM OXIDE

Magnesium salt, laxative. Trade names: Mag-ox 400, Maox 420, Uro-Mag.

MAGNESIUM SULFATE (EPSOM SALTS)

Magnesium salt, antacid, laxative. Can also be used as an anticonvulsant.

MAGNETIC RESONANCE IMAGING

A technology allowing the imaging of a body without radiation hazard.

MAILLARD REACTION

A nonenzymatic browning reaction of reducing sugars, in which they condense with amino acids. It is a sequence of reactions resulting in the formation of a mixture of insoluble dark-brown polymeric pigments, known as melanoidins. In the early steps of the reaction, a complex mixture of carbonyl compounds and aromatic substances is formed. These products are water soluble and mostly colorless. They are called premelanoidins. Animal studies have indicated that large intakes of premelanoidins inhibit growth, disturb reproduction, and cause liver damage. Further, certain types of allergic reactions have been attributed to Maillard reaction products. Maillard reactions can be prevented by using the additive power of the carbonyl group in reducing sugars. Regulation of temperature, pH, and water content can additionally inhibit Maillard reactions. Maillard reactions account for the browning of bread during baking and the browning of meat through exposure to high heat. Foods prepared in this manner provide very little premelanoidins.

MALABSORPTION

A condition where nutrients are not absorbed normally. May be due to a nutrient intolerance or some other disease that causes the intestinal cells to lose their absorptive capacity.

MALAISE

A feeling of illness or depression.

MALATE

A four-carbon intermediate in the citric acid cycle.

MALATE ASPARTATE SHUTTLE

A shuttle for moving reducing equivalents into the mitochondria from the cytosol (see Figure 28); has rate-limiting properties in gluconeogenesis.

MALIGNANCY

Uncontrolled growth of cells; cancer.

MALNUTRITION

Inadequate or unbalanced intake of essential nutrients. The physical signs associated with malnutrition are listed in Table 37.

MALTITOL

An alcohol of maltose.

MALTOSE

A disaccharide consisting of two molecules of glucose joined by a 1,4 linkage.

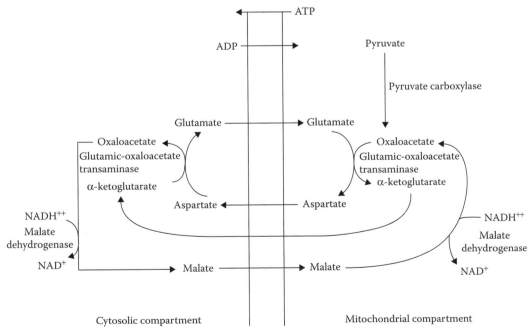

FIGURE 28   Malate aspartate cycle.

TABLE 37
Physical Signs That Are Often Associated with Malnutrition

Area of Body Examined	Normal Appearance	Common Signs of Malnutrition	Other Causes of These Clinical Signs
Appearance in general	Normal weight for age, sex, and height. Alert and emotionally stable. No areas of edema.	Significantly overweight or underweight. Apathetic or hyperirritable. Loss or slowness of ankle or knee reflexes. Pitting edema.	Nonnutritional metabolic disorders. Endocrine disease.
Eyes	Shiny and free from areas of abnormal pigmentation, opacity, vascularization, and dryness.	Paleness, dryness, redness, or pigmentation of membranes (conjunctiva). Foamy patches or conjunctiva (Bitot's spots). Dullness, softness, or vascularization of the cornea. Redness or fissures on eyelids.	Exposure to environmental or chemical irritants. Tissue changes accompanying aging.
Face	Skin is clear and uniform in color, free of all except minor blemishes. Free of swollen or lumpy areas.	Skin has lighter (depigmentation) and darker (over cheeks and under eyes) areas. Greasy scales around nose and lips. Swollen or lumpy areas.	Poor hygiene. Cushing's disease (moon face).
Glands	No swollen areas on face or neck.	Swelling of parotids (enlarged jowls) or thyroid (front of neck near its base).	Mumps. Inflammation, tumor, or hyperfunction of the thyroid.
Gums	Red; free from bleeding or swelling.	Receded. "Spongy" and bleeding. Swelling of the gingiva.	Medication. Periodontal disease. Poor oral hygiene.
Hair	Shiny, firmly attached to scalp (not easily plucked without pain to patient).	Dullness; may be brittle and easily plucked without pain. Sometimes lighter in color than normal (depigmentation may be bandlike when hair is held up to a source of light).	Endocrine disorders.
Lips	Smooth, not chapped, cracked, or swollen.	Swollen, red, corners, cracked (cheilosis).	Herpes (blisters). Exposure to strong sunshine, dry or cold climates.
Muscles	Muscles are firm and of normal size.	Wasting and flabbiness of muscle. Bleeding into muscle.	Wasting diseases. Trauma.
Nails	Firm, pink.	Spoon-shaped nails. Brittle and ridged nails.	Cardiopulmonary disease.
Organs, internal	Normal heart rate and rhythm. Normal blood pressure. Internal organs cannot be palpated (except the liver in children).	Racing heartbeat (over 100 beats/min). Abnormal rhythm of heart. High blood pressure. Palpable enlargement of liver or spleen.	Rheumatic fever. Nonnutritional diseases of the heart, liver, spleen, and kidneys.
Skeleton	Bones have normal sizes and shapes.	Softening, swelling, or distorted shapes of bones and joints.	Nonnutritional connective tissue disorders. Changes with age in porosity.
Skin	Smooth, free of rashes, swellings, and discoloration.	Roughness (follicular hyperkeratosis), dryness, or flakiness. Irregular pigmentation, black and blue marks, "crazy pavement" lesions. Symmetrical, reddened lesions. Looseness of skin (lack of subcutaneous fat).	Secondary syphilis. Poor or improper hygiene. Environmental irritants. Trauma. Anticoagulant therapy.

TABLE 37 (*Continued*)
Physical Signs That Are Often Associated with Malnutrition

Area of Body Examined	Normal Appearance	Common Signs of Malnutrition	Other Causes of These Clinical Signs
Teeth	Enamel is unbroken and unspotted. None or a few small cavities.	Caries. Mottled or darkened areas of enamel.	Developmental abnormalities. Stains from foods or cigarettes.
Tongue	Normal size of papillae (no atrophy or hypertrophy). Color is uniform and deep red. Sense of taste is normal.	Atrophy of papillae (the tongue is smooth) or hypertrophy of papillae. Irregularly shaped and distributed white patches. Swollen, scarlet, magenta (purple-colored), or raw tongue.	Dietary irritants. Colors or dyes from food. Nonnutritional anemias. Antibiotics. Uremia. Malignancy.

Source: Adapted from Ensminger et al. 1994. *Foods and Nutrition Encyclopedia.* 2nd ed., 1351–2. Boca Raton, FL: CRC Press.

MANGANESE

An essential mineral that serves as a cofactor for the enzymes pyruvate carboxylase (converts pyruvate to oxaloacetate) and superoxide dismutase. The latter enzyme also requires copper as a cofactor. (See Minerals.)

MANNITOL

An alcohol of mannose. Also an osmotic diuretic if consumed in sufficient quantity.

MANNOSE

A six-carbon sugar that can be converted to fructose via phosphorylation and isomerization.

MAO

Monoamine oxidase. A copper-containing enzyme that catalyzes the removal of oxygen from epinephrine, tyramine, and serotonin, inactivating them and reducing neuronal activity. Inhibitors of MAO are valuable drugs for treating depression.

MAPLE SYRUP URINE DISEASE

A rare genetic disease due to a mutation in the genes that code for the branched-chain amino acid dehydrogenases. Characterized by mental retardation, ketoacidosis, and early death. The urine of such patients smells like maple syrup, hence the name.

MARASMUS

Condition caused by deficient energy and protein intake. Also called protein calorie malnutrition (PCM). Although children of all ages and adults can suffer from a deficiency of both energy and protein, the marasmic child is usually less than one year old. In developing countries, a common cause for marasmus is the cessation of breast-feeding. Milk production by the mother may have stopped because of the mother's poor health, the mother may have died, or there may be a desire on the part of the mother to bottle-feed her infant rather than breast-feed. This decision to bottle-feed may be made for a variety of reasons. The mother may view bottle-feeding as a status symbol, she may be forced to work to earn a living and may be unable to have her baby with her, or she may not be able to lactate. While under optimal conditions of economics and sanitation the bottle-fed child may be well fed, in emerging nations this is not always true. The mother may not be able to buy the milk formula in sufficient quantities to adequately nourish the child, she may overdilute the milk, or she may use unsafe water and unsanitary conditions to prepare the formula for the child. This, plus the insufficient nutrient content of the milk formula, often precipitously leads to the development of marasmus, a form of starvation characterized by growth failure with prominent ribs, a characteristic monkey-like face, and matchstick limbs with little muscle or adipose tissue development; tissue wastage but not edema is present. Whereas the kwashiorkor child has a poor appetite, the marasmus child is eager to eat. The child is mentally alert but not irritable. Anemia and diarrhea are present for the same reasons as in kwashiorkor. The skin and hair appear to be of normal color.

The treatment of both kwashiorkor and marasmic children must be approached with due care and caution. Because their enzymes for digestion and their protein absorption and transport systems are less active, feeding these children with large quantities of good-quality protein would be harmful. Their diets must be gradually enriched with these proteins to allow their bodies sufficient time to develop the appropriate metabolic pathways to handle a better diet. Giving these children solutions of either predigested proteins or amino acids may be of benefit initially, but these solutions, too, must be used with care. If the amino acids in excess of immediate use are deaminated and if the pathway for synthesizing urea is not fully functional, ammonia can accumulate in the child and become lethal.

Not only must one be concerned about the enzymes of the malnourished child, but also keep in mind that the protein-depleted child is unable to synthesize adequate amounts of the protein hormones that regulate and coordinate his/her use of dietary nutrients. In addition, protein deprivation affects the structures of the cell hormone receptor sites, thus further dampening the effectiveness of those hormones produced. Children with marasmus or kwashiorkor have been shown to have decreased blood sugar levels, decreased serum insulin and growth hormone levels, and, in marasmus, decreased thyroid hormone levels. Additional hormonal changes have been observed, but their relevance to treatment has not been ascertained. Most probably these changes in the levels of the protein-, peptide-, or amino acid–derived hormones are reflective of reduced synthesis of them as a result of a shortage of incoming amino acids. Changes in the steroid hormones probably reflect the response of the child to the stress of deprivation.

MASTITIS

Inflammation of the mammary gland.

MATRIX

Center or formative section of a tissue such as bone.

MCARDLE'S DISEASE

One of the glycogen storage diseases that develops because of a mutation in the gene for muscle phosphorylase; characterized by exercise intolerance.

MCV

Mean corpuscular volume. The ratio of the volume of packed cells to the volume of the blood sample; an indirect measure of the number of red blood cells in a blood sample.

MEAN

Average value for a group of values.

MEAN ARTERIAL PRESSURE

The average of the diastolic and systolic pressures.

MECHANICAL SOFT DIET

Diet characterized by foods that have been altered in texture or form to make them easier to chew and swallow.

MECONIUM

Stool produced by the fetus typically expelled during the first days of life.

MEDIAN

Value where half the values fall below and half fall above this value.

MEDICAL NUTRITION THERAPY

An integral part of the medical treatment for a specific disease state that improves the outcome and speeds up recovery. Components of medical nutrition therapy include nutrition screening, nutrition assessment, and nutrition treatment.

MEDICINAL PLANTS

Plants that "may have" medicinal value. Some are recognized remedies while others are folklore. Table 38 lists some of these plants. Excess intake of some of these may be toxic. Plants and their commercial preparations are highly variable in their active ingredient content.

MEDIUM-CHAIN TRIGLYCERIDES

Fatty acids containing 8–12 carbon atoms.

MEGADOSE

Very large dose.

MEGALOBLAST

Large immature red blood cell.

MEGALOBLASTIC ANEMIA

Anemia characterized by an abundance of large immature nucleated red blood cells. A typical feature of folacin deficiency.

TABLE 38
Plants Used as Herbal Remedies

Common and Scientific Names	Description	Production	Part(s) of Plant Used	Reported Uses
Agrimony *Agrimonia gryposepala*	Small yellow flowers on a long spike; leaves hairy and at least 5 inch (13 cm) long, narrow and pointed; leaf edges toothed; a perennial.	Needs good soil and sunshine; grows in New England and middle Atlantic states.	Whole plant including roots.	A tonic, alterative, diuretic, and astringent; infusions from the leaves for sore throats; treatment of kidney and bladder stones; root for jaundice.
Aletris root (whitetube stargrass) *Aletris farinosa*	Grasslike leaves in a flat rosette around a spike-like stem; white to yellow tubular flowers along stem.	Moist locations in woods, meadows, or bogs; New England to Michigan and Wisconsin; south to Florida and west to Texas.	Leaves; roots.	Poultice of leaves for sore breast; liquid from boiled roots for stomach pains; tonic, sedative, and diuretic.
Alfalfa *Medicago sativa*	Very leafy plant growing 1–2 feet (30–61 cm) high; small green leaves; bluish purple flowers; deep roots.	A legume cultivated widely in the United States.	Leaves.	Powdered and mixed with cider vinegar as a tonic; infusions for a tasty drink; leaves may also be used green.
Aloe vera *Aloe barbadensis*	A succulent plant with leathery sword-shaped leaves, 6–24 inch (15–61 cm) long.	A semidesert plant that grows in Mexico and Hawaii; temperature must remain above 50°F (10°C); can be a house plant.	Mucilaginous juice of the leaves.	Effective on small cuts and sunburn; speeds healing; manufactured product for a variety of cosmetic purposes.
Angelica *Angelica atropurpurea*	Shrub growing to 8 feet (2.4 m) high; stem purplish with three-toothed leaflets at tip of each leaf stem; white or greenish flowers in clusters at end of each stalk.	Grows in rich low soil near streams and swamps and in gardens; from New England, west to Ohio, Indiana, Illinois, and Wisconsin; south to Delaware, Maryland, West Virginia, and Kentucky.	Roots; seeds.	Small amount of dried root or seeds for relief of flatulence; roots for the induction of vomiting and perspiration; roots for treatment of toothache, bronchitis, rheumatism, gout, fever, and to increase menstrual flow.
Anise (anise seed) *Pimpinella anisum*	Annual plant, 1–2 feet (30–61 cm) high; belongs to carrot family; small white flowers on long, hairy stalk; lower leaves egg shaped; upper leaves feathery.	Grown all over the world; grows wild in countries around the Mediterranean; much is imported to United States.	Seed.	As a hot tea to relieve flatulence or for colic.
Asafetida *Ferula sp.*	A coarse plant growing to 7 feet (2.1 m) high with numerous stem leaves; pale green-yellow flowers; flowers and seeds borne in clusters on stalks; large fleshly root; tenacious odor.	Indigenous to Afghanistan, but some species grow in other Asiatic countries.	Gummy resin from the root.	As an antispasmodic; to ward off colds and flu by wearing in a bag around the neck.

Plant	Description	Habitat	Parts Used	Uses
Bayberry (Southern wax myrtle) *Myrica cerifera*	Perennial shrub growing to 30 feet (9.2 m) high; waxy branchlets; narrow evergreen leaves tapering at both ends; yellowish flowers; fruits are grayish berries.	Grows in the coastal regions of New Jersey, Delaware, and Maryland to Florida, Alabama, Mississippi, and Arkansas.	Root bark; leaves and stems.	Decoction of root bark to treat uterine hemorrhage, jaundice, dysentery, and cankers; leaves and stems boiled and used to treat fevers; decoction of boiled leaves for intestinal worms.
Bearberry *Arctostaphylos uva-ursi*	Creeping evergreen shrub with stems up to 6 inch (15 cm) high; reddish bark; bright green leaves, 1 inch (3 cm) long; white flowers with red markings, in clusters; smooth red fruits.	Grows in well-drained soils at higher altitudes; from Oregon, Washington, and California to Colorado and New Mexico.	Leaves.	As a diuretic; boiled infusions used as a drink to treat sprains, stomach pains, and urinary problems; poison oak inflammations treated with leaf decoction by pioneers.
Black cohosh *Cimicifuga racemosa*	Perennial shrub growing to 9 feet (2.7 m) or more in height; leaf has 2–5 leaflets; plant topped with spike of slender candlelike white or yellowish flowers; rhizome gnarled and twisted.	Grows throughout the eastern United States; commercial supply from Blue Ridge Mountains.	Rhizomes and roots.	Infusion and decoctions used to treat sore throat, rheumatism, kidney trouble, and general malaise; also used for "women's ailments" and malaria.
Black walnut *Juglans nigra*	A tree growing up to 120 feet (36.6 m) high; leaflets alternate 12–23 per stem, finely toothed and about 3–3.5 inch (8–9 cm) long; nut occurs singly or in clusters with fleshy, aromatic husk.	Native to a large section of the rich woods of the eastern and Midwestern United States.	Bark; nut husk; leaves.	Inner bark used as a mild laxative; husk of nut used for treating intestinal worms, ulcers, syphilis, and fungus infections; leaf infusion for bedbugs.
Blackberry (brambleberry, dewberry, raspberry) *Rubus* spp.	Shrubby or viny thorny perennial; numerous species; large white flowers; red or black fruit.	Grows wild or in gardens throughout the United States; grows wild in old fields, waste areas, forest borders, and pastures.	Roots; root bark, leaves; fruit.	Infusion made from roots used to dry up runny noses; infusion from root bark to treat dysentery; fruit used to treat dysentery in children; leaves also used in similar manner.
Blessed thistle *Cnicus benedictus*	Annual plant growing to 2 feet (61 cm) high; spiny tooth, lobed leaves; many-flowered yellow heads.	Grows along roadsides and in waste places in eastern and parts of the southwestern United States.	Leaves and flowering tops in full bloom; seeds.	Infusions from leaves and tops for cancer treatment, to induce sweating, as a diuretic, to reduce fever, and for inflammations of the respiratory system; infusion of tops as Indian contraceptive; seeds induce vomiting.

(Continued)

TABLE 38 (*Continued*)
Plants Used as Herbal Remedies

Common and Scientific Names	Description	Production	Part(s) of Plant Used	Reported Uses
Boneset *Eupatorium perfoliatum*	Perennial bush growing to 5 feet (1.5 m) in height; heavy stems with leaves opposite; purplish to white flowers borne in flat heads.	Commonly found in wet areas such as swamps, rich woods, marshes, and pastures; grows from Canada to Florida and west to Texas and Nebraska.	Leaves; flowering tops.	Infusions made from leaves used for laxative and treatment of coughs and chest illnesses; a cold remedy; Negro slaves and Indians used it to treat malaria.
Borage *Borago officinalis*	Entire plant not over 1 feet (30 cm) high; nodding heads of starlike flowers grow from clusters of hairy obovate leaves.	Introduced in the United States from Europe; occasionally grows in waste areas in northern states; cultivated widely in gardens.	Leaves.	Most often used as an infusion to increase sweating, as a diuretic, or to soothe intestinal tract; can be applied to swellings and inflamed areas for relief.
Buchu Rutaceae	Low shrubs with angular branches and small leaves growing in opposition; flowers from white to pink.	Grown in rich soil in the warm climate of South Africa.	Dried leaves.	Prepared as tincture or infusion; used for genitourinary diseases, indigestion, edema, and early stages of diabetes.
Buckthorn *Rhamnus purshiana*	Deciduous tree growing to 25 feet (7.6 m) high; leaves 2–6 inch (5–15 cm) long; flowers small greenish yellow; fruit globular and black, about 1/4 inch (6 mm) across.	Grows usually with conifers along canyon walls, rich bottom lands, and mountain ridges in the western United States.	Bark; fruit.	Bark used as a laxative and tonic; fruit (berries) used as a laxative.
Burdock *Arctium minus*	Biennial or perennial growing to 5–8 feet (1.5–2.4 m) high; large leaves resembling rhubarb; tube-shaped white and pink to purple flowers in heads; brown, bristled burrs contain seeds.	Grows in wastelands, fields, and pastures throughout the United States.	Root.	Infusion of roots for coughs, asthma, and to stimulate menstruation; tincture of root for rheumatism and stomachache.
Calamus (sweet flag) *Acorus calamus*	Perennial growing 3–5 feet (1.0–1.5 m) high; long narrow leaves with sharp edges; aromatic leaves; flower stalk 2–3 inch (3–8 cm) long and clublike; greenish yellow flowers.	Grows in swamps and edges of streams and ponds from New England west to Oregon and Montana, and from Texas east to Florida and north.	Rhizomes.	Root chewed to clear phlegm (mucous) and ease stomach gas; infusions to treat stomach distress; considered useful as tonic and stimulant.

Plant	Description	Distribution	Part Used	Uses
Catnip *Nepeta cataria*	Perennial growing to 3 feet (1 m) in height; stem downy and whitish; leaves heart shaped opposite coarsely toothed and 2–3 inch (3–8 cm) long; tubular and whitish with purplish marked flowers in compact spikes.	Grows wild along fences, roadsides, waste places, and streams in Virginia, Tennessee, West Virginia, Georgia, New England, Illinois, Indiana, Ohio, New Mexico, Colorado, Arizona, Utah, and California; readily cultivated in gardens.	Entire plant.	Infusions for treating colds, nervous disorders, stomach ailments, infant colic, and hives; smoke relieves respiratory ailments; poultice to reduce swellings.
Celery *Apium graveolens*	A biennial producing flower stalk second year; terminal leaflet at end of stem; fruit brown and round.	Cultivated in California, Florida, Michigan, New York, and Washington.	Seeds.	As an infusion to relieve rheumatism and flatulence (gas); to act as a diuretic; to act as a tonic and stimulant; oil from seeds used similarly.
Chamomile *Anthemis nobilis*	Low-growing, pleasantly strong-scented, downy, and matlike perennial; daisylike flowers with white petals and yellow center.	Cultivated in gardens; some are wild growing, which escaped from gardens.	Leaves and flowers.	Powdered and mixed with boiling water to stimulate stomach, to remedy nervousness in women, and stimulate menstrual flow; poultice to relieve pain; chamomile tea known to be soothing; sedative; completely harmless.
Chaparral *Croton corynbulosus*	Shrubby perennial plant of the Spurge family.	Grows in dry rock areas from Texas west.	Flowering tips.	Infusions act as laxative; some claim it useful for cancer treatment.
Chickweed *Stellaria media*	Annual growing, 12–15 inch (30–38 cm) high; stems matted to somewhat upright; upper leaves vary but lower leaves ovate; white, small individual flowers.	Grows in shaded areas, meadows, wasteland, cultivated land, thickets, gardens, and damp woods in Virginia to South Carolina and southeast.	Entire plant in full bloom.	Poultice made to treat sores, ulcers, infections, and hemorrhoids.
Chicory *Cichorium intybus*	Easily confused with its close relative the dandelion; in bloom bears blue or soft pink blooms not resembling dandelions.	Introduced from Europe, now a common wild plant in the United States; some grown in gardens.	Roots; leaves.	No great medicinal value; some mention of diuretic, laxative, and tonic use; mainly added to give coffee a distinctive flavor.
Cinnamon *Cinnamomum zeylanicum*	An evergreen bush or tree growing to 30 feet (9 m) high.	A native plant of Sri Lanka, India, and Malaysia; tree kept pruned to a shrub; bark of lower branches peeled and dried.	Bark.	Treatment for flatulence, diarrhea, vomiting, and nausea.

(Continued)

TABLE 38 (Continued)
Plants Used as Herbal Remedies

Common and Scientific Names	Description	Production	Part(s) of Plant Used	Reported Uses
Cleaver's herb (Catchweed bedstraw) *Galium aparine*	Annual plant; weak, reclining bristled stem with hairy joints; leaves in whorls of eight; white flowers in broad, flat cluster; bristled fruit.	Grows in rich woods, thickets, seashores, waste areas, and shady areas from Canada to Florida and west to Texas.	Entire plant during flowering.	To increase urine formation; to stimulate appetite; to reduce fever; to remedy vitamin C deficiency; also used to remove freckles.
Cloves *Syzygium aromaticum*	Dried flower bud of a tropical tree, which is a 30-feet (9 m) high red-flowered evergreen.	Tree native to Molucca, but widely cultivated in the tropics; flower-bud picked before flower opens, and dried.	Flower bud.	To promote salivation and gastric secretion; to relieve pain in stomach and intestines; applied externally to relieve rheumatism, lumbago, toothache, muscle cramps, and neuralgia; clove oil used, too; infusions with clove powder relieves nausea and vomiting.
Colt's foot (Canada wild ginger) *Asarum canadense*	Low-growing stemless perennial; heart-shaped leaves; flowers near root, brown and bell shaped.	Found in moist woods from Maine to Georgia and west to Ohio.	Roots; leaves.	Infusion of root to relieve flatulence; powdered root to relieve flatulence, induce sweating, and to relieve aching head and eyes; leaves substitute for ginger.
Comfrey *Symphytum officinale*	A perennial that reaches about 2 feet (61 cm) in height; leaves are large and broad at base but lancelike at terminal; fine hair on leaves; tail-shaped head of white to purple flowers at terminal.	Prefers a moist environment; a European plant now naturalized in the United States.	Roots; leaves.	Numerous uses including treatments for pneumonia, coughs, diarrhea, calcium deficiency, colds, sores, ulcers, arthritis, gallstones, tonsils, cuts and wounds, headaches, hemorrhoids, gout, burns, kidney stones, anemia, and tuberculosis; used as a poultice, infusion, powder, or in capsule form.
Dandelion *Taraxacum officinale*	Biennial growing 2–12 inch (5–30 cm) high; leaves deeply serrated forming a basal rosette in spring; yellow flower but turns to gray on maturing.	Weed throughout the United States; the bane of lawns.	Flowers; roots; green leaves.	Root uses include diuretic, laxative, and tonic uses, and used to stimulate appetite; infusion from flower for heart troubles; paste of green leaves and bread dough for bruises.

Plant	Description	Distribution	Part Used	Uses
Echinacea (purple echinacea) *Echinacea purpurea*	Perennial from 2–5 feet (0.6–1.5 m) high; alternate lance-shaped leaves; leaf margins toothed; top leaves lack stems; purple to white flower.	Grows wild on road banks; prairies; and dry, open woods in Ohio to Iowa, south to Oklahoma, Georgia, and Alabama.	Roots.	Treatment of ulcers and boils, syphilis, snakebites, skin diseases, and blood poisoning; used as powder and in capsules.
Eucalyptus *Eucalyptus globulus*	Tall, fragrant tree growing up to 300 feet (92 m) high; reddish brown stringy bark.	Native to Australia but grown in other semitropical and warm temperate regions.	Leaves and oil distilled from leaves.	Antiseptic value; inhaled freely for sore throat; asthma relief; local application to ulcers; used on open wounds.
Eyebright (Indian tobacco) *Lobelia inflata*	Branching annual, growing to 3 feet (1 m) high with leaves 1–3 inch (3–8 cm) long; small violet to pinkish white flowers in axils of leaves; seed capsules at base of flower containing many tiny brown seeds.	Roadside weed of the eastern United States, west to Kansas.	Entire plant in full bloom or when seeds are formed.	Treatment of whooping cough, asthma, epilepsy, pneumonia, hysteria, and convulsion; alkaloid extracted for use in antismoking preparations.
Fenugreek *Trigonella foenum-graceum*	Annual plant similar to clover in size.	Native to the Mediterranean regions and northern India; widely cultivated; easily grown in home gardens.	Seed.	Poultice for wounds; gargle for sore throat.
Flax (linseed) *Linum usitatissimum*	Herbaceous annual; slender upright plant with narrow leaves and blue flowers; grows to about 2 feet (61 cm) high.	Originated in the Mediterranean region; cultivated widely for fiber and oil.	Seed.	Ground flaxseed mixed with boiling water for poultice on burns, boils, carbuncles, and sores; used internally as a laxative.
Garlic *Allium sativum*	Annual plant growing to 12 inch (30 cm) high; long, linear, narrow leaves; bulb composed of several bulblets.	Throughout the United States under cultivation; some wild.	Entire plant when in bloom; bulbs.	Fresh poultice of the mashed plant for treating snakebite, hornet stings, and scorpion stings; eaten to expel worms; treat colds, coughs, hoarseness, and asthma; bulb expressed against the gum for toothache.
Gentian (Sampson snakeroot) *Gentiana villosa*	Perennial with stems growing 8–10 inch (20–25 cm) high; opposite ovate, lance-shaped leaves; pale blue flowers.	Grows wild in swampy areas Florida west to Louisiana, north to New Jersey, Pennsylvania, Ohio, and Indiana.	Rhizomes and roots.	Treatment of indigestion, gout, and rheumatism; induction of vomiting; aid to digestion; a tonic.
Ginger *Zingiber officinale*	Perennial plant; forms irregular-shaped rhizomes at shallow depths.	Native to southeastern Asia; now grown all over the tropics.	Rhizome.	An expectorant; treatment of flatulence, colds, and sore throats.

(Continued)

TABLE 38 (Continued)
Plants Used as Herbal Remedies

Common and Scientific Names	Description	Production	Part(s) of Plant Used	Reported Uses
Ginseng *Panax quinquefolia*	Hollow stems solid at nodes; leaves alternate; root often resembles shape of a man; small, inconspicuous flowers; vivid, shiny, scarlet berries.	Grows in eastern Asia, Korea, China, and Japan; some grown in the United States.	Root.	As a tonic and stimulant; treatment of convulsions, dizziness, vomiting, colds, fevers, headaches, and rheumatism; commonly believed to be an aphrodisiac.
Goldenrod *Solidago odora*	Grows 18–36 inch (46–91 cm) high with narrow leaves scented like anise; inconspicuous head with 6–8 flowers.	Grows throughout the United States.	Leaves.	Infusions from dried leaves as aromatic stimulant, a carminative, and a diuretic.
Goldenseal *Hydrastis canadensis*	Perennial growing to about 1 feet (30 cm) high; one stem with 5–7 lobed leaves near the top; several single leafstalks topped with petalless flowers; raspberry-like fruit but inedible.	Grows in rich, shady woods of southeastern and the midwestern United States; grown under cultivation in Washington.	Roots, leaves, and stalks.	Root infusion as an appetite stimulant and tonic; root powder for open cuts and wounds; chewing root for mouth sores; leaf infusion for liver and stomach ailments.
Guarana *Paullinia cupana*	Climbing shrub of the soapberry family; yellow flowers; pear-shaped fruit; seed in three-sided, three-celled capsules.	Grows in South America, particularly Brazil and Uruguay.	Seeds.	Stimulant; seeds high in caffeine.
Hawthorn *Crataegus oxycantha*	Hardy shrub or tree depending on growth conditions; small, berry fruit; cup-shaped flowers with five parts; thorny stems.	Originally grown throughout England in hedges; also grows wild; some introduced in the United States.	Berry.	Tonic for heart ailments such as angina pectoris, valve defects, rapid and feeble heart beat, and hypertrophied heart; reverses arteriosclerosis.
Hop *Humulus lupulus*	Twining, perennial growing 20 feet (6 m) or more; 3 smooth-lobed leaves 4–5 inch (10–13 cm) long; membranous, conelike fruit.	Grows throughout the United States; often a cultivated crop.	Fruit (hops).	Straight hops or powder used; hot poultice of hops for boils and inflammations; treatment of fever, worms, and rheumatism; as a diuretic; as a sedative.

Plant	Description	Distribution	Parts Used	Uses
Horehound (white horehound) *Marrubium vulgare*	Shrub growing to 3 feet (1 m) in height; fuzzy ovate-round leaves that are whitish above and gray below; foliage aromatic when crushed.	Grows wild throughout most of the United States in pastures, old fields, and waste places, except in arid southwest.	Leaves and small stems; bark.	Decoctions to treat coughs, colds, asthma, and hoarseness; other uses include treatment for diarrhea, menstrual irregularity, and kidney ailments.
Huckleberry (sparkleberry) *Vaccinium arboreum*	Shrub or tree growing to 25 feet (7.6 m) high; leathery; shiny; thick leaves; white flowers; black berries; other species.	Grows wild in woods, clearings, sandy and dry woods in Virginia, Georgia, Florida, Mississippi, Indiana, Illinois, Missouri, Texas, and Oklahoma.	Leaves, root bark, and berries.	Decoctions of leaves and root bark to treat sore throat and diarrhea; drink from berry for treating chronic dysentery.
Hyssop *Hyssopus officinalis*	Hardy, fragrant, bushy plants belonging to the mint family; stem woody; leaves hairy, pointed, and about 1/2 inch (20 mm) long; blue flowers in tufts.	Grows in various parts of Europe including the Middle East; some grown in the United States.	Leaves.	Infusions for colds, coughs, tuberculosis, and asthma; an aromatic stimulant; healing agent for cuts and bruises.
Juniper (common juniper) *Juniperus communis*	Small evergreen shrub growing 12–30 feet (3.7–9.2 m) high; bark of trunk reddish brown and tends to shred; needles straight and at right angles to branchlets; dark, purple, fleshy berrylike fruit.	Widely distributed from New Mexico to the Dakotas and east; dry areas.	Fruit (berries).	Used as a diuretic, to induce menstruation, to relieve gas, and to treat snakebites and intestinal worms.
Lemon balm *Melissa officinalis*	Persistent perennial growing to 1 feet (30 cm) high; light green, serrated leaves; lemon smell and taste to crushed leaves.	Wild in much of the United States; grown in gardens.	Leaves.	Infusion used as a carminative, diaphoretic, or febrifuge.
Licorice (wild licorice) *Glycyrrhiza lepidota*	Erect perennial growing to 3 feet (1 m) high; pale yellow to white flowers at end of flower stalks; brown seed pods resemble cockleburs.	Grows wild on prairies, lakeshores, and railroad right-of-ways throughout much of the United States.	Root.	Caution: Licorice raises the blood pressure of some people dangerously high, due to the retention of sodium. Root extract to help bring out phlegm (mucus); treatment of stomach ulcers, rheumatism, and arthritis; root decoctions for inducing menstrual flow, treating fevers, and expulsion of afterbirth.

(Continued)

TABLE 38 (Continued)
Plants Used as Herbal Remedies

Common and Scientific Names	Description	Production	Part(s) of Plant Used	Reported Uses
Marshmallow *Althaea officinalis*	Stems erect and 3–4 feet (0.9–1.2 m) high with only a few lateral branches; roundish, ovate-cordate leaves 2–3 inch (5–8 cm) long and irregularly toothed at margin; cup-shaped, pale-colored flowers.	Introduced into the United States from Europe; now found on banks of tidal rivers and brackish streams; grows wild in salt marshes, damp meadows, by ditches, by the sea, and banks of tidal rivers from Denmark south.	Root.	Primarily a demulcent and emollient; used in cough remedies; good poultice made from crushed roots.
Motherwort *Leonurus cardiaca*	Perennial growing 5–6 feet (1.5–1.8 m) high; lobed, dented leaves, 5 inch (13 cm) long; very fuzzy white to pink flowers.	Grows wild in pastures, waste places, and roadsides from northeastern states west to Montana and Texas, south to North Carolina and Tennessee.	Entire plant above ground.	Used as a stimulant, tonic, and diuretic; Europeans used this for asthma and heart palpitation; usually taken as an infusion.
Mullien (Aaron's rod) *Verbascum thapsus*	At base a rosette of woody, lance-shaped, oblong leaves with a diameter of up to 2 feet (61 cm); yellow flowers along a clublike spike arising from the rosette to a height of up to 7 feet (2.1 m).	Grows wild throughout the United States in dry fields, meadows, pastures, rocky or gravelly banks, burned areas, etc.	Leaves; roots; flowers.	Infusions of leaves to treat colds and dysentery; dried leaves and flowers serve as a demulcent and emollient; leaves smoked for asthma relief; boiled roots for croup; oil from flowers for earache; local applications of leaves for hemorrhoids, inflammations, and sunburn.
Nutmeg *Muristica fragrans*	Evergreen tree growing to about 25 feet (7.6 m) high; grayish-brown, smooth bark; fruit resembles yellow plum, the seed of which is known as nutmeg.	Native to the Spice Islands of Indonesia; now cultivated in other tropical areas.	Seed.	For the treatment of nausea and vomiting; grated and mixed with lard for hemorrhoid ointment.
Papaya *Carica papaya*	Small tree seldom above 20 feet (6.1 m) high; soft, spongy wood; leaves as large as 2 feet (61 cm) in diameter and deeply cut into seven lobes; fruit oblong and dingy green-yellow.	Originated in the South American tropics; now cultivated in tropical climates.	Leaves.	Dressing for wounds and an aid for digestion; contains proteolytic enzyme, papain, used as a meat tenderizer.

Plant	Description	Distribution	Parts Used	Uses
Parsley *Petroselinum crispum*	Biennial that is usually grown as an annual; finely divided, often curled, fragrant leaves.	Originated in the Mediterranean area; now grown worldwide.	Leaves; seeds; roots.	As a diuretic with aromatic and stimulating properties.
Passion flower (maypop passion-flower) *Passiflora incarnata*	Perennial vine growing to 30 feet (9.2 m) in length; alternate leaves composed of 3–5 finely toothed lobes; showy, vivid, purple, flesh-colored flowers; smooth, yellow ovate fruit 2–3 inch (5–8 cm) long.	Grows wild in the West Indies and the southern United States; cultivated in many areas.	Flowering and fruiting tops.	Crushed parts for poultice to treat bruises and injuries; other uses include treatment of nervousness, insomnia, fevers, and asthma.
Peppermint *Mentha piperita*	Perennial growing to about 3.5 feet (1 m) high; dark, green, toothed leaves; purplish flowers in spikelike groups.	Originated in temperate regions of the Old World where most is still grown; grows in shady, damp areas in many areas of the United States; grown in gardens.	Flowering tops; leaves.	Infusions for relief of flatulence, nausea, headache, and heartburn; fresh leaves rubbed into skin to relieve local pain; extracted oil contains medicinal properties.
Plantain *Plantago* sp.	Low perennial with broad leaves; flowers on erect spikes.	Grows wild throughout the United States in poor soils, fields, lawns, and edges of woods.	Leaves; seeds; root.	Infusion of leaves for a tonic; seeds for laxative; soaking seeds provides sticky gum for lotions; fresh, crushed leaves to reduce swelling of bruised body parts; fresh, boiled roots applied to sore nipples.
Pleurisy root (butterfly milkweed) *Asclepias tuberosa*	Leafy perennial growing to 3 feet (1 m) high; alternate leaves that are 2–6 inch (5–15 cm) long and narrow; bright orange flowers in a cluster; root spindle-shaped with knotty crown.	Grows in sandy, dry soils; pastures, roadsides, and gardens; south to Florida and west to Texas and Arizona.	Root.	Small doses of dried root as a diaphoretic, diuretic, expectorant, and alternative; ground roots fresh or dried for poultice to treat sores.
Queen's delight *Stillingia sylvatica*	Perennial growing to 3 feet (1 m) high; contains milky juice; leathery, fleshy, stemless leaves; yellow flowers.	Grows wild in dry woods, sandy soils, and old fields; Virginia to Florida, Kansas, and Texas, north to Oklahoma.	Root.	Treatment of infectious diseases; as an alterative.

(Continued)

TABLE 38 (Continued)
Plants Used as Herbal Remedies

Common and Scientific Names	Description	Production	Part(s) of Plant Used	Reported Uses
Red clover *Trifolium pratense*	Biennial or perennial legume less than 2 feet (61 cm) high; three oval-shaped leaflets form leaf; flowers globe shaped and rose to purple colored.	Throughout the United States; some wild, some cultivated.	Entire plant in full bloom.	Infusions to treat whooping cough; component of salves for sores and ulcers; flowers as sedative; to relieve gastric distress and improve the appetite.
Rosemary *Rosmarinus officinalis*	Low-growing perennial evergreen shrub; leaves about 1 inch (3 cm) in height; orange-yellow flowers; white, shiny seeds.	Native to the Mediterranean region; now cultivated in most of Europe and the Americas.	Leaves.	Used as a tonic, astringent, diaphoretic, stimulant, carminative, and nervine.
Saffron (safflower) *Carthamus tinctorius*	Annual with alternate spring leaves; grows to 3 feet (1 m) in height; orange-yellow flowers; white, shiny seeds.	Wild in Afghanistan; cultivated in the United States, primarily in California.	Flowers; seeds; entire plant in bloom.	Paste of flowers and water applied to boils; flowers soaked in water to make a drink to reduce fever, as a laxative, to induce perspiration, to stimulate menstrual flow, and to dry up skin symptoms of measles.
Sage (garden sage) *Salvia officinalis*	Fuzzy perennial belonging to the mint family; leaves with toothed edges; terminal spikes bearing blue or white flowers in whorls.	Originated in the Mediterranean area where it grows wild and is cultivated; grown throughout the United States, some wild.	Leaves.	Treatment for wounds and cuts, sores, coughs, colds, and sore throat; infusions used as a laxative and to relieve flatulence; major use for treatment of dyspepsia.
Sarsaparilla *Smilax* sp.	Climbing evergreen shrub with prickly stems; leaves round to oblong; small, globular berry for fruit.	Grown in tropical areas of Central and South America and in Japan and China.	Root.	Primarily an alterative; regarded as an aphrodisiac; for colds and fevers; to relieve flatulence; best used as an infusion.
Sassafras *Sassafras album*	Tree growing to 40 feet (12.2 m) high; leaves may be three-lobed, two-lobed, mitten shaped, or unlobed; yellowish-green flowers in clusters; pea-sized, one-seeded berries in fall.	Originated in the new world; grows in New England, New York, Ohio, Illinois, and Michigan, south to Florida and Texas; grows along roadsides, in woods, along fences, and in fields.	Root bark.	Sassafras was formerly used for medical purposes, but the use of the roots was banned by the Food and Drug Administration (FDA) because of their carcinogenic qualities.

Plant	Description	Habitat	Part Used	Uses
Saw palmetto *Serenoa serrulata*	Low-growing fan palm; whitish bloom covers sawtoothed, green leaves; flowers in branching clusters; fruit varies in size and shape.	Grows in warm, swampy, low areas near the coast.	Fruit (berries).	To improve digestion; to treat respiratory infections; as a tonic and as a sedative.
Senna (wild senna) *Cassia marilandica*	Perennial growing to 6 feet (1.8 m) in height; alternate leaves with leaflets in pairs of 5–10; bright yellow flowers.	Grows along roadsides and in thickets from Pennsylvania to Kansas and Iowa, south to Texas and Florida.	Leaves.	Infusions primarily employed as a laxative.
Skullcap *Scutellaria lateriflora*	Perennial growing 1–2 feet (30–61 cm) high; toothed, lance-shaped leaves; blue or whitish flowers.	Native to most sections of the United States; prefers moist woods, damp areas, meadows, and swampy areas.	Entire plant in bloom.	Powdered plant primarily a nervine.
Spearmint *Mentha spicata*	Perennial resembling other mints; grows to 3 feet (1 m) in height; pink or white flowers borne in long spikes.	Throughout the United States in damp places; cultivated in Michigan, Indiana, and California.	Above ground parts.	Primarily a carminative; administered as an infusion through extracted oils.
Tansy *Tanacetum vulgare*	Perennial growing to 3 feet (1 mg) in height; pungent fernlike foliage with tops of composite heads of buttonlike flowers.	Grown or escaped into the wild in much of the United States.	Leaves and flowering tops.	Infusions used as stomachic, emmenagogue, or to expel intestinal worms; extracted oil induces abortion often with fatal results; poultice for sprains and bruises.
Valerian *Valeriana officinalis*	Coarse perennial growing to 5 feet (1.5 m) high; fragrant, pinkish-white flowers opposite pinnate leaves.	Native to Europe and Northern Asia; cultivated in the United States.	Root.	As a calmative and as a carminative.
Witch hazel *Hamamelis virginiana*	Crooked tree or shrub 8–15 feet (2.4–4.6 m) in height; roundish to oval leaves; yellow, threadlike flowers; fruits in clusters along the stem eject shiny, black seeds.	Found in damp woods of North America from Nova Scotia to Florida and west to Minnesota and Texas.	Leaves, bark, and twigs.	Twigs, leaves, and bark basis for witch hazel extract, which is included in many lotions for bruises, sprains, and shaving; bark sometimes applied to tumors and skin inflammations; some preparations for treating hemorrhoids.
Yerba santa *Eriodictyon californicum*	Evergreen shrub with lance-shaped leaves.	Part of flora of the west coast of the United States.	Leaves.	As an expectorant; recommended for asthma and hay fever.

Source: Adapted from Ensminger et al. 1994. *Foods and Nutrition Encyclopedia.* 2nd ed., 1432–41. Boca Raton, FL: CRC Press.

MELANIN

Skin pigment.

MELANOCORTIN 4-RECEPTOR (MC4R)

A protein that binds melanocortin; the gene for this receptor has several variants. If there is an insufficient number of normal receptors, obesity can result.

MELATONIN

Hormone produced by the pineal gland in response to darkness. Its production and release is suppressed by light. The function of melatonin in humans is unclear. It may have a role in human sleep-wake cycles.

MELOXICAM

Nonsteroidal anti-inflammatory; analgesic. Trade name: Mobic.

MEMBRANE COMPOSITION

There are three major classes of lipids in membranes: (1) glycolipids, (2) cholesterol, and (3) phospholipids. Glycolipids have a role in the cell surface–associated antigens as well as cell-surface receptors, whereas cholesterol serves to regulate fluidity. Phospholipids have fatty acids attached at carbons 1 and 2. It is usual to find a saturated fatty acid attached at carbon 1 and an unsaturated fatty acid at carbon 2. In addition, phosphatidylethanolamine and phosphatidylserine usually have fatty acids that are more unsaturated than PI and phosphatidylcholine. Less than 10% of the membrane phospholipid is PI. Plasma membranes have no cardiolipin, and the mitochondrial membranes have very little phosphatidylserine. Several of these phospholipids have important roles in the signal transduction processes that mediate the action of a variety of hormones. Phosphatidylinositol and its role in the PI cycle is one of the most important. Phosphatidylcholine and phosphatidylethanolamine also play a role in these systems. The PIP cycle functions in moving the calcium ion from its intracellular store to the inner aspect of the cell membrane where it stimulates protein kinase C. Phosphatidylinositol also serves to anchor glycoproteins to the membrane. Glycoproteins are tethered to the external aspect of the plasma membrane and play a role in the cell recognition process. Antigens, pathogens, and foreign proteins are recognized by these structures.

MEMBRANE-AFFECTING BACTERIAL TOXINS

See also Food-Borne Illness. An example of bacteria producing these toxins is *Staphylococcus aureus*. They are nonmotile, gram-positive, nonspore-forming, facultative anaerobic bacteria, which produce several enzymes and toxins. The enzymes include coagulase (both free and bound to cell membrane staphylokinase), hydraluronidase, phosphatase, proteinase, lipase, and gelatinase. The toxins produced by *Staphylococcus aureus* are aexotoxin (lethal, dermonecrotic, hemolytic, and leucolytic), b exotoxin (hemolytic), g exotoxin (hemolytic), d exotoxin (dermonecrotic and hemolytic), leucocidin (leucolytic), exfoliative toxin (causing the scalded skin syndrome in skin infections), and enterotoxins.

Enterotoxins, which are simple proteins with molecular weights of 30,000–35,000 Da, can be specified as enterotoxin type A, B, C, D, or E. Characteristics of enterotoxins are as follows:

- Heat stability (enterotoxin B is the most heat stable: heating for 87 minutes at 99°C destroys the activity of type B, whereas only 1 minute at 100°C destroys 100% of the activity of type A and 80% of the activity of type D)

- Resistance to proteolytic enzymes such as trypsin, chymotrypsin, and papain
- Resistance to irradiation (type B only)

It has been observed that the type A strain is the most common, accounting for about 50% of the total number of enterotoxin-producing strains. The next most common type is D, whereas type B is less common. Strains producing both types A and D together are also significant in number (27%). The estimated toxic dose of enterotoxin for humans is probably <1 mg. Concerning the enterotoxin levels in foods involved in poisoning outbreaks (canned prawns: 6–9 mg/100 g; trifles: 5 mg/100 g; tongue and beef: 4 mg/100 g; ham: 5–8 mg/100 g; cold chicken: 2–4 mg/100 g; vanilla cake: <1 mg/100 g; torta cream cake: 2 mg/100 g; ham and potato: 2.5 mg/100 g), consumption of less than 100 g of food will have enough toxin to elicit poisoning. Symptoms of enterotoxin poisoning, developing after 0.5–6 hours following the consumption of contaminated food, include vomiting, diarrhea, and, in severe cases, enteritis. Other symptoms are salivation, nausea, abdominal cramps, prostration, headache, muscular cramps, sweating, fever or hypothermia, hypotension, and presence of mucus and blood in the vomitus and stools. The disease is rarely fatal.

Factors affecting growth of *Staphylococcus aureus* and production of enterotoxins include the following:

- Substrates and nutritional requirements (amino acids: arginine and cystine; vitamins: thiamin, nicotinic acid, biotin, and pantothenic acid; metals and other minerals: calcium, magnesium, and potassium; energy sources)
- Temperature (growth of staphylococci and toxin production occur between 10°C and 45°C; the optimum temperature is 35°C–37°C)
- Acidity (toxin production occurs between pH 5 and pH 9)
- Effects of salts (*Staphylococcus aureus* is very salt resistant: growth can occur in the presence of NaCl levels up to 14%)
- Effect of moisture content (aerobic growth occurs with a water activity between 0.86 and 0.99) and drying (*Staphylococcus aureus* is resistant to drying or a dry environment)
- Effects of other microorganisms growing with *Staphylococcus aureus* on specific substrates (*Staphylococcus aureus* cannot compete effectively with other microorganisms growing on food)
- Other inhibitors (antibiotics such as streptomycin inhibit toxin production without interfering with the growth)

Sources of enterotoxins of *Staphylococcus aureus* include nose and throat discharges; hands and skin; and infected cuts, wounds, burns, boils, pimples, acne, and feces. The principal food types in which bacterial contamination of *Staphylococcus aureus* occurs are cooked ham and other meat products; cream-filled pastry; potato, ham, poultry, and fish salads; milk, cheese, and shrimp; and other low-acid foods stored and served between 5°C and 55°C. Prevention of Staphylococcal food poisoning focuses on three factors:

(1) The human contaminator (adequate personal hygiene, cleanliness, and good disinfection practice)
(2) The food product (heating)
(3) The storage and handling of food products prior to consumption (refrigerated storage and, if possible, avoidance of preparation of food products in multiple steps, in large quantities, and far in advance)

MEMBRANES

The physical boundaries of cells and cell compartments. Membranes exist as a lipid bilayer because phospholipids have amphipathic characteristics. They have both polar (the phosphorylated substituent at carbon 3) and nonpolar (the fatty acids) regions. The polar region is hydrophilic and is positioned such that it is in contact with the aqueous media around and within the cells. The nonpolar or fatty acid region is oriented toward the center of the bilayer so that it is protected from contact with the contents of the cell and the fluids that surround it.

MENADIONE

Synthetic vitamin K; vitamin K_3.

MENAQUINONE

Vitamin K_2; form found in animal cells.

MENARCHE

Beginning of estrus cycles.

MENKES DISEASE

A rare genetic disorder of copper absorption. The defect is in the mechanism for copper absorption by the enterocyte. Symptoms are those of copper deficiency. The mutation is in the ATP7A gene that encodes the copper transporter P-type ATPase.

MENOPAUSE

Cessation of estrus cycles.

MERCURY

A toxic mineral that may be a contaminant of ocean fish and fish oils. Halibut, tilefish, king mackerel, tuna, and swordfish contain more mercury than perch, flounder, and tilapia.

MESSENGER RNA (mRNA)

A single strand of purine and pyrimidine bases synthesized in the nucleus so that its base sequence complements DNA. The mRNA leaves the nucleus, attaches to the ribosome, and provides the code for the synthesis of a single protein. Each protein has its own mRNA template. (See Protein Synthesis.)

METABOLIC ACIDOSIS

Acid-base imbalance associated with shock, diabetes, starvation, alcoholism, renal failure, or severe diarrhea and characterized by shortness of breath, lethargy, confusion, drowsiness, flushed and warm skin, hypotension, stupor, and coma.

METABOLIC ALKALOSIS

Acid-base imbalance associated with vomiting and gastric drainage, prolonged diuretic therapy, Cushing's syndrome, or excessive ingestion of bicarbonate and characterized by slow and shallow respiration, dizziness, paresthesia, confusion, agitation, seizures, and coma.

METABOLIC CONTROL

The regulation of the rates at which metabolic pathways function and interact.

METABOLIC REACTION

A food-intolerance reaction resulting from the effect of a food product on a metabolic abnormality of the host. Examples include the problems associated with missing or deficient digestive enzyme activity.

METABOLIC SYNDROME

Syndrome featuring hypertension, diabetes, and obesity.

METABOLIC WATER

Water formed as a result of metabolic reactions.

METABOLISM

The sum of all the anabolic and catabolic reactions that take place in the body.

METABOLITE

An intermediate formed in the course of a metabolic pathway.

METABOLIZABLE ENERGY (ME)

The energy in food corrected for the energy lost in feces, urine, and combustible gas:

$$ME = IE - (FE + UE + GE)$$

METALLOENZYME

An enzyme containing a mineral as an integral part of its structure.

METALLOPEPTIDASES

Mammalian cell-surface enzymes that participate in the postsecretory processing and metabolism of neuropeptides and peptide hormones.

METALLOTHIONEIN

A carrier for certain minerals such as zinc.

METASTASIS

Migration of abnormal proliferative cells as in cancer.

MET-ENKEPHALIN

A hormone produced by the pars distalis of the anterior pituitary. It arises from the same gene product as ACTH. The function of this hormone in humans is unclear.

METFORMIN

A drug used as a hypoglycemic agent. It is a biguanide. Trade names: Glucophage and Glucophage XR.

METHIONINE

An essential amino acid (see Table 5). Methionine serves as an essential methyl donor for the synthesis of many compounds. Sulfur is conserved through its interconversion to cysteine, as shown in Figure 29.

METHOTREXATE, METHOTREXATE SODIUM

An antimetabolite that interferes with the action of the vitamin, folic acid. This drug also suppresses the immune system and serves as an antineoplastic drug. Trade names: Folex PFS, Mexate-AQ, Rheumatrex.

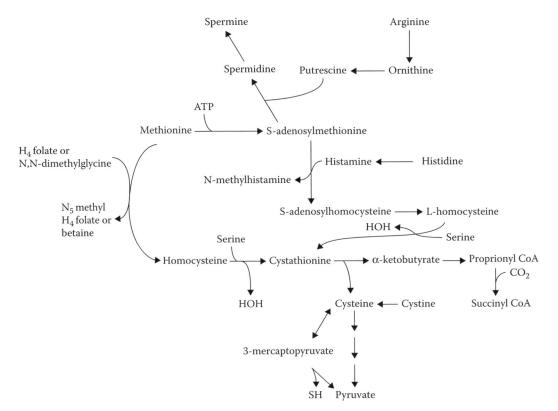

FIGURE 29   Conservation of SH groups via methionine cysteine interconversion.

METHYLDOPA, METHYLDOPA HYDROCHLORIDE

A drug that is an antihypertensive and an anticholinergic compound. Trade names: Aldomet, Apo-Methyldopa, Dopamet, Novo-Medopa.

METHYLMALONIC ACIDEMIA

Accumulation of methyl malonic acid in the blood; can be due to a genetic error, but also is a characteristic of vitamin B_{12} deficiency.

METHYLSELENOL

A selenium metabolite having anticancer activity.

METOCLOPRAMIDE HYDROCHLORIDE

A derivative of para-amino benzoic acid used as an antiemetic. It is also a gastrointestinal tract (GI) stimulant. Trade names: Apo-Metaclop, Clopra, Maxidon, MetaclopramideIntensol, Octamide, Raclomide, Raglan.

METOLAZONE

A quinazoline derivative that acts as a diuretic and an antihypertensive. Trade names: Mykrox, Zaroxolyn.

METOPROLOL SUCCINATE OR TARTRATE

A beta blocker and antihypertensive. Trade names: Toprol-XL, Apo-Metoprolol, Lopressor.

METYRAPONE

A compound that inhibits the production of the adrenal steroids, the glucocorticoids.

MGA

Measured genotype analysis.

MICELLES

See Lipid Absorption.

MICROANGIOPATHY

Thickening of the capillary basement membrane.

MICROCYTIC HYPOCHROMIC ANEMIA

Anemia characterized by a low number of small red blood cells that contain less than the normal amount of hemoglobin (see Table 9).

MICROFLORA

Advantageous bacteria that thrive in the gastrointestinal tract.

MICRONUTRIENTS

A group of nutrients (vitamins and minerals) required in small amounts.

MICROSATELLITE MARKER

A dispersed group of 2–5 base sequences that are repeated up to 50 times. May occur at 50–100 locations in the genome. Used in linkage analysis.

MICROSATELLITE POLYMORPHISM

Heterozygosity of a certain microsatellite marker in an individual.

MICROVASCULAR

Capillaries; vessels of a diameter sufficient for the passage of red blood cells one at a time.

MID-ARM CIRCUMFERENCE

An anthropometric measure used to calculate total arm area as part of an estimate of body fat and muscle mass.

MIGLITOL

An α-glucosidase inhibitor that may have use as a hypoglycemic agent. Trade name: Glyset.

MILK ALKALI SYNDROME

Condition resulting from excessive ingestion of milk and absorbable antacids, which causes increased serum calcium and renal dysfunction.

MILLIEQUIVALENT

A measurement of the concentration of electrolytes in solution that is determined by multiplying the milligrams per liter by the valence of the chemical and dividing by the molecular weight of the substance:

$$mEq/L = (mg/L) \cdot valence/molecular\ weight$$

A measurement of the osmotic activity of a solution that is determined by dividing the milliequivalent value by its valence.

MINERALCORTICOID

See Aldosterone.

MINERALS

Minerals are essential for the growth and maintenance of cells and metabolic systems. They are divided into three categories: (1) macrominerals (calcium, phosphorus, sodium, chlorine, and magnesium), (2) microminerals (iron, zinc, and copper), and (3) the ultratrace minerals (chromium, fluorine, silicon, arsenic, boron, vanadium, nickel, cadmium, lithium, lead, selenium, iodine, molybdenum, manganese, and cobalt). Some of the ultratrace minerals are very toxic, that is, arsenic, cadmium, and lead. Almost all of the minerals can be toxic if consumed in large amounts. However, many are poorly absorbed and this protects the body somewhat from toxic intakes. Sodium and potassium salts are readily soluble in water and thus available for uptake from the intestine. Several other elements, such as iron, calcium, and phosphorus, are present in complex salts that are relatively insoluble. These elements are not easily absorbed from the gut. After intake, the major part of insoluble salts appears in the feces. Minerals are important constituents of bones and teeth. Minerals may be integral parts of biologically important compounds such as hemoglobin and cytochromes. Minerals also serve as required cofactors for enzymatic reactions. Minerals may be divided into two groups based on the levels at which they occur in the body: (1) elements that are present in considerable amounts (e.g., iron, calcium, sodium, potassium, chlorine, magnesium, and phosphorus; combined mass: ±3 kg), and (2) elements that are required in very small amounts only, the so-called trace elements (e.g., zinc, iodine, selenium, copper, manganese, fluorine, chromium, and molybdenum; combined mass: ±30 g). Mineral-mineral interactions occur that can reduce or increase availability. An example of positive interactions is that of calcium and phosphorus. When present in equal amounts both are better absorbed than when one is present in great excess of the other. Example of negative effects is the negative effect of copper on zinc absorption. The individual minerals are described next.

Calcium (Ca)

The primary function of calcium is to build the bones and teeth and to maintain the bones. Calcium also functions in blood clotting; muscle contraction and relaxation, especially the heart muscles; nerve transmission; cell wall permeability; enzyme activation; and the secretion of a number of hormones and hormone-releasing factors. Deficiency symptoms include stunting of growth, poor-quality bones and teeth, and malformation of bones (rickets). Osteomalacia is the adult counterpart of rickets.

Osteoporosis, a condition of too little calcium in the bone, results when bone resorption exceeds bone formation. Hypercalcemia can occur and is characterized by high serum calcium levels. Tetany and kidney stones are sometimes related to abnormal calcium metabolism.

Regarding toxicity, normally, the small intestine prevents excess calcium from being absorbed. However, a breakdown of this control may raise the level of calcium in the blood and lead to calcification of the kidneys and other internal organs.

High calcium intake may cause excess secretion of calcitonin and very dense bones. High calcium intakes have also been reported to cause kidney stones. Good food sources include cheeses, wheat-soy flour, blackstrap molasses, milk, and milk products. Calcium is the most abundant mineral in the body. It comprises about 40% of the total mineral present; 99% of it is in the bones and teeth.

Generally, nutritionists recommend a calcium–phosphorus ratio of 1.5:1 in infancy, decreasing to 1:1 at 1 year of age, and remaining at 1:1 throughout the rest of life; but they consider ratios between 2:1 and 1:2 to be satisfactory.

Phosphorus (P)

Essential for bone formation and maintenance; important in the development of teeth; essential for normal milk secretion; important in building muscle tissue. Phosphorus is a component of nucleic acids (RNA and DNA), which are important in genetic transmission and control of cellular metabolism: energy utilization, phospholipid formation; amino acid metabolism; protein formation; and enzyme systems.

Deficiency symptoms include general weakness, loss of appetite, muscle weakness, bone pain, and loss of calcium. Severe and prolonged deficiencies of phosphorus may be manifested by rickets, osteomalacia, and other phosphorus-related diseases.

Regarding toxicity, there is no known phosphorus toxicity per se. However, excess phosphate consumption may cause hypocalcemia (a deficiency of calcium in the blood). Phosphorous is present in cocoa powder, cottonseed flour, fish flour, peanut flour, pumpkin and squash seeds, rice bran, rice polish, soybean flour, sunflower seeds, wheat, and bran. Phosphorus comprises about one-fourth the total mineral matter in the body. Eighty percent of the phosphorus is in the bones and teeth in inorganic combination with calcium. Normally, 70% of the ingested phosphorus is absorbed.

Generally, nutritionists recommend a calcium–phosphorus ratio of 1.5:1 in infancy, decreasing to 1:1 at 1 year of age, and remaining at 1:1 throughout the rest of life; but they consider ratios between 2:1 and 1:2 as satisfactory.

SODIUM (NA)

Helps to maintain the balance of water, acids, and bases in the fluid outside the cells. A constituent of pancreatic juice, bile, sweat, and tears. Associated with muscle contraction and nerve functions. Plays a specific role in the absorption of carbohydrates. Deficiency symptoms include reduced growth, loss of appetite, loss of body weight due to loss of water, reduced milk production in lactating mothers, muscle cramps, nausea, diarrhea, and headache. Excess perspiration and salt depletion may be accompanied by heat exhaustion.

Regarding toxicity, salt may be toxic when a high intake is accompanied by a restriction of water. Table salt, processed meat products, and pickled/cured products are good source of sodium. Deficiencies of sodium may occur when there has been heavy and prolonged sweating, diarrhea, vomiting, or adrenal cortical insufficiency. In such cases, additional sodium should be provided.

CHLORINE (CL)

Plays a major role in the regulation of osmotic pressure, water balance, and acid-base balance. Required for the production of hydrochloric acid in the stomach; this acid is necessary for the proper absorption of vitamin B_{12} and iron, for the activation of the enzyme that breaks down starch, and for suppressing the growth of microorganisms that enter the stomach with food and drink.

Severe deficiencies may result in alkalosis (an excess of alkali in the blood), which is characterized by slow and shallow breathing, listlessness, muscle cramps, loss of appetite, and, occasionally, convulsions. Deficiencies of chloride may develop from prolonged and severe vomiting, diarrhea, pumping of the stomach, and injudicious use of diuretic drugs.

Regarding toxicity, an excess of chlorine ions is unlikely when the kidneys are functioning properly. Food sources include table salt (sodium chloride) and foods that contain salt. Persons whose sodium intake is severely restricted (owing to diseases of the heart, kidney, or liver) may need an alternative source of chloride; a number of chloride-containing salt substitutes are available for this purpose.

MAGNESIUM (MG)

Constituent of bones and teeth. Essential element of cellular metabolism, often as an activator of enzymes involved in phosphorylated compounds and of high-energy phosphate transfer of ADP and ATP. Magnesium is involved in activating certain peptidases in protein digestion. It also relaxes nerve impulse, functioning antagonistically to calcium, which is stimulatory.

A deficiency of magnesium is characterized by muscle spasms (tremor, twitching) and rapid heartbeat; confusion, hallucinations, and disorientation; and lack of appetite, listlessness, nausea, and vomiting.

Magnesium toxicity is characterized by slowed breathing, coma, and sometimes death.

Rich food sources of magnesium include coffee (instant), cocoa powder, cottonseed flour, peanut flour, sesame seeds, soybean flour, spices, wheat bran, and wheat germ. Overuse of such substances as "milk of magnesia" (magnesium hydroxide) or Epsom salts (magnesium sulfate) may lead to deficiencies of other minerals or even to toxicity.

POTASSIUM (K)

Involved in the maintenance of proper acid-base balance and the transfer of nutrients in and out of individual cells. Relaxes the heart muscle—an action opposite to that of calcium, which is stimulatory. Required for the secretion of insulin by the pancreas and for enzyme reactions involving phosphorylation.

Potassium deficiency may cause rapid and irregular heartbeats and abnormal electrocardiograms; muscle weakness, irritability, and occasionally paralysis; and nausea, vomiting, diarrhea, and swollen abdomen also develop. Extreme and prolonged deficiency of potassium may cause hypokalemia, culminating in the heart muscle stopping.

Acute toxicity from potassium (known as hyperkalemia) can result when kidneys are not functioning properly. The condition may prove fatal due to cardiac arrest. Good food sources include dehydrated fruits, molasses, potato flour, rice bran, seaweed, soybean flour, spices, sunflower seeds, and wheat bran. Potassium is the third most abundant element in the body, after calcium and phosphorus, and it is present in twice the concentration of sodium.

COBALT (CO)

The only known function of cobalt is as an integral part of vitamin B_{12}, an essential vitamin in the formation of red blood cells. A cobalt deficiency as such has never been reported in humans. The signs and symptoms that are sometimes attributed to cobalt deficiency are actually due to a lack of vitamin B_{12}, characterized by pernicious anemia, poor growth, and, occasionally, neurological disorders. Cobalt is present in many foods.

COPPER (CU)

Copper facilitates the absorption of iron from the intestinal tract and the release from it from storage in the liver and the reticuloendothelial system. Copper is essential for the formation of hemoglobin, although it is not a part of hemoglobin as such. It is a constituent of several enzyme systems and is important for the development and maintenance of vascular and skeletal structures (blood vessels, tendons, and bones).

It is important for the structure and function of the central nervous system. Required for normal pigmentation of hair. It is a component of important copper-containing proteins. It also has a role in reproduction.

Deficiency is most apt to occur in malnourished children, premature infants fed exclusively on modified cow's milk, and infants breast-fed for an extended period of time. Deficiency leads to a variety of abnormalities, including anemia, skeletal defects, demyelination, degeneration of the nervous system, defects in pigmentation and structure of the hair, reproductive failure, and pronounced cardiovascular lesions.

Copper is relatively nontoxic to monogastric species, including humans. The recommended copper intake for adults is in the range of 2–3 mg/day. Daily intakes of more than 20–30 mg over extended periods are expected to be unsafe. Good food sources include black pepper, blackstrap molasses, brazil nuts, cocoa, liver, and oysters (raw). Most cases of copper poisoning result from drinking water or beverages that have been stored in copper tanks and/or pass through copper pipes. Dietary excesses of calcium, iron, cadmium, zinc, lead, silver, and molybdenum plus sulfur reduce the utilization of copper.

Fluorine (F)

Constitutes 0.02%–0.05% of the bones and teeth. Necessary for sound bones and teeth. Assists in the prevention of dental caries.

Deficiency symptoms include excess dental caries. Also, there is indication that a deficiency of fluorine results in osteoporosis in the aged. Signs of toxicity include deformed teeth and bones, and softening, mottling, and irregular wear of the teeth.

Fluorine is found in many foods, but seafood and dry tea are the richest food sources. Fluoridation of water supplies to bring the concentration of fluoride to 1 ppm. Large amounts of dietary calcium, aluminum, and fat lower the absorption of fluorine. Fluoridation of water supplies (1 ppm) is the simplest and most effective method of providing added protection against dental caries.

Iodine (I)

The sole function of iodine is to make the iodine-containing thyroid hormones. Iodine deficiency is characterized by goiter (enlargement of the thyroid gland at the base of the neck), coarse hair, obesity, and high blood cholesterol. Iodine-deficient mothers may give birth to infants with a type of dwarfism known as cretinism, a disorder characterized by malfunctioning of the thyroid gland, goiter, mental retardation, and stunted growth. A similar disorder of the thyroid gland known as myxedema may develop in adults.

Regarding toxicity, long-term intake of iodine in excess may disturb the utilization of iodine by the thyroid gland and result in goiter. Among natural foods, the best sources of iodine are kelp, seafood, and vegetables grown in iodine-rich soils and iodized salt. Stabilized iodized salt contains 0.01% potassium iodide (0.0076%), or 76 mcg of iodine per gram. Certain foods (especially plants of the cabbage family) contain goitrogens, which interfere with the use of thyroxine and may produce goiter. Fortunately, goitrogenic action of these compounds is prevented by cooking.

Iron (Fe)

Iron (heme) combines with protein (globin) to make hemoglobin, the iron-containing compound in red blood cells that transports oxygen. Iron is also a component of enzymes that are involved in energy metabolism.

Deficiency symptoms include iron-deficiency (nutritional) anemia, the symptoms of which are paleness of skin and mucous membranes, fatigue, dizziness, sensitivity to cold, shortness of breath, rapid heartbeats, and tingling of the fingers and toes.

An excess of iron in the diet can tie up phosphorus in an insoluble iron-phosphate complex, thereby creating a deficiency of phosphorus. Red meat, egg yolk, and dark green, leafy vegetables are rich sources of iron. About 70% of the iron is present in the hemoglobin, the pigment of red blood cells. The other 30% is present as a reserve store in the liver, spleen, and bone marrow.

Manganese (Mn)

Manganese is important for the formation of bone and for the growth of other connective tissues. It also has a role in blood clotting, insulin action, and cholesterol synthesis. It is an activator of various enzymes in the metabolism of carbohydrates, fats, proteins, and nucleic acids.

No clear deficiency disease in humans has been reported. Toxicity in humans as a consequence of dietary intake has not been observed. However, it has occurred in workers (miners and others) exposed to high concentrations of manganese dust. The symptoms resemble those found in Parkinson's and Wilson's diseases. Good food sources include rice (brown), rice bran and polish, walnuts, wheat bran, and wheat germ. In average diets, only about 45% of the ingested manganese is absorbed. The manganese content of plants is dependent on the manganese content of the soil.

MOLYBDENUM (MO)

Component of three different enzyme systems involved in the metabolism of carbohydrates, fats, proteins, sulfur-containing amino acids, nucleic acids (DNA and RNA), and iron. Molybdenum is a component of the enamel of teeth.

Naturally occurring deficiency in humans is not known. Molybdenum-deficient animals are especially susceptible to the toxic effects of bisulfite, characterized by breathing difficulties and neurological disorders.

Severe molybdenum toxicity in animals (molybdenosis), particularly cattle, occurs throughout the world wherever pastures are grown on high-molybdenum soils. The symptoms include diarrhea, loss of weight, fading of hair color, and symptoms of copper deficiency. The concentration of molybdenum in food varies considerably, depending on the soil in which it is grown.

Most of the dietary molybdenum intake is derived from organ meats, whole grains, leafy vegetables, legumes, and yeast. The utilization of molybdenum is reduced by excess copper, sulfate, and tungsten.

SELENIUM (SE)

Component of the enzyme glutathione peroxidase, the metabolic role of which is to suppress free radical formation and resultant tissue damage.

There are no clear-cut deficiencies of selenium because this mineral is very closely related to vitamin E and it is difficult to distinguish deficiency due to selenium alone.

Regarding toxicity, poisonous effects of selenium are manifested by abnormalities of the hair, nails, and skin; garlic odor of the breath; intensification of selenium toxicity by arsenic or mercury; and higher than normal rates of dental caries. The selenium content of plant and animal products is affected by the selenium content of the soil and animal feed, respectively. The high-selenium areas of the United States are in the Great Plains and the Rocky Mountain states, especially in parts of the Dakotas and Wyoming. Good food sources include Brazil nuts, butter, flour, fish, and lobster.

ZINC (ZN)

Needed for normal skin, bones, and hair. A component of several different enzyme systems that are involved in digestion and respiration. Required for the transfer of carbon dioxide in red blood cells, for proper calcification of bones, for the synthesis and metabolism of proteins and nucleic acids, for the development and functioning of reproductive organs, for wound and burn healing, for the functioning of insulin, and for normal taste acuity.

Deficiency symptoms include loss of appetite, stunted growth in children, skin changes, impaired male sexual development, loss of taste sensitivity, lightened pigment in hair, white spots on the fingernails, and delayed healing of wounds. In the Middle East, pronounced zinc deficiency in humans has resulted in hypogonadism and dwarfism. In pregnant animals, experimental zinc deficiency has resulted in malformation and behavioral disturbances in offspring.

Regarding toxicity, ingestion of excess soluble salts may cause nausea, vomiting, and diarrhrea. Good food sources include beef, liver, oysters, spices, and wheat bran. The biological availability of zinc in different foods varies widely; meats and seafood are much better sources of available zinc than vegetables. Zinc availability is adversely affected by phytates (found in whole grains and beans), high calcium, oxalates (in rhubarb and spinach), high fiber, copper (from drinking water conveyed in copper piping), and ethylene diamine tetra acetic acid (EDTA, an additive used in certain canned foods).

MITOCHONDRIA

Organelle in the cell; contains the citric acid cycle and respiration coupled with ATP synthesis; involved in fatty acid oxidation. Cells vary in the number of mitochondria they contain. Liver cells contain 800–1200; ova contain up to 20,000.

MITRAL INSUFFICIENCY

Failure of the mitral valve of the heart to close completely causing blood to flow backward from left ventricle to left atrium during ventricular contraction.

MITRAL STENOSIS

Failure of the mitral valve of the heart to open completely from severe narrowing of the mitral valve orifice.

MITRAL VALVE PROLAPSE

A form of mitral insufficiency that occurs when one or more of the mitral leaflets of this valve protrudes into the left atrium during systole, leading to blood regurgitation from the left ventricle into the left atrium.

MOBILE GLUCOSE TRANSPORTERS

Glucose-specific transport proteins sequestered in the cell, which, when needed, migrate to the cell surface, bind to glucose, and transport it through the plasma membrane to its site of use. There are several different proteins involved. They are identified as GLUT 1, 2, 3, and 4.

MOLYBDENUM

An essential mineral; serves as a cofactor for xanthine oxidase, aldehyde oxidase, and sulfate oxidase. High intakes of molybdenum increase copper excretion.

MONOAMINE OXIDASE (MAO) INHIBITORS

Group of medications used to treat depression. Consumption with tyramine-containing foods can cause severe hypertension.

MONOCYTE

A relatively large mononuclear leukocyte.

MONOGLYCERIDE (MONOACYLGLYCEROL)

A glycerol having only one fatty acid esterified to it.

MONOMERIC FORMULA

Specialized formulation of hydrolyzed macronutrients.

MONOSACCHARIDE

A simple sugar containing only one saccharide unit.

MONOSODIUM GLUTAMATE (MSG)

An additive involved in idiosyncratic food intolerance reactions. Salts of glutamic acid are used as flavorings, for instance in Chinese food, soup, meat products, and heavily spiced foods. The "Chinese restaurant syndrome" is well-known. Symptoms can include tightness of the chest, headache, nausea, vomiting, abdominal cramps, and even shock. In asthmatic patients, this additive may cause bronchoconstriction. The first symptoms may appear after 15 minutes after consumption, while an interval of 24 hours has also been described. The mechanism underlying this syndrome is not known.

MONOUNSATURATED FATTY ACID

A fatty acid having only one double bond; a common one is oleic acid (16 carbons; one double bond). Olive oil contains oleic acid.

MORBIDITY

Illness leading to death.

MORTALITY

Cause of death.

MOTILIN

A gastrointestinal hormone that plays a role in controlling the motility of the small intestine during periods without food.

mTOR

Transduction pathway in liver for amino acid sensing.

MUCOPOLYSACCHARIDE

A group of complex carbohydrates containing hexosamine; a thick gelatinous material.

MUCOSA

Mucus-secreting membrane.

MUCUS

A polypeptide containing a carbohydrate, usually a hexosamine.

MUCUS MEMBRANE

A membrane lining the cavities and canals of the body kept moist by the secretion of mucus.

MULTIPAROUS

A woman who has had more than one pregnancy.

MULTIPLE SCLEROSIS

A chronic disease characterized by demyelination of nerve fibers with accompanying motor and sensory deficits.

MUSCULAR DYSTROPHY

An inherited disorder characterized by a gradual muscle wasting and loss.

MUSCULIN

A hormone released by skeletal muscle that may have effects on the endocrine pancreas to restrain the size of the beta cell mass and to tonically inhibit insulin biosynthesis and release.

MUSH

A hot cereal made by boiling cornmeal in water.

MUTAGENS

Chemicals that cause changes in the base sequence of DNA.

MUTATION

When the sequence of bases in the DNA is disturbed by a deletion, repetition, or substitution of one or more of the bases, the code is said to be mutated and the protein coded by this sequence will not be synthesized in its normal amino acid sequence. The amino acid sequence determines the shape and function of the protein. Many mutations occur that have an effect on this sequence but have no effect on function because the substitution or deletion does not occur in the active or working part of the protein molecule.

MUTTON

Meat from mature sheep.

MUTUAL SUPPLEMENTATION

Food blends that provide the optimal array of essential amino acids.

MYASTHENIA GRAVIS

Autoimmune disease characterized by chronic, progressive muscle fatigue and weakness, especially in the face and throat.

MYCOTOXINS

See also Food-Borne Illness. Secondary metabolites of fungi, which can induce acute as well as chronic toxic effects (i.e., carcinogenicity, mutagenicity, teratogenicity, and estrogenic effects) in animals and humans. According to their habitat, mycotoxin-producing fungi can be classified as fungi infecting living plants (e.g., *Aspergillus flavus*, *Claviceps purpurea*, and *Fusarium graminearum*), fungi infecting stored food products (e.g., *Aspergillus flavus*, *Aspergillus ochraceus*, *Aspergillus parasiticus*, *Fusarium graminearum*, *Penicillium expansum*, and *Penicillium viridicatum*), and fungi infecting decaying organic matter (e.g., *Fusarium graminearum*). Some important mycotoxins are aflatoxins, sterigmatocystin, ochratoxins, patulin, trichothecenes, zearalenone, and ergot alkaloids. Toxic syndromes resulting from the intake of mycotoxins by animals and humans are known as mycotoxicoses. Well-known examples of mycotoxicoses include "holy fire" in Europe caused by the mold *Claviceps purpurea*, "alimentary toxic aleukia" in the Soviet Union caused by *Fusarium* spp., and "yellow rice disease" in Japan caused by *Penicillium* spp. Factors affecting mold growth, mycotoxin production, and infection of foods and feeds are as follows:

- Moisture (growth—in general, water activity ≥0.80)
- Temperature (growth—psychrophilemolds [optimum temperature: <10°C]; mesophilemolds [optimum temperature: 10°C –40°C]; and thermophile molds [optimum temperature: >40°C])
- Mechanical, insect, and mold damage
- Time (in general, there is a lag between mold growth and mycotoxin production)
- Types of substrates and nutritional factors
- Atmospheric oxygen and carbon dioxide levels (molds are highly aerobic and require a minimum amount of atmospheric oxygen for growth and efficient mycotoxin production)
- Chemical treatment
- Presence of other molds
- Geographical location

Thus, mycotoxin contamination of food and feed depends on the environmental conditions that lead to mold growth and toxin production. The detectable presence of live molds in food does not automatically indicate that mycotoxins have been produced. On the other hand, the absence of viable molds in foods does not necessarily mean that there are no mycotoxins. The latter could have been formed at an earlier stage, prior to food processing. Because of their chemical stability, several mycotoxins persist during food processing, while the molds are destroyed. Since the discovery of the aflatoxins, probably no commodity can be regarded as absolutely free from mycotoxins. Also, mycotoxin production can occur in the field or during harvest, processing, storage, and shipment of a given commodity.

MYELIN

The fatty coating of nerves.

MYOCARDIAL INFARCTION

Heart attack. Occurs when one or more of the coronary vessels is occluded and heart muscle fails to receive sufficient oxygen and dies. The term infarction refers to the fact that the depolarization of the muscle just prior to contraction (a part of the pumping action of the heart) cannot spread across this dead part of the muscle. The presence of this infarction can be detected by an electrocardiograph, which documents the depolarization and repolarization of the heart muscle.

MYOCARDIUM

Heart muscle.

MYOGLOBIN

Iron-containing globulin in muscle.

MYOSIN

Muscle cell protein that (with actin) plays a role in muscle contraction and relaxation.

MYRISTICIN

A methylenedioxyphenyl substance. It is found in nutmeg and mace, and in lesser quantities in black pepper, parsley, celery, dill, and carrots. Nutmeg produces effects similar to alcoholic intoxication. Reportedly, these spices have been frequently used as narcotics by prison inmates. Around 5–15 g of nutmeg powder can produce euphoria, hallucinations, and narcosis. The side effects, however, are very unpleasant and severe: headache, nausea, abdominal pain, delirium, hypotension, depression, acidosis, stupor, shock and, in large doses, liver damage and death.

MYXEDEMA

Advanced deficiency of thyroxine in adults.

N

NAD, NADH, NADP, NADPH

Niacin-containing coenzymes that function as carriers for hydrogen ions in dehydrogenase catalyzed reactions.

NA⁺K⁺ PUMP

An energy-dependent pump that operates to keep Na^+ on the outside of cells and K^+ on the inside of cells.

NALOXONE

A specific inhibitor of the analgesic properties of the endorphins.

NAPTHAQUINONE

A derivative of quinone that has some vitamin K activity.

NASOGASTRIC TUBE

The tube inserted through the nose and ending in the stomach that carries liquid nourishment.

NATEGLINIDE

A hypoglycemic agent. Trade name: Starlix.

NATIONAL CENTER FOR HEALTH STATISTICS (NCHS) (U.S.)

An agency that collects data on the causes of death and disease in the United States as well as in other countries.

NATIONAL HEALTH EXAMINATION SURVEY (NHANES) (U.S.)

Data collected at intervals to document the usual types and amounts of food consumed as related to a variety of measurements of body size and body function. Assessments of health status are part of this survey.

NATIONAL RESEARCH COUNCIL (NRC)

A division of the U.S. National Academy of Sciences established in 1916 to promote the effective utilization of scientific and technical resources.

NATIONAL SCIENCE FOUNDATION (NSF) (U.S.)

A U.S. government funding organization for the basic sciences.

NATIONWIDE FOOD CONSUMPTION SURVEY (NFCS) (U.S.)

Data collected by scientists in the U.S. Department of Agriculture to document the kinds and amounts of food consumed in the United States.

NATURALLY OCCURRING TOXICANTS

Products of the metabolic processes of animals, plants, and microorganisms from which the food products are derived.

NAUSEA

Upset stomach associated with the urge to vomit.

N-CORRECTED METABOLIZABLE ENERGY (MnE)

Metabolizable energy corrected for total nitrogen (TN) retained or lost from tissues: $MnE = ME - (k \times TN)$. For birds or monogastric animals, gaseous energy loss is usually not considered. The correction for mammals is generally $k = 7.45$ kcal/g nitrogen retained in the body tissues (TN). The factor of 8.22 kcal/g TN is used for birds representing the energy equivalent of uric acid per gram of nitrogen. A number of different values for k have been suggested and used.

NDP CAL %

Net protein calories percent. The percent of the total energy value of the diet provided by the protein.

NECROSIS

Cellular changes that occur and are indicative of cellular death.

NEONATAL HEMORRHAGING

Excessive blood loss by the neonate.

NEONATAL JAUNDICE

An accumulation of bilirubin under the skin of the newborn infant giving the infant a yellowish hue.

NEONATE

A newborn animal. In the human, a neonate is an infant of < 4 weeks of age.

NEOPLASTIC DISEASES

Proliferative disorders characterized by an uncoordinated and uncontrolled growth of cells.

NEPHRON

The basic structural unit of the kidney. The unit functions to filter waste products from the blood for excretion in the urine. This unit reabsorbs water and conserves sodium under the influence of antidiuretic hormone (ADH). The nephron consists of a tuft of capillaries known as the glomerulus and the renal tubule. The average adult human kidney contains about one million glomeruli.

NEPHROSCLEROSIS

Hardening of the vessels (arteries) of the kidney.

NEPHROTIC SYNDROME

Kidney damage characterized by increased permeability in renal tubules and loss of protein in the glomerular filtrate.

NEURAL TUBE DEFECT

Occurs early in embryonic development; can be spina bifida (inadequate closure of the end of the spinal cord) or hydrocephali (infant head enlargement due to fluid accumulation); in some instances may be related to inadequate folate intake prior to and in the early stages of pregnancy. Females contemplating pregnancy should consume 400 μg folate/day.

NEURITIS

Inflammation of nerve endings.

NEUROPEPTIDE Y (NPY)

One of the most abundant peptides found in the central and peripheral nervous system. Serves as a vasoconstrictor in conjunction with norepinephrine. It is released by the GI tract and signals hunger. It plays an unknown role in the placenta where its level rises early in pregnancy and remains high for the duration of the pregnancy. Leptin reduces its synthesis.

NEUROTENSIN

A blood-borne cytokine that is an appetite suppressant.

NEUROTRANSMITTER

A chemical signal for nerve action. Serotonin, epinephrine, and acetylcholine, for example, are neurotransmitters.

NEUTROPENIA

Elevated levels of neutrophils in blood.

NFκB

A signal peptide that is active in the inflammatory cascade. The inflammatory pathway includes cytokines, chemokines, and interferons, all of which drive the immune response to a variety of antigens and inflammatory signals.

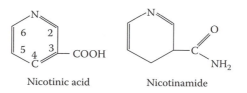

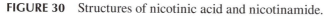

Nicotinic acid   Nicotinamide

FIGURE 30   Structures of nicotinic acid and nicotinamide.

NFCS

See Nationwide Food Consumption Survey.

NHANES

See National Health Examination Survey.

NIACIN (B₃)

A vitamin that serves as an essential component of the coenzymes NAD and NADP and can be synthesized from tryptophan. It exists as nicotinamide (the active form of the vitamin) and nicotinic acid. Nicotinic acid and nicotinamide (Figure 30) are widely distributed in nature.

In order to have vitamin activity, there must be a pyridine ring substituted with a β carboxylic acid or corresponding amide, and there must be open sites at pyridine carbons 2 through 6.

Nicotinic acid is an amphoteric molecule and forms salts with acids and bases. Its carboxyl group can form esters and anhydrides and can be reduced. Both the acid and amide forms are very stable in the dry form, but when the amide form is in solution, it is readily hydrolyzed to the acid form.

Several substituted pyridines can antagonize the biological activity of niacin. These include pyridine 3-sulfonic acid, 3-acetylpyridine, isonicotinic acid hydrazide, and 6-aminonicotinamide. HPLC is the analytical method of choice for this vitamin which does not occur in large amounts in the free form. Most often, it occurs as the coenzyme NAD$^+$ or NADP$^+$. Chemical analysis using the Koenig reaction, which opens up the pyridine ring with cyanogen bromide, followed by reaction with an aromatic amine to form a colored product, is used. The most widely used method employs a chromophore-generating base, p-methylaminophenol sulfate, sulfanilic acid, or barbituric acid. The color intensity so developed is dependent on the concentration of the vitamin.

SOURCES

This vitamin is widely distributed in the human food supply. Especially good sources are whole grain cereals and breads, milk, eggs, meats, and vegetables that are richly colored.

ABSORPTION AND METABOLISM

In contrast to thiamin and riboflavin, niacin is not absorbed via an active process. Rather, both nicotinic acid and nicotinamide cross the intestinal cell by way of simple diffusion and facilitated diffusion. There are species differences in the mechanism of absorption. After absorption, the vitamin circulates in the blood as its free form. The form that is not converted to NAD$^+$ or NADP$^+$ is metabolized further and excreted in the urine. The excretory metabolites are N^l-methylnicotinamide, nicotinuric acid, nicotinamide-N^l-oxide, N^l-methylnicotinamide-N^l-oxide, N^{l}methylnicotinamide-N^l oxide, N^l-methyl-4-pyridone-3-carboxamide, and N^l-methyl-2-pyridone-5-carboxamide. Niacin can be synthesized from tryptophan in a ratio of 60 molecules of tryptophan to 1 of nicotinic acid.

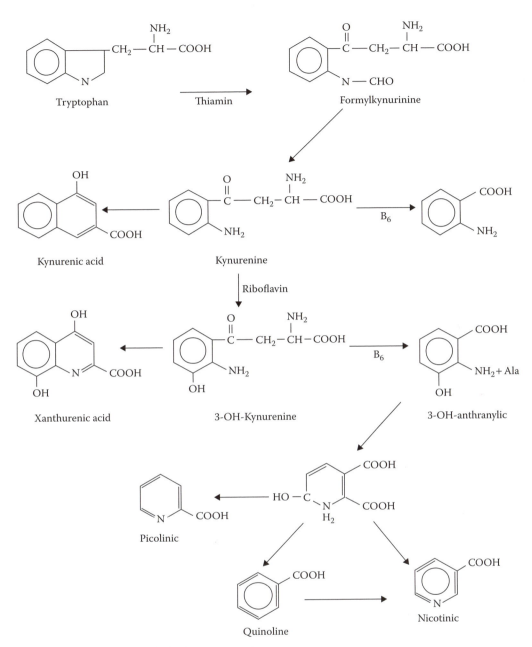

FIGURE 31 Synthesis of niacin from tryptophan.

The pathway for conversion is shown in Figure 31. Note the involvement of thiamin, pyridoxine, and riboflavin in this conversion.

FUNCTION

The main function of this vitamin is as part of the coenzymes NAD+ and NADP+. Both the coenzymes function in the maintenance of the redox state of the cell. These coenzymes are loosely bound to the dehydrogenase enzyme during the catalytic cycle and therefore serve more as substrates than as prosthetic groups. They act as electron acceptors during the enzymatic removal of hydrogen atoms from specific substrate molecules. One hydrogen atom of the substrate is transferred as a hydride ion to the nicotinamide portion of the oxidized NAD^+ or $NADP^+$ forms of these coenzymes to yield the reduced forms. The other hydrogen ion remains loosely associated. Thus, the reduced coenzyme is represented as $NADH^+H^+$ or $NADPH^+H^+$. Most enzymes are specific for NAD or NADP, and these enzymes are members of the oxidoreductase family of enzymes. Some will use either, that is, glutamate dehydrogenase. Most of the NAD- or NADP-linked enzymes are involved in catabolic pathways, that is, glycolysis or the pentose phosphate shunt. NAD turns over quite rapidly in the cell. Its degradation is shown in Figure 32. NAD^+ acts as a substrate for a variety of ADP-ribosylation reactions including poly- and mono-ADP-ribosylation of proteins, formation of cyclic ADP-ribose, and generation of O-acetyl-ADP-ribose in deacetylation reactions. These non-redox reactions are critical in the regulation of cellular metabolism, and they are sensitive to niacin status. Ribosylation reactions are essential to and regulate the chromatin structure. Altered chromatin structure means that there is a loss in genomic stability in niacin-deficient states, and thus, cell division, differentiation, and apoptosis are affected.

Beyond its use in biological systems as a precursor of NAD^+ or $NADP^+$, nicotinic acid has a pharmacological use. When consumed in pharmacological doses, it is degraded as though it was benzoic acid. Nicotinic acid, the drug, is used as a lipid-lowering drug. Large intakes (1 g/day) lower serum cholesterol. However, large doses also result in flushing due to its effect on vascular tone. Nicotinic acid elicits a fibrinolytic activation of very short duration. Both nicotinic acid and nicotinamide can

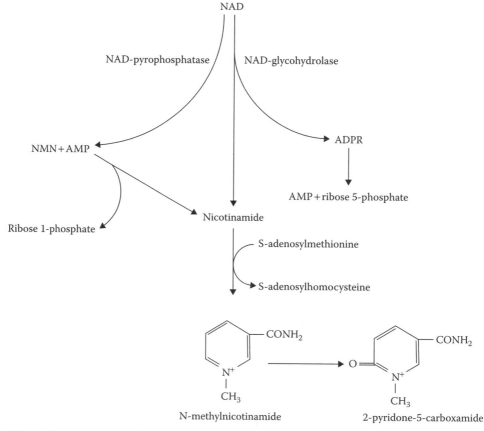

FIGURE 32 Degradation of NAD.

be toxic if administered at levels greater than 10 μmoles/kg. Chronic administration of 3 g/day to humans results in a variety of symptoms including headache, heartburn, nausea, hives, fatigue, sore throat, dry hair, inability to focus the eyes, and skin tautness. In experimental animals, nicotinic acid supplements result in a reduction in adipocyte free fatty acid release by streptozotocin-diabetic rats, an inhibition of adipocyte adenylate cyclase activity in normal hamsters, and degenerative changes in the heart muscle of normal rats. All of these responses were those that characterize a defense against a toxic exposure to nicotinic acid rather than a response to a normal intake level.

DEFICIENCY

Pellagra has been well described as the niacin deficiency disease. It is characterized by skin lesions that are blackened and rough especially in areas exposed to sunlight and abraded by clothing. The typical skin lesions of pellagra are accompanied by insomnia, loss of appetite, weight loss, soreness of mouth and tongue, indigestion, diarrhea, abdominal pain, burning sensations in various parts of the body, vertigo, headache, numbness, nervousness, apprehension, mental confusion, and forgetfulness. Many of these symptoms can be related to niacin deficiency–induced deficits in the metabolism of the central nervous system. This system has, as its choice metabolic fuel, glucose. Glycolysis with its attendant need for NAD^+ as a coenzyme is appreciably less active. As the deficient state progresses, numbness followed by a paralysis of the extremities occurs. The more advanced cases are characterized by tremor and a spastic or ataxic movement that is associated with peripheral nerve inflammation. Death from pellagra ensues if the patient remains untreated.

More subtle biochemical changes have also been reported in experimental niacin deficiency. It is well known that NAD is the substrate for poly (ADP-ribose) polymerase, an enzyme associated with DNA repair. In the deficient state this repair does not occur readily, and one of the characteristics of niacin deficiency is an increase in DNA strand breaks. If niacin deficiency accompanies conditions known to increase oxidative damage, via free radical attack, to DNA, then the two conditions are additive with respect to cell damage and subsequent tissue pathology. Such has been proposed as a mechanism for the induction of cancer in susceptible cells.

Early indications of niacin deficiency include a reduction in the levels of urinary niacin metabolites, especially those that are methylated (N^I methyl-nicotinamide and N^I-methyl-2-pyridone-5-carboxamide). Since the discovery early in the twentieth century of the curative power of nicotinic acid and nicotinamide, pellagra is very rare. The exception is in the alcoholic population. This population frequently substitutes alcoholic beverages for food and thereby is at risk for multiple nutrient deficiencies including pellagra. The metabolism of ethanol is NAD dependent. This dependency drives up the need for niacin in the face of inadequate intake, setting the stage for alcoholic pellagra. In part, the CNS symptoms of alcoholism are those of pellagra as described above.

There is another very small population at risk for developing niacin deficiency. This group carries a mutation in the gene for tryptophan transport (Hartnup's disease). Its symptoms, apart from tryptophan inadequacy effects on protein synthesis, are very similar to those of niacin deficiency. This is because of the use of tryptophan as a precursor of nicotinic acid. If niacin supplements are given to people with Hartnup's disease, these pellagra-like symptoms disappear.

Because tryptophan can be converted to nicotinic acid, the DRI for niacin is stated in terms of niacin equivalents. A niacin equivalent is equal to 1 mg niacin or 60 mg of tryptophan. The need is related to energy intake as well, particularly the carbohydrate intake. However, the DRI takes into account varying diet composition as well as individual differences in nutrient need. Age and gender also influence need. Go to http://www.nap.edu for niacin DRI.

NIACINAMIDE

See Niacin.

NICK TRANSLATION

A technique for labeling DNA based on the ability of the DNA polymerase from *E. coli* to degrade a strand of DNA that has been nicked and then resynthesized; if a radioactive nucleotide is used, the rebuilt strand becomes labeled and can be used as a probe.

NICKEL

A mineral that may or may not be essential to humans. It is needed in trace amounts by growing chicks.

NICOTINIC ACID

See Niacin.

NIEMANN-PICK DISEASE

A genetic disease in which a mutation in the gene for sphingolipid-degrading enzyme (sphingomyelinase) has occurred. The disease is characterized by CNS degeneration and very early (under 3 years) death.

NIFEDIPINE

A calcium channel blocker that can reduce angina pain. It can also be used as an antihypertensive agent. Trade names: Adalet, Adalet CC, Apo-Nifed, Nifedical XL, Nu-Nifed, Procardia, Procardia XL.

NIGHT BLINDNESS

First symptom of vitamin A deficiency. The individual is unable to adapt to changes in light intensity. It is reversible if the vitamin is provided.

NIH

The National Institutes of Health (U.S.). Located primarily in Bethesda, Maryland. One of the largest U.S. government–funded health and disease research centers.

NISOLDIPINE

A calcium channel blocker that is used as an antihypertensive drug. Trade name: Sular.

NITRATE (NO_3^-)

The principal natural source of nitrate in the biosphere is microbial nitrification. This process is responsible for the nitrate conversion of ammonia in fertilizers, used either as such or in the form of urea, derived from the decomposition of human and animal waste matter. The nitrification reaction is a two-step process: (1) $2NH_4^+ + 3O_2$ becomes $2NO^{2-} + 2H2O + 4H^+$ (by chemoautotrophic nitrifiers, for example, species of *Nitrosomonas*, *Nitrospira*, and *Nitrosolobus*); and (2) $NO^{2-} + 1/2 O_2$ becomes NO_3^- (by nitrite oxidizers, for example, species of *Nitrobacter*, *Nitrospira*, and *Nitrococcus*). Counteracting the accumulation of nitrate in the biosphere are the denitrifying bacteria and fungi, which are capable of reducing nitrate to nitrite, or in some cases to ammonia. Because contamination with nitrogen compounds results in an increase in the nitrate concentration of groundwater, levels of nitrate in drinking water and foods (of plant origin) can be increased as well. Nitrate has been reported to occur in several foods, such as vegetables (e.g., asparagus, beets, beans, broccoli, cabbage, carrots, celery, corn, cucumbers, eggplant, lettuce, melons, onion, peas, sweet peppers, pickles, potatoes, pumpkin, spinach, sauerkraut, and tomatoes), breads, all fruits, juices, cured meats, milk and milk products, and water. Since the nitrate content of the reported foods varies greatly, the level of consumption is also important. Foodstuffs contributing most to the total nitrate intake include potatoes (14.2 mg/person/day), lettuce (18.9 mg/person/day), and celery (16.0 mg/person/day). Oral toxicity of nitrate can be due to the nitrate ion per se or to the microbial conversion of nitrate to nitrite in situ in the food and in the mouth or gastrointestinal tract. In general, nitrate has a low oral toxicity because it is rapidly excreted in the urine. Repeated large doses of nitrate can cause dyspepsia, mental depression, headache, and weakness. The intake of nitrate via food consumption is estimated at 1.4–2.5 mg/kg/day and from water at 0.3 mg/kg/day. The acceptable daily intake of nitrate is 3.64 mg/kg/day.

NITRITE (NO_2^-)

Produced by bacterial reduction of nitrate, which may be present as a contaminant or food additive. The toxicological significance of nitrate lies in its easy conversion to nitrite by nitrifying bacteria that may be present in foodstuffs, the saliva, and in the gastrointestinal tract. Populations that are particularly at risk are those that lack the NADH-dependent methemoglobin reductase activity (e.g., infants under 1 year of age, subjects with hereditary familial methemoglobinemia), those lacking erythrocyte glucose-6-phosphate dehydrogenase activity (e.g., certain Mediterranean and Middle Eastern populations), pregnant women, and those with decreased stomach acidity as a result of diseases such as pernicious anemia, chronic gastritis, stomach ulcer, and cancer. An important toxic effect of nitrite is methemoglobinemia (i.e., an increased level of methemoglobin in the blood). Iron in hemoglobin is in the ferrous state (Fe^{2+}). When it is oxidized (e.g., by nitrite) to the ferric state (Fe^{3+}), hemoglobin is transformed to methemoglobin, which is incapable of transporting oxygen. There is normally a small amount of methemoglobin (1.7%) in the blood, and this level is maintained by methemoglobin reductase in the presence of NADH. At levels below 5%, no symptoms have been observed. Levels of 5%–20% are associated with mild cyanosis; 20%–40% with marked cyanosis, fatigue, and dyspnea; 40%–60% with severe cyanosis, tachypnea, serious cardiopulmonary signs, tachycardia, and depression; and >60% with ataxia, coma, and death. Another important effect of nitrite is the formation of nitrosamine.

NITROGEN

An essential element that is a component of amino acids.

NITROGEN BALANCE

When the intake of nitrogen (from protein) is equal to the excretion of nitrogen in the urine and feces, the individual is in nitrogen balance. Negative nitrogen balance is when excretion exceeds intake. Positive balance is when intake exceeds excretion. This happens in growth while the former happens in tissue wasting or when intake is of poor quality or quantity of protein.

NITROGLYCERIN

A vasodilator used to ease the pain of angina pectoris (pain in the chest due to insufficient oxygen supply to the heart).

NITROPRUSSIDE SODIUM

A vasodilator that is used as an antihypertensive agent. Trade name: Nitropress.

NITROSAMINES

Formed outside or inside the body from precursors like amines, amides, and nitrites. The fundamental requirements are a secondary amino nitrogen and nitrous acid. Three types of nitrosamines can be distinguished: (1) dialkyl nitrosamines (e.g., dimethylnitrosamine, diethylnitrosamine), (2) cyclic nitrosamines (e.g., N-nitrosopiperidine, N-nitrosopyrrolidine), and (3) acylalkyl nitrosamines or nitrosamides (different types of nitrosoureas, thioureas, carbamates, carboxamides, and guanidines). The conditions in the alimentary tract from the mouth to the anus are conducive to nitrosamine formation. The most important factor inhibiting nitrosamine formation is ascorbic acid, which rapidly reacts with nitrite to form nitric oxide and dehydroascorbic acid. Other inhibitors are gallic acid, sodium sulfite, cysteine, tannins, and urea. Occurrence of different nitrosamines has been reported in several foodstuffs: dimethylnitrosamine (e.g., fried bacon, luncheon meat, salami, sausages, fish [raw sable, salmon, and shad; smoked sable and salmon; smoked and nitrate or nitrite-treated sable, salmon, shad and salted marine fish], fish sauce, cheese, baby foods, dried shrimps, shrimp sauce, squid, uncooked canned meats, uncooked ham and other pork products, uncooked beef products, light and dark beers, and Scotch whisky); diethylnitrosamine (e.g., fried bacon, luncheon meat, salami, and wheat flour); nitrosopiperidine (e.g., fried bacon); and nitrosopyrrolidine (e.g., fried bacon, fish sauce, dried shrimps, and squid). In animals, a large number of N-nitroso compounds have been shown to be carcinogenic. Factors enhancing the carcinogenicity of N-nitroso compounds are hormones, other carcinogens or toxicants, viral or bacterial infections, metals, and nutritional factors. The inhibitory factors can be identified as those that decrease the metabolism of the carcinogen (e.g., aminoacetonitrile [affects dimethylnitrosamine], dibenamine [affects dimethylnitrosamine], and phenobarbitone [affects diethylnitrosamine]); and those that retard or interfere with the formation of the carcinogen (e.g., ascorbic acid, tannins, sulfite, and cysteine). Since no animal species that has been tested so far is resistant to dimethylnitrosamine or diethylnitrosamine, it is expected that humans are not resistant to the nitrosamines either. When the amounts of total nitrosamines in food, water, and other sources are added to those formed throughout the alimentary tract, the total nitrosamine load could be considerable.

NITROUS OXIDE (N_2O)

An inhalation anesthetic.

NOCTURIA

Excessive urination during the night.

NONCALORIC SWEETENERS

Non-nutritive sweeteners, cyclamate, saccharine, and aspartame, compounds that elicit the sweet taste without contributing to the energy intake.

NONESSENTIAL AMINO ACIDS (NEAA)

Those amino acids that the body can synthesize in sufficient quantity to meet its need.

NONEXPERIMENTAL STUDIES

Studies in which the exposure is "chosen" by the subjects themselves. The investigator confines himself or herself to observe the subjects and to collect data on their exposure and disease, without interfering with their way of life. Also known as observational studies. In general, four types of nonexperimental studies can be identified: (1) cross-sectional studies (possibilities: estimation of prevalence of exposure or disease; limitations: distinction between cause and effect is difficult); (2) follow-up or cohort studies (possibilities: (a) a large number of exposures and diseases can be studied, (b) exposure is determined before onset of the disease, and (c) estimation of the incidence of the disease; limitations: (a) during the follow-up period the investigators must keep track of all study subjects, (b) expensive [in terms of time and money], and (c) only suitable for frequently occurring diseases); (3) case-control studies (possibilities: (a) a large number of exposures can be studied, (b) the number of study subjects may be relatively small, and (c) suitable for rare diseases; limitations: exposure is determined after onset of the disease and reporting of exposure by the respondents might be affected by the disease), and (4) ecological studies (possibilities: can be used when information is only available on an aggregated level; limitations: ecological fallacy). The rank order from weak suggestions to strong evidence of a causal relation in the studies would be ecological studies, cross-sectional studies, case-control studies, and finally follow-up or cohort studies.

NONHEME IRON

Iron in the body not associated with the heme of hemoglobin. Some of the cytochromes have iron as part of their structures.

NONIMMUNOLOGICAL DEFENSE MECHANISM

One of the defense mechanisms is the digestive tract, which forms a physical barrier against unwanted effects of food. The mucus membrane of the gut forms a protective barrier against penetration of pathogenic microorganisms and allergens. Also, the secretion of certain enzymes and gastric acid (which may lead to degradation of unwanted substances) and the enteric motility (which prevents excessive proliferation of bacteria in the small intestine as well as absorption of macromolecules through the digestive mucosa) contribute to the nonimmunological defense.

NONINSULIN-DEPENDENT DIABETES MELLITUS (NIDDM)

Outdated term for type 2 Diabetes Mellitus.

NONINVASIVE TECHNIQUE

A medical treatment or procedure that does not involve surgery. X-rays, for example, are in this category of techniques.

NONSTEROIDAL ANTI-INFLAMMATORY DRUGS (NSAID)

Aspirin, indomethacin, and phenylbutazone. These drugs block the action of cyclooxygenase by acetylating the enzyme. While occasional use of these drugs for the occasional injury or headache is harmless, long-term, chronic use can result in untoward effects. Long-term, chronic use of aspirin, for example, can affect vascular competence and blood clotting. People consuming large amounts of aspirin over long periods of time may find an increase in bruises (subcutaneous hemorrhages). Small contact injuries that normally would not result in a bruise will do so in these people. Gastric bleeding is another possible complication with long-term, chronic aspirin ingestion. Aplastic anemia can result from long-term phenylbutazone therapy.

NONTROPICAL SPRUE

Malabsorption/diarrhea due to localized reaction to certain foods. See Absorption; Gluten-Sensitive Enteropathy.

NO-OBSERVED-EFFECT LEVEL (NOEL)

The highest concentration of a substance that may be administered to a test animal in any way without causing that animal to be distinguishable from a control to which the substance is not administered.

NOREPINEPHRINE

A neurotransmitter released in response to stress; part of the "fight or flight" response. Acts as a vasoconstrictor. Produced by the adrenal medulla and the sympathetic nervous system. It is released by the nerve endings and crosses the nerve junctions to stimulate subsequent neural fibers.

NORMAL CLINICAL VALUES FOR BLOOD

Ranges of values for nutrients and metabolites in blood (Table 39).

NORTHERN BLOT

A method for transferring RNA from an agarose gel to a nitrocellulose filter on which the RNA can be detected using a suitable probe.

NOSOCOMIAL INFECTION

Infection that originated in a hospital.

NOSTRUM

Folk remedy that may be ineffective in treatment of a clinical condition.

NOVEL FOOD

A food that the consumer has never eaten or a food newly developed by food manufacturers.

NPU

Net protein use. A measure of the biological value of a dietary protein based on the amount of protein retained in the body as a percentage of that consumed.

TABLE 39
Normal Clinical Values for Blood

Component	Common Units or SI Units
Ammonia	22–39 mmol/L
Calcium	8.5–10.5 mg/dL or 2.25–2.65 mmol/L
Carbon dioxide	24–30 meq/L or 24–29 mmol/L
Chloride	100–106 meq/L or mmol/L
Copper	100–200 mg/dL or 16–31 mmol/L
Iron	50–150 mg/dL or 11.6–31.3 mmol/L
Lead	50 mg/dL or less
Magnesium	1.5–2.0 meq/L or 0.75–1.25 mmol/L
Partial pressure CO_2	35–40 mm Hg
pH	7.35–7.45
Phosphorus	3.0–4.5 mg/dL or 1–1.5 mmol/L
P O_2	75–100 mm Hg
Potassium	3.5–5.0 meq/L or 2.5–5.0 mmol/L
Sodium	135–145 meq/L or 135–145 mmol/L
Acetoacetate	<2 mmol
Ascorbic acid	0.4–15 mg/dL or 23–85 mmol/L
Bilirubin	0.4–0.6 mg/dL or 1.71–6.84 mmol/L
Carotinoids	0.8–4.0 mg/mL
Creatinine	0.6–1.5 mg/dL or 60–130 mmol/L
Lactic acid	0.6–1.8 meq/L or 0.44–1.28 mmol/L
Cholesterol	120–220 mg/dL or 3.9–7.3 mmol/L
Triglycerides	40–150 mg/dL or 6–18 mmol/L
Pyruvic acid	0–0.11 meq/L or 79.8–228.0 mmol/L
Urea nitrogen	8–25 mg/dL or 2.86–7.14 mmol/L
Uric acid	3.0–7.0 mg/dL or 0.18–0.29 mmol/L
Vitamin A	0.15–0.6 mg/dL
Albumin	3.5–5.0 g/dL
Insulin	6–20 mU/dL
Glucose	80–120 mg/dL or 4–6 mmol/L

NUCLEAR FACTOR-κB (NFκB)

A transcription factor in apoptosis genes. Hyperhomocysteinemia activates this factor in endothelial cells via oxidative stress.

NUCLEIC ACIDS

Chains of nucleotides whose function is to store and transmit the genetic information from one generation to the next. A nucleotide contains a ribose, one to three phosphate groups, and either a purine (adenine or guanine) or a pyrimidine (cytosine, uracil, or thymine).

NUCLEOSOME

The structural subunit of chromatin, consisting of ~200 bp of DNA and an octamer of histones.

NUCLEUS

An organelle in the cell containing DNA, the genetic material plus the enzymes, coenzymes, and cofactors needed to synthesize mRNA, which transfers genetic messages from the DNA to the ribosome where proteins are synthesized.

NULL MUTATION

A mutation that completely eliminates the function of a gene, usually because it has been deleted.

NUTRIENT DENSITY

The nutrient composition of food expressed in terms of nutrient quantity per 1000 kcal or 4200 kJ.

NUTRIENT REQUIREMENTS

The amounts of nutrients absolutely required by an individual to avoid the symptoms of deficiency disease and to optimize health and well-being.

NUTRIENT-RICH FOOD INDEX

A system for ranking and/or classifying foods based on their nutritive value.

NUTRIENTS

The chemical substances present in food that are utilized by the body as components for synthesizing needed materials and for fuel.

NUTRITION SCREENING

Process of identifying characteristics associated with dietary and nutritional problems.

NUTRITION THERAPY

A component of medical treatment that includes enteral and parenteral nutrition as well as disease-specific therapeutic diets.

NUTRITION TREATMENT

Intervention, management, and counseling of individuals on appropriate food choices to meet their nutrient needs.

NUTRITIONAL ADEQUACY

A measure of the health and well-being of the individual in relation to the intake of essential nutrients.

NUTRITIONAL ASSESSMENT

Measurement of indicators of dietary status and nutrition-related health status of individuals or populations.

NUTRITIONAL STATUS

The health of the individual with respect to nutrient intake.

NUTRITIVE VALUE OF FOODS

The content of essential nutrients as assessed in an analytical laboratory. The nutrient content of many foods humans consume can be found in the Tables of Composition compiled by the U.S. Department of Agriculture (http://www.nal.usda.gov/fnic/foodcomp/data/foods). Other tables are also available.

O

OBESITY

Excess body fat (more than 20% of the body weight as fat), accompanied by biomarkers of inflammation. Obesity may be the result of an interaction between genetics and lifestyle choices. There are social and cultural influences that can ensure or potentiate genetic tendencies to develop obesity. Anthropologists and medical historians have identified examples of cultural groups that consider excess body fat to be a mark of beauty as well as an indication of economic status within their society.

A number of genetically obese rats, mice, dogs, and desert animals have been described. In these animals, there are mutations in the genes for cytokines that signal hunger or satiety. Leptin and its receptor are implicated in animals whose chief characteristic is hyperphagia (excess food intake). Other errors in the perception of hunger and/or satiety by the brain have also been identified. Hyperphagia may also characterize some genetically obese humans. Yet there are obese people who are not hyperphagic. There are those who cannot dissipate their surplus intake energy as heat, that is, thermogenesis. (See BAT Thermogenesis.) These individuals do not tolerate cold well either. The common thread to these two conditions is the apparent inability of tissues to regulate the degree of uncoupling of its mitochondria so as to release more heat and synthesize less ATP. This ATP is used for the synthesis of macromolecules.

TREATMENT OF OBESITY

In almost no other area of medicine have there been so many failures as have occurred in the treatment of obesity. Surgical procedures such as the gastric bypass, exercise regimens, diet regimens, and diet and exercise protocols have been devised to help excessively fat people lose their excess fat store. Unfortunately, 90% of all those who lose weight regain it. The individual must constantly monitor both food intake and physical activity in order to sustain the weight loss.

Exercise on a regular basis stimulates muscle protein development as well as increases energy expenditure. Exercise can be a useful adjunct to energy intake restriction because it redirects energy loss from the lean body mass. In the sedentary individual, weight loss occurs at the expense of both fat and protein components of the body. In the exercising, food-restricted individual, the weight loss is primarily fat loss. Further, mild to moderate exercise seems to suppress food intake. Thus, food restriction together with exercise are additive in a beneficial way with respect to the loss and regain of body fat.

OBLIGATORY LOSS

Usually refers to the excretion of the products of one-way reactions, for example, the loss of nitrogen in creatinine and the product of the conversion of creatine to creatinine.

OCHRATOXINS

Mycotoxins produced by *Aspergillus ochraceus*, *Aspergillus* spp., and *Penicillium viridicatum*. They can be categorized as ochratoxin A, B, and C and 4-hydroxyochratoxin A. Ochratoxin A, the most important ochratoxin, is a fairly stable substance that is not easily metabolized. It is a potent hepatotoxin (in rats, ducklings, and Babcock cockerels) and a nephrotoxin (in rats and pigs). Theprimary target organ is the developing central nervous system (CNS). Furthermore, it was reported to be teratogenic in mice and rats, whereas it was noncarcinogenic to rats by both oral and subcutaneous administration. Ochratoxin A production in cereals is favored under humid conditions at moderate temperatures. Occurrence of ochratoxin A has been reported in grains and, following transfer, in the organs and blood of a number of animals, especially pigs.

ODDS RATIO (OR)

A good approximation of the relative risk. It compares the ratio of exposed/unexposed individuals among the diseased with the ratio of exposed/unexposed individuals among the controls. The odds ratio is a measure that is used in case-control studies, where cases and controls are selected at the same time.

ODYNOPHAGIA

Pain associated with swallowing.

OILS

Lipids that are liquid at room temperature (20°C–22°C). Usually of vegetable origin with the exception of the marine oils. These are fats extracted from sea creatures and are rich in long-chain polyunsaturated fatty acids. Although the tropical oils such as coconut oil are called oils, they are solids at room temperatures common to North America. In the tropics, these lipids are liquid.

OLESTRA

A synthetic fat that is a sucrose polyester. It has the texture of fat but does not have the energy value of fat.

OLFACTION

The sense of smell.

OLIGURIA

Decreased urine production.

OLMESARTAN MEDOXOMIL, OLMESARTAN MEDOXOMIL HYDROCHLORIDE

An angiotensin receptor antagonist that works as an antihypertensive. When joined with a thiazide, it is also a diuretic. Trade names: Benicar, Benecar HCT.

OMEGA-3 FATTY ACIDS, ω-3 FATTY ACIDS, N-3 FATTY ACIDS

See Fatty Acids. Fatty acids having a double bond in the omega-3 (N-3) position. The numbers begin at the methyl end of the molecule. The fatty acid can have more than one double bond.

OMEGA-6 FATTY ACIDS, ω-6 FATTY ACIDS, N-6 FATTY ACIDS

See Fatty Acids. Fatty acids having a double bond in the omega-6 (N-6) position. More than one double bond can occur in these fatty acids.

OMEPRAZOLE

A proton pump inhibitor and gastric acid production suppressor. Trade names: Losec, Prilosec.

ONCOGENES

Part of the DNA that contains genes responsible for cell division and tissue growth. When their expression is uncontrolled, cancer develops. When a normal cell escapes its usual constraint in terms of growth and function, it does so through the action of oncogenes that encode altered forms of hormones or receptors or transcription factors that in turn distort the cell and its function. More than 50 oncogenes have been identified. The effect of oncogene products arises through their differences from their corresponding normal cellular proteins. They may have different rates of synthesis and/or degradation, altered cellular functions, or be resistant to the normal control mechanisms in place that regulate cell function. In order for the cell to become a cancer cell, it must have at least five independent oncogenic events. This is due to the broad spectrum of control mechanisms and the complex cellular processes and signaling mechanisms within the cell. It also explains why the risk of cancer increases with age since time and oncogenic events are needed for the full expression of the cancerous state.

ONCOGENESIS

The process to converting a normal cell to a cancer cell.

ONCOTIC PRESSURE

The pressure exerted by the plasma proteins on the walls of the vascular system. These proteins are too large to pass through the capillaries, hence this pressure is noted only in the large vessels.

OOCYTE

An egg produced by the ovary.

OOGENESIS

The production of oocytes by the ovary of the female.

OPHTHALMIA

Inflammation of the conjunctiva (membrane that lines the eyelid) of the eye.

OPIOID RECEPTORS

Structures on the surface of neuronal cells that mediate the function of opiates. Both naturally produced opiates (endorphins) and drugs are bound by these receptors and when bound analgesia is produced.

OPSIN

A protein that combines with retinal (vitamin A aldehyde) to form rhodopsin (visual purple). Rhodopsin bleaches upon exposure to bright light and breaks apart. It is reformed and this process is called the visual cycle. The cycle does not function in the vitamin A–deficient individual and night blindness results.

ORAL

Pertaining to the mouth.

ORGANELLE

A discrete structure within the cell.

ORGANIC

Substances containing carbon that originate from living creatures.

ORGANIC FOOD

A term usually taken to mean a food grown without the aid of fertilizers, herbicides, and pesticides. This is a misnomer since all foods are comprised of organic molecules and hence are organic. Foods that are labeled organic must follow the FDA guidelines for such labeling.

ORGANOGENESIS

The development of specific organs in the course of embryonic and fetal development.

ORGANOLEPTIC

Features of a food perceived by the senses of taste, smell, sound, vision, and tactile, or feel.

ORI

Origin of replication in prokaryotes.

ORNITHINE CYCLE

Part of the Urea Cycle. See Metabolic Maps, Appendix 2.

OROTIC ACID

Metabolic intermediate in the synthesis of prymidines.

ORTHOSTATIC HYPOTENSION

Hypotension that results from standing and is often associated with dehydration.

OSMOLALITY

Quantity of solutes per liter of solution, which contributes to the pressure of that solution on a membrane.

OSMORECEPTORS

Structures in the hypothalamus that detect changes (elevations) in blood tonicity. When tonicity is increased a signal is generated that inhibits water loss.

OSMOSIS

The passage of solvents across a membrane so as to equalize the concentrations of solutes on each side of the membrane.

OSMOTIC EFFECT

The effects of solutes on water passage.

OSMOTIC PRESSURE

The pressure that must be applied to prevent the passage of a solvent. Only those solutes that cannot pass through a membrane can contribute to osmotic pressure.

OSSIFICATION

The process of bone formation.

OSTEOARTHRITIS

Degenerative bone and joint disease due to wear and tear; age-associated condition.

OSTEOBLASTS

Bone-forming cells.

OSTEOCALCIN

A protein whose synthesis is dependent on vitamin K and which acts to promote mineral deposition in bone. This protein contains numerous glutamic acid residues, which are carboxylated post-translationally through the action of the vitamin K-dependent epoxide cycle.

OSTEOCLASTS

Cells responsible for bone remodeling. These cells mobilize bone mineral.

OSTEOMALACIA

A condition characterized by a weakening and softening of the bone and in which the bending of long bones can develop. Associated with vitamin D deficiency.

OSTEOPENIA

Decreased bone mass.

OSTEOPOROSIS

Disease in which the bone loses its mineral content and becomes porous; associated with aging, particularly in females lacking estrogen.

OVALBUMIN

Egg albumin; the major protein in egg white.

OVERHYDRATION

Extracellular fluid volume excess.

OVERWEIGHT

A body weight in excess of that thought to be normal for height.

OVOLACTOVEGETARIAN

An individual who includes fruits, milk, vegetables, milk products, eggs, and cheese in the diet but not meat.

OVOMUCOID

A minor protein in egg white that contains carbohydrate as part of its structure.

OXALATES

See Type B Antinutritives.

OXALIC ACID

A two-carbon dicarboxylate found in foods especially rhubarb, spinach, parsley, cocoa, and tea. It can bind divalent minerals and make them biologically unavailable.

OXALOACETATE

A labile metabolic intermediate. (See Citric Acid Cycle.)

OXIDASE

An enzyme group responsible for oxygen removal; it catalyzes oxidation/reduction reactions using oxygen as the electron acceptor.

OXIDATION

The removal of electrons using oxygen as the electron acceptor. The process may not always involve an enzyme. It may occur spontaneously, and when this occurs, it is called autoxidation. In food, autoxidation occurs and is responsible for the deterioration of food quality. The discoloration of red meat upon exposure to air at room temperature is an indication of the autoxidation process. The off odor that accompanies this discoloration is the result of the autoxidation of the fatty acids in the meat fat. In living systems, the process of autoxidation is suppressed to a large extent because the products of this oxidation, fatty acid peroxides, can be very damaging. Peroxides denature proteins, rendering them inactive and attacking the DNA in the nucleus and mitochondria, resulting in base pair deletions or breaks in the DNA, which, in turn, result in mutations or errors in this DNA. In the nucleus, these breaks or deletions can be repaired. In the aging animal, the repair mechanism loses its efficiency. One of the characteristics of aged cells is the loss of its DNA repair ability. Mitochondria have little DNA repair capability, so base pair deletions, substitutions, or insertions occurring as a result of free radical attack cannot be reversed. Fortunately, there are many mitochondria in each cell so that if a few are damaged in this way, the effect is not as devastating as happens with unrepaired DNA damage in the nucleus.

To prevent widespread damage to cellular proteins and DNA by these radicals, there is a potent antioxidation system in all cells. This antioxidation system includes the selenium-containing enzyme glutathione peroxidase, catalase, and superoxide dismutase (SOD). These enzymes are listed in Table 40. These enzymes are found in the peroxisomes. SOD is also found in the mitochondria. All of these components serve to suppress free radical formation. The free radical chain reaction is shown in Figure 33.

Free radicals can form when the oxygen atom is excited by a variety of drugs and contaminants and by ultraviolet light. The excited oxygen atom is called singlet oxygen (O_2^-). Pollutants such as the oxides of nitrogen or carbon tetrachloride can provoke this reaction. In vivo, the detoxification reactions catalyzed by the cytochrome P450 enzymes generate free radicals. In the respiratory chain of the mitochondria, the possibility of oxygen radical production exists, and it is for this reason the mitochondria possess a particularly potent peroxide suppressor, SOD. SOD in the mitochondria requires the manganese ion as a cofactor. The cytosol also has SOD, but this enzyme requires the copper and zinc ions. Both forms of the enzyme catalyze

TABLE 40
Antioxidant Enzymes Found in Mammalian Cells

Enzyme	Required Mineral Cofactor	Reaction Catalyzed
Superoxide dismutase	CuZn	$2\,O_2^{-\cdot} + 2\,H^+ \rightarrow + H_2O_2$
Glutathione peroxidase	Se	$H_2O_2 + 2\,GSH \rightarrow GSSG + 2\,H_2O$
		$ROOH + 2\,GSH \rightarrow GSSG + ROH + H_2O$
Catalase	Fe	$2\,H_2O_2 \rightarrow 2\,H_2O + O_2$
Glutathione S-transferases		$ROOH + 2\,GSH \rightarrow GSSG + ROH + H_2O$

$$2\,O_2^{-\cdot} + 2\,H^+ \xrightarrow{\text{SOD}} H_2O_2 + O_2$$

$$2\,H_2O_2 \xrightarrow{\text{Catalase}} 2\,H_2O + 1/2\,O_2$$

$$H_2O_2 + R(OH)_2 \xrightarrow{\text{Peroxidase}} H_2O + RO_2$$

$$H_2O_2 + 2\,GSH \xrightarrow{\text{GSH-Px}} GSSG + 2\,H_2O$$

NADPH   NADP

NAD   NADH

SOD	Superoxide dismutase (requires Mg^{++} or Cu^{++} or Mn^{++} or Cu^{++} and Zinc)
GSH-Px	Glutathione peroxidase (requires Se)
GSH	Reduced glutathione
GSSG	Oxidized glutathione
H_2O_2	Hydrogen peroxide

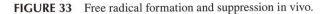

FIGURE 33   Free radical formation and suppression in vivo.

the reaction: $O_2^- \cdot + O_2^- \cdot + 2\ H^+ \rightarrow H_2O_2 + O_2$. Two superoxides and two hydrogen ions are joined to form one molecule of hydrogen peroxide and a molecule of oxygen. In turn, the peroxide can be converted to water through the action of the enzyme catalase. Peroxides can also be "neutralized" through the action of glutathione S-transferase. This reaction requires two moles of reduced glutathione and produces two molecules of oxidized glutathione and two molecules of water. Fatty acid radicals can also be neutralized by glutathione peroxidase, producing a molecule of an alcohol with the same chain length as the fatty acid. Glutathione S-transferase can duplicate the action of glutathione peroxidase. In addition to the reactions that counteract the in vivo formation of oxygen radicals or fatty acid peroxides, certain of the vitamins have this role as well. Ascorbic acid has an antioxidant function as it can donate reducing equivalents to a peroxide converting it to an alcohol. β-carotene can quench singlet oxygen and thus convert it into O_2. Vitamin E is perhaps the best known antioxidant vitamin, and its action is similar to that of ascorbic acid. It donates reducing equivalents to a peroxide converting it to an alcohol.

Although the foregoing paragraphs have emphasized the negative aspects of the partial reduction products of oxygen, there is some evidence that peroxide formation has some benefit. For example, leukocytes produce peroxides as a means of killing invading bacteria. Other examples no doubt will emerge as scientists struggle to understand the role of peroxidation (and the peroxisomes) in mammalian metabolism.

OXIDATION/REDUCTION

Reactions in which electrons are lost by one reactant and gained by another.

OXIDATIVE DEAMINATION

The removal of an amino group together with the loss of electrons that are accepted by oxygen.

OXIDATIVE DECARBOXYLATION

The removal of a carboxyl group together with the loss of electrons accepted by oxygen.

OXIDATIVE PHOSPHORYLATION (OXPHOS)

See Metabolic Maps, Appendix 2. Two processes whereby water and ATP are synthesized simultaneously: (1) respiration joins hydrogen and oxygen ions to make water, and (2) ATP synthesis uses some of the energy so released to synthesize ATP. These coupled processes occur in the mitochondria of the cell.

OXIDATIVE RANCIDITY

Caused by products from reactions of fatty acids with atmospheric oxygen. Oxidation of fats and oils usually results in the formation of a variety of toxic substances. Three types of oxidation can be identified: (1) autoxidation, (2) photooxidation, and (3) enzymatic oxidation.

OXYCODON HYDROCHLORIDE

An opioid analgesic that can become habit-forming. Trade names: Oxycontin, Oxy-FAST, OxyIR, Roxicodone, Intensol, Supeudol.

OXYTOCIN

Hormone that stimulates uterine contractions as part of the parturition process. There is also a synthetic preparation called Pitocin that is used to stimulate uterine contractions and lactation.

OXYTOCIN RECEPTORS

Structures on/in the plasma membranes of mammary cells and uterine cells that bind oxytocin and transmit a signal (via the inositol signaling pathway) into these cells, which initiates contraction of the uterus or the mammary lacteals.

P

PABA (PARA-AMINOBENZOIC ACID)

A growth factor for bacteria; an integral part of folacin.

PACEMAKER

Electrical device used to maintain a normal sinus rhythm of myocardial contraction by electrically stimulating the heart muscle.

PANCREATIN

Extract of pancreas; contains pancreatic enzymes.

PANCREATITIS

Inflammation of the pancreas; associated with alcoholism or biliary tract obstruction. If untreated, the exocrine pancreas becomes necrotic and characteristic disturbances in digestion occur together with progressive decline of health. This can be life threatening.

PANCREOZYMIN

A hormone (also called cholecystokinin) secreted by endocrine cells lining the duodenum. Its release is stimulated by the presence of lipid in the chyme. It signals the exocrine pancreas to release pancreatic enzymes (pancreatic juice) and stimulates the release of bile from the gall bladder.

PANTOTHENIC ACID

An essential B vitamin that is an integral part of coenzyme A (CoA). CoA is essential for the synthesis of fatty acids. In food, pantothenic acid is found in a free form and also as part of phosphopantetheine. Pantothenic acid is the trivial name for the compound dihydroxy-β, β-dimethyl butyryl-β-alanine. It has two metabolically active forms: CoA and as part of acyl carrier protein (ACP). Pantothenic acid exists as the free acid or as a calcium salt. It is the condensation product of β-alanine and a hydroxyl and methyl substituted butyric acid, pentoic acid. Its structure is shown in Figure 34.

It is an unstable pale yellow oil, commercially available as a white, stable, crystalline calcium or sodium salt. When dry, the salt is stable to air and light but is hygroscopic. The salt is soluble in water and glacial acetic acid. The vitamin is stable in neutral solution but is readily destroyed by heat and either alkaline or acidic pH. When heated, there is hydrolytic cleavage of the molecule yielding β-alanine and 2,4 dihydroxy-3, 3-dimethyl butyrate.

SOURCES

Pantothenic acid is widely distributed in nature. Excellent food sources are organ meats, mushrooms, avocados, broccoli, and whole grains.

ABSORPTION AND METABOLISM

Absorption occurs via facilitated diffusion and travels in the blood within the erythrocytes as well as in the plasma. Large doses of pantothenic acid are rapidly excreted in the urine, indicating little storage and little degradation.

FUNCTION

Pantothenic acid's main function is as a component of CoA. Unlike most vitamin coenzymes, pantothenic acid does not comprise the functional unit of CoA; instead, it provides the backbone for its derivative, pantotheine, whose sulfhydryl (SH) group forms the reactive site. The structure of CoA is shown in Figure 35 and its synthesis in Figure 36.

The function of CoA is to serve as a carrier of acyl groups in enzymatic reactions involving fatty acid oxidation, fatty acid synthesis, pyruvate oxidation, and biologic acetylations. It cannot cross the cell membrane and must, therefore, be synthesized in cells. Acetyl CoA (active acetate) is formed during the oxidation of pyruvate or fatty acids. It may also be generated from free acetate in the presence of the enzyme acetyl CoA synthetase. Acetyl CoA may then react with an acyl group acceptor such as choline to yield acetylcholine or oxaloacetate for citrate synthesis in the citric acid

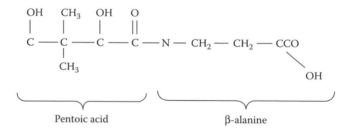

FIGURE 34   Structure of pantothenic acid.

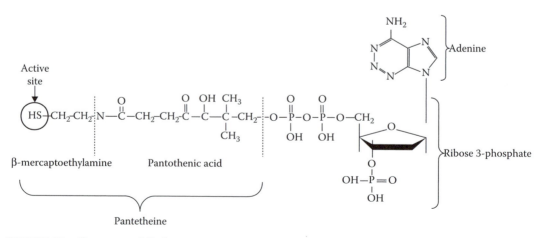

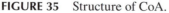

FIGURE 35   Structure of CoA.

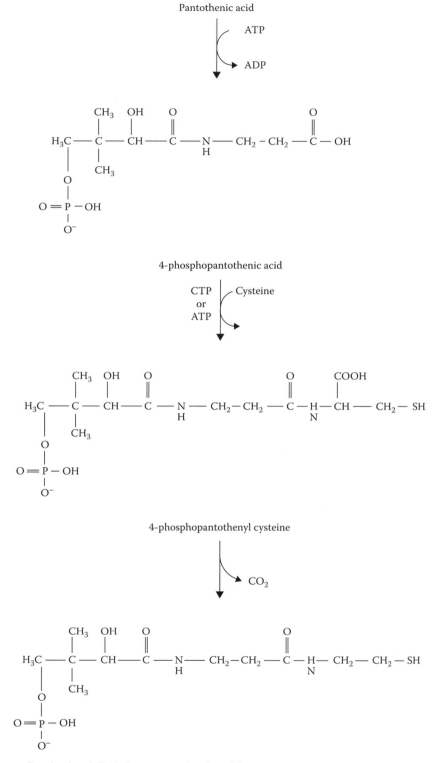

FIGURE 36 Synthesis of CoA from pantothenic acid.

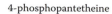

4-phosphopantetheine

ATP

PP$_i$

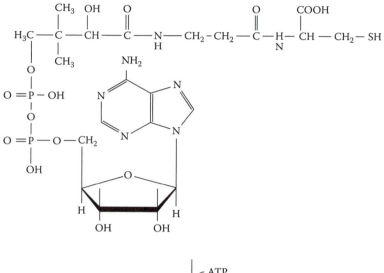

ATP

ADP

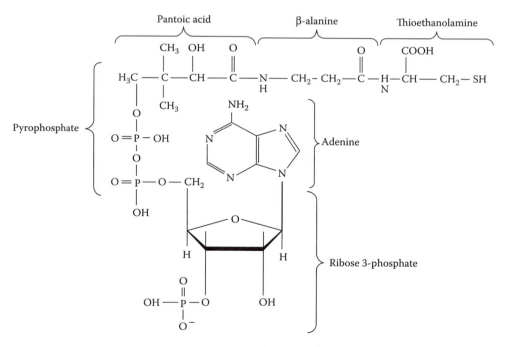

Coenzyme A

FIGURE 36 *(Continued)*

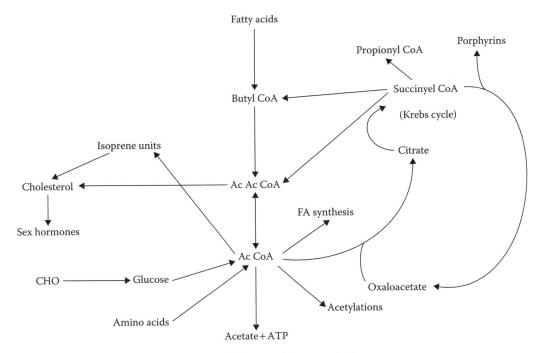

FIGURE 37 Central role of acetyl CoA in intermediary metabolism.

cycle (Figure 37). The SH group of the β-mercaptoethylamine is the site at which acyl groups are linked for transport by the coenzyme. The ability of the CoA SH to form thioesters with carboxylic acids is responsible for the vital role of the coenzyme in numerous metabolic processes.

All known acyl derivatives of CoA are thiol esters. These acyl derivatives of CoA may participate in a number of metabolic reactions: condensation, addition, acyl group interchanges, and nucleophilic attack. These reactions fall into three general categories:

1. Acetylation of choline and certain aromatic amines such as sulfonamides.
2. Oxidation of fatty acids, pyruvate, α ketoglutarate, and acetaldehyde.
3. Synthesis of fatty acids, cholesterol, sphingosine, citrate, acetoacetate, porphyrin, and sterols.

Thus, CoA serves not only as an acetyl donor/acceptor but also as an acyl donor/acceptor. CoA serves as a central integrator of intermediary metabolism as illustrated in Figure 37.

Fatty acid synthesis in the cytoplasm involves an additional role of pantothenic acid in the form of a cofactor 4′-phosphopantetheine. This cofactor is bound to a protein commonly called ACP. ACP plus 4′-phosphopantetheine appears to be involved in fatty acid synthesis. The acyl intermediates formed during fatty acid synthesis are esterified to the SH group. Phosphopantetheine is a cofactor bound to the GTP-dependent acyl CoA synthetase. Thus, 4′-phosphopantotheine serves in a capacity analogous to CoA during fatty acid oxidation. Carnitine reacts with fatty acyl CoA esters to form carnitine esters capable of crossing the mitochondrial membrane. CoA does not travel across membranes and thus must be synthesized within each cell as the need for it arises.

Deficiency Symptoms

Deficiency symptoms are species specific. Pantothenic acid deficiency has not been described in humans as a single entity. If it occurs, it is accompanied by other deficiency disorders as well. The exception to this is in patients treated with the pantothenic acid antagonist, ω-methyl pantothenic acid. In these patients, neurological symptoms (parasthesia of toes and feet), depression, fatigue, insomnia, vomiting, and muscle weakness have been reported. Changes in glucose tolerance, increased sensitivity to insulin, and decreased antibody production have also been noted.

PAPAIN

A proteolytic enzyme found in papaya.

PARABIOSIS

The circulatory system of one animal is joined with that of another animal. The two animals must be very closely related in order for both to survive.

PARACRINES, PARACRINE SYSTEM

The hormone secreted by one cell is transmitted a very short distance to the cell it affects. Usually these cells are adjacent to each other.

PARALYTIC SHELLFISH TOXINS (PSTs)

Neurotoxins that are among the most potent of the known low–molecular weight toxins. Paralytic shellfish poisoning is attributed to the consumption of shellfish that have become contaminated with a toxin or group of toxins on the ingestion of toxic plankton, in particular, toxic dinoflagellates. The shellfish involved are pelecypods, a family of mollusks, including mussels and clams. The paralytic toxins from dinoflagellates can be categorized in two groups: (1) water-soluble toxins, responsible for almost all types of paralytic shellfish poisoning in humans, and (2) lipid-soluble toxins, found in oysters and clams. So far, seven different kinds of paralytic shellfish toxins have been identified and characterized: (1) saxitoxin, (2) neosaxitoxin (1-hydroxysaxitoxin), (3) gonyautoxin-I (11-a-neosaxitoxin sulfate), (4) gonyautoxin-II (11-a-saxitoxin sulfate), (5) gonyautoxin-III (11-b-saxitoxin sulfate), (6) gonyautoxin-IV (11-b-neosaxitoxin sulfate), and (7) gonyautoxin-V (structure unknown).

Two major effects of the paralytic shellfish toxins are noted: (1) effects on peripheral and central nervous system, and (2) systemic effects. The initial symptoms (within 30 minutes) of paralytic shellfish poisoning in humans include tingling, burning sensation, and numbness (lips, gums, tongue, face, and fingertips). Then, similar sensations spread to the neck, arms, and legs, and general muscular incoordination ensues. Other symptoms may also be present, such as weakness, dizziness, malaise, prostration, headache, salivation, rapid pulse, intense thirst, dysphagia, perspiration, anuria, impairment of vision, or even temporary blindness. Depending on the amount of toxin ingested, death following respiratory paralysis may occur within 2–12 hours. The risk of contamination and poisoning is highest during a so-called red tide. In many parts of the world, the sea sometimes suddenly becomes colored as a result of dinoflagellate bloom. This phenomenon is referred to as red tide, although the bloom may also be yellow or brown. In spite of the frequent occurrence of red tide and the high toxicity of the paralytic shellfish toxins, intoxication rarely happens. This is largely due to the strict regulations set by many countries and the awareness of people in coastal areas of the risks associated with eating shellfish during red tides. Although ordinary cooking destroys up to 70% of the toxin(s) and panfrying even more, there may be sufficient toxin left in the mollusks to cause serious poisoning.

PARATHORMONE (PARATHYROID HORMONE)

A hormone synthesized and released by the parathyroid glands located in the thyroid gland. This hormone is involved in the regulation of blood calcium levels through its action to increase the rate of conversion of $25(OH)D_3$ to $1\alpha\ 25(OH)_2D_3$ in kidney tissue, and thus increase the levels of this form of the vitamin in blood. This increases blood levels of calcium. The hormone also increases the extent of osteoclastic and osteocytic osteolysis (bone resorption and remodeling). Parathyroid hormone increases the urinary excretion of phosphate and hydroxyproline-containing peptides, thus reducing urinary calcium excretion.

PARATHYROID HORMONE RECEPTOR

Structure on the surface of bone and kidney cells that binds parathyroid hormone and signals these cells to respond to this hormone.

PARATHYROIDECTOMY

Removal of parathyroid glands.

PARENTERAL NUTRITION

Nutritional support furnished through the vascular system.

PARESTHESIA

A sensation of burning, numbness, or tingling usually associated with damage to sensory nerves.

PARIETAL CELLS

Stomach cells that secrete hydrochloric acid.

PARKINSON'S DISEASE

Disease of the nervous system characterized by palsy. The syndrome may be the result of arterio-sclerotic changes in the basal ganglia characterized by arrhythmic muscular tremors and rigidity of movement.

PARS DISTALIS

Cells in the anterior pituitary that produce thyroid-stimulating hormone, luteotropic hormone, adrenocorticotrophic hormone (ACTH), prolactin, lipotropin, β-endophin, and follicle-stimulating hormone.

PARS INTERMEDIA

Cells in the anterior pituitary that secrete melanotropic hormone, as well as ACTH. These cells are intermixed with those of pars distalis.

PARS TUBERALIS

Cells in the anterior pituitary with no discernable function.

PARTURITION

Birth.

PARTS PER MILLION (PPM)

Expression of concentration of a solute in a solution.

PASSIVE DIFFUSION

A process for the passage of solutes across a membrane that does not involve a carrier or energy.

PASTEURIZATION

Process of heating a liquid to destroy harmful organisms.

PATHOGENS

Microorganisms that cause disease.

PATULIN

A mycotoxin produced by *Penicillium urticae, Penicillium patulum, Penicillium expansum*, 12 other species of *Penicillium, Aspergillus*, and *Byssochlamys nivea*. It is a wide-spectrum toxicant that is poisonous to mammals, plants, and many lower forms of life. Patulin is stable under conditions required for fruit juice production and preservation. In experimental animals, it has been shown to cause hemorrhages, formation of edema, and dilatation of the intestinal tract. In subchronic studies, hyperemia of the epithelium of the duodenum and kidney function impairment were observed as main effects. Factors involved in fungal growth and patulin production include moderate temperature, high moisture content, and a pH between 3 and 5. Occurrence of patulin is mainly reported in fruits, such as apples, peaches, pears, apricots, and cherries. Patulin is an indicator of poor manufacturing practice (use of moldy raw material) and can pose a serious threat to human and animal health.

PBB

Polybrominated biphenyl; an environmental contaminant.

PBI TEST

A test that measures thyroid activity by measuring the amount of protein-bound iodine in the blood.

PCB (POLYCHLORINATED BIPHENYL)

A plasticizer and insulator material used in the electronics industry found to be a very long-lived toxic environmental contaminant.

PCOS (POS)

Polycystic ovary syndrome. A syndrome characterized by menstrual irregularities, hyperandrogenism, infertility, polycystic ovaries, and (sometimes) obesity, glucose intolerance, mild to moderate acne, hirsutism, and hyperpigmentation. Not all of the latter characteristics are present in all females with PCOS.

PECTIN

A type of water-soluble fiber found in many fruits. When hydrolyzed it forms a gel.

PEDIATRICS

A specialty having to do with children.

PELLAGRA

Niacin deficiency disorder.

PENTOSE

A five-carbon sugar found in plums and cherries.

PENTOSE PHOSPHATE PATHWAY

See Hexose Monophosphate Shunt and Metabolic Maps, Appendix 2.

PENTOSURIA

A rare genetic disease due to a mutation in the gene for the NADP-linked enzyme xylose or xylulose dehydrogenase and characterized by the presence of xylose or xylulose in the urine instead of xylitol. This has no clinical significance.

PEP

Phosphoenolpyruvic acid; a key intermediate in glucose synthesis and in glycolysis.

PEPCK

Phosphoenolpyruvate carboxykinase; rate-limiting enzyme in gluconeogenesis.

PEPSIN

A protein digestive enzyme released by gastric cells as pepsinogen and activated by hydrochloric acid.

PEPSINOGEN

The inactive precursor form of pepsin.

PEPTIC ULCER

Chronic lesions found in the gastrointestinal tract in locations exposed to hydrochloric acid or pepsin. The most common locations are the duodenum and stomach. Lesions are due to a penicillin-sensitive organism, *Helicobacter pylori*.

PEPTIDE BOND

The bond formed between the amino group of one amino acid and the carboxyl group of another. A molecule of water is formed as a by-product of this reaction.

PEPTIDES

Single chains of amino acids joined together by peptide bonds. (See Protein Structure.)

PEPTONES

A secondary protein derivative formed during protein digestion in the stomach.

PER OS

By mouth.

PERCUTANEOUS TRANSLUMINAL CORONARY ANGIOPLASTY (PTCA)

See Cardiovascular Tests and Therapies.

PERICARDITIS

Inflammation of the sac enclosing the heart and its vessels, known as the pericardium.

PERINATAL

Period of time occurring before and immediately after birth.

PERIODONTAL DISEASE

Inflammation of the gums.

PERIPHERAL VASCULAR DISEASE

Atherosclerotic changes in the vessels of the limbs.

PERISTALSIS

The rhythmic contractions of the smooth muscles which surround the gastrointestinal tract.

PERITONEAL DIALYSIS

Therapy useful in treating renal failure in which toxic substances are removed from the body by using the peritoneum as a semipermeable membrane.

PERNICIOUS

Adjective that describes a fatal (usually) disease.

PERNICIOUS ANEMIA

Disease of vitamin B_{12} deficiency. Characterized by low numbers of red blood cells that are poorly formed and by demyelination of the sheaths of nerve tracts.

PEROXIDATION

Oxidation to the point of forming peroxides. (See Oxidation.)

PEROXISOMAL FATTY ACID OXIDATION

Peroxisomal oxidation in the kidney and liver is an important aspect of drug metabolism. The peroxisomes are a class of subcellular organelles that are important in protection against oxygen toxicity. They have a high level of catalase activity. The peroxisomal fatty acid oxidation pathway differs in three important ways from the mitochondrial pathway. First, the initial dehydrogenation is accomplished by a cyanide-insensitive oxidase that produces H_2O_2. This H_2O_2 is rapidly extinguished by catalase. Second, the enzymes of the pathway prefer long-chain fatty acids and are slightly different in structure from those (with the same function) of the mitochondrial pathway. Third, β-oxidation in the peroxisomes stops at eight carbons rather than proceeding all the way to acetyl CoA. The peroxisomes also serve in the conversion of cholesterol to bile acids and in the formation of ether lipids (plasmalogens).

PESTICIDES

See Contamination with Organic Chemicals under Contamination of Food. Chemicals used to reduce the population of plant and animal insects, fungi, molds, and parasites.

PETECHIAE

Minute hemorrhagic spots in the skin.

PGI, PGE

Prostaglandins in the I or E series.

pH

The numerical representation of the hydrogen ion concentration in a solution. A low pH represents an acid solution while a high pH represents a basic or alkaline solution. Physiological pH is 7.4.

PHARMACOLOGICAL REACTION

A food-intolerance reaction resulting from the pharmacological effect of a food component. A well-known example is caffeine, a methylxanthine derivative present in coffee. Its biological action includes stimulation of the heart muscle, the central nervous system, and the production of gastrin. Symptoms associated with a high coffee intake are restlessness, tremors, weight loss, palpitations, and alterations in mood. Other biologically active substances are histamine, tyramine, phenylethylamine, and histamine releasers.

PHENANTHRENE

The basic ring structure of the steroid class of compounds.

PHENFORMIN

A biguanide derivative that serves as an oral hypoglycemic agent useful in managing type 2 diabetes mellitus.

PHENOL OR PHENYL OXIDASES

Copper-containing enzymes responsible for the browning of fruit at the cut surface. These enzymes can be inhibited by ascorbic acid or by heating.

PHENOTYPE

A category or group to which an individual is assigned based on one or more inherited characteristics; the overt expression of the genotype.

PHENTOLAMINE

A drug that blocks the action of vasopressin in terms of its stimulatory effect on glycogenolysis.

PHENYLALANINE

An essential amino acid containing a phenyl group and alanine; a precursor to tyrosine. (See Amino Acids, Table 5.)

PHENYLETHYLAMINE

A biologically active substance, which can be involved in the pharmacological reactions of food intolerance. It occurs in chocolate, old cheese, and red wine and can provoke migraine attacks. It is the amine form of phenylalanine, which forms when phenylalanine hydroxylase does not metabolize all of the phenylalanine present.

PHENYLKETONURIA (PKU)

A genetic disease due to a mutation in the gene for the enzyme phenylalanine hydroxylase. Several variants have been described. The phenotypic expression of the genotype includes mental retardation. Expression can be prevented by early diagnosis and use of a low phenylalanine diet.

PHEOCHROMOCYTOMA

A tumor of the adrenal medulla chromaffin cell characterized by hypersecretion of epinephrine with intermittant to permanent hypertension. Death can occur if not recognized and the tumor removed.

PHOSPHATASE

An enzyme that catalyzes the removal of a phosphoryl group from a substrate.

PHOSPHATE

A molecule (PO_4) containing phosphorus and oxygen.

PHOSPHATIDYLCHOLINE

A phospholipid commonly known as lecithin.

PHOSPHATIDYLETHANOLAMINE

A phospholipid in membranes; an important component (cephalin) of the brain lipids.

PHOSPHATIDYLINOSITOL

A phospholipid in the plasma membrane that is an important component of the second-messenger system called the PIP cycle. (See Inositol.)

PHOSPHOCREATINE

See Creatine Phosphate.

PHOSPHOGLUCONATE PATHWAY

See Hexose Monophosphate Shunt.

PHOSPHOGLYCERIDE

A lipid containing a glycerol backbone, one or two fatty acids, and a phosphate group.

PHOSPHOLIPID

A family of compounds containing a glycerol or sphingosine backbone plus one or two fatty acids and a phosphate group linked to one of the following: choline, inositol, ethanolamine, or serine.

PHOSPHOLIPASE A$_2$

Enzyme responsible for the release of arachidonic acid from membrane phospholipids.

PHOSPHOLIPASE C

A membrane-bound enzyme responsible for the hydrolysis of phosphatidylinositol 4,5-diphosphate (PIP_2) to form two second messengers, diacylglyceride (DAG), and inositol 1,4,5-triphosphate (IP_3).

PHOSPHORUS

An essential mineral component of bone tissue, where it occurs in the mass ratio of 1 phosphorus to 2 calcium, and also an essential ingredient of intermediary metabolism and membranes. Phosphorus is present in nearly all foods. In a number of species, excess phosphorus, that is, a calcium–phosphorus ratio of 0.5, leads to a decrease in the blood calcium level and secondary hyperparathyroidism with loss of bone. The phosphorus levels in normal diets are not likely to be harmful.

PHOSPHORYLASE KINASE

An enzyme that specifically phosphorylates SER 14 of glycogen phosphorylase b. This is one of the early steps in glycogen degradation.

PHOSPHORYLATION

The addition of a phosphate group.

PHOTOOXIDATION

Oxidative degradation of a substance by photoreaction. (Poly)unsaturated fatty acids can undergo two types of photooxidation: (1) a free-radical chain reaction, which starts from the excited state of another molecule, and (2) a singlet oxygen ($1O_2$) reaction in which the absorption of photons by molecules of another food component is followed by energy transfer to ground-state oxygen, leading to the formation of singlet oxygen. Photooxidation of foods can be prevented by using packaging materials that absorb the photochemically active light and by removing endogenous photosensitizers and oxygen from the food.

PHOTOSYNTHESIS

The process whereby plants convert CO_2 and water into carbohydrates with the energy provided by ultraviolet light.

PHYLLOQUINONE

Vitamin K from plant sources.

PHYSIOLOGICAL FUEL VALUE

The energy provided by food with a correction for the energy lost through digestion and absorption.

PHYTIC ACID

A component of plants that can bind divalent ions. Phytate is a form of inositol that is phosphorylated in all six positions of the carbons; when calcium and magnesium are bound, it becomes an insoluble salt called phytin. (See Type B Antinutritive.) Phytates bind zinc and can impair growth in children fed plant-based diets without meat, milk, and eggs.

PHYTOBEZOAR

A mass of food in the stomach, usually vegetable type food, that does not pass into the intestine.

PHYTOCHEMICALS

Nutritionally important chemicals found in plant products.

PHYTOESTROGENS

Estrogen-like compounds present in plant foods, particularly foods from soybeans.

PHYTOSTEROL

A sterol related to cholesterol found in plants.

PICA

Habitual consumption of nonfood items such as laundry starch, clay, paint chips, and other items.

PIGMENTATION

Coloration of skin related to the amount of melanin present.

PINEAL GLAND

A gland that receives light information by way of the eyes and sympathetic nerves. It produces melatonin, serotonin, and acetylserotonin. It is located in the brain between the thalamus and the mesencephalon.

PINEAL HORMONES

Melatonin, serotonin, acetylserotonin.

PINOCYTOSIS

Engulfing process in which cells absorb or ingest nutrients and fluid before hydrolysis.

PITUITARY GLAND

The master endocrine gland located at the base of the brain; secretes a number of tropic hormones that activate other endocrine organs. ACTH is an example. The pituitary gland also releases growth hormone as well as a number of other hormones that have direct action on metabolic processes.

PLACEBO

An inert preparation given for its psychological effect.

PLACENTA

The organ that surrounds the unborn child and serves as a barrier between the mother and child. It is permeable to a large number of solutes. The umbilical cord connects the placenta to the child.

PLACENTAL HORMONES

Chorionic proopiomelanocortin, chorionic thyrotropin, chorionic ACTH, and other chorionic tropic hormones.

PLANT HORMONES

Gibberellins, kinins, auxins. These stimulate plant growth and development.

PLANTAIN

Banana.

PLASMA

The fluids surrounding the red blood cells.

PLASMALOGENS

An acetyl phosphatide.

PLASMID

A small extrachromosomal circular molecule that replicates independently of the host DNA.

PLATELETS

Small, rod-shaped blood cells that, when meshed together, help form a clot.

PLP

Pyridoxal phosphate; a coenzyme required in amino acid metabolism that contains the vitamin pyridoxine in the aldehyde form.

PLUMBISM

Consumption of paint chips. If the paint contains lead oxide as the pigment, lead intoxication can develop. This is characterized by anemia, low serum iron and copper values, growth depression, ataxia, kidney damage, coma, convulsions, and death.

PNEUMOTHORAX

Collection of air or gas in the pleural space between the visceral and parietal pleurae of the lungs.

POACH

A method of cooking using water heated to a temperature just below boiling.

POISONOUS PLANTS

Plants that contain toxic materials sufficient to cause serious symptoms. Examples are listed in Table 41.

TABLE 41
Some Important Poisonous Plants of North America

Common Name	Scientific Name	Description	Toxic Parts	Geographical Distribution	Poisoning	Symptoms	Remarks
Baneberry	*Actaea* sp.	Perennial herb growing to 3 ft (1 m) tall from a thick root; compound leaves; small, white flowers; white or red berries with several seeds borne in short, terminal clusters.	All parts, but primarily roots and berries.	Native in rich woods occurring from Canada south to Georgia, Alabama, Louisiana, Oklahoma, and the Northern Rockies; red-fruited western baneberry from Alaska to central California, Arizona, Montana, and South Dakota.	Attributed to a glycoside or essential oil, which causes severe inflammation of the digestive tract.	Acute stomach cramps, headache, increased pulse, vomiting, delirium, dizziness, and circulatory failure; only six berries can cause symptoms persisting for hours.	Treatment may be a gastric lavage or vomiting; bright red berries attract children.
Buckeye; horse chestnut	*Aesculus* sp.	Shrub or tree; deciduous, opposite, palmately divided leaves with five to nine leaflets on a long stalk; red, yellow, or white flowers; two- to three-valved, capsule fruit; with thick, leathery husk enclosing one to six brown shiny seeds.	Leaves, twigs, flowers, and seeds.	Various species throughout the United States and Canada; some cultivated as ornamentals, others growing wild.	Toxic parts contain the glycoside, esculin.	Nervous twitching of muscles, weakness, lack of coordination, dilated pupils, nausea, vomiting, diarrhea, depression, paralysis, and stupor.	By making a "tea" from the leaves and twigs or by eating the seeds, children have been poisoned. Honey collected from the buckeye flower may also cause poisoning. Roots, branches, and fruits have been used to stupefy fish in ponds. Treatment usually is a gastric lavage or vomiting.
Buttercup	*Ranunculus* sp.	Annual or perennial herb growing to 16–32 in. (41–81 cm) high; leaves alternate entire to compound, and largely basal; yellow flowers borne singly or in clusters on ends of seed stalks; small fruits, one-seeded pods.	Entire plant	Widely distributed in woods, meadows, pastures, and along streams throughout temperate and cold locations.	The alkaloid, protoanemonin, which can injure the digestive system and ulcerate the skin.	Burning sensation of the mouth, nervousness, nausea, vomiting, low blood pressure, weak pulse, depression, and convulsions; sap and leaves may cause dermatitis.	Cows poisoned by buttercups produce bitter milk or milk with a reddish color.

(Continued)

TABLE 41 (Continued)
Some Important Poisonous Plants of North America

Common Name	Scientific Name	Description	Toxic Parts	Geographical Distribution	Poisoning	Symptoms	Remarks
Castor bean	Ricinus communis	Shrub-like herb 4–12 ft. (1.2–3.7 m) tall; simple, alternate, long-stalked leaves with 5 to 11 long lobes that are toothed on margins; fruits oval, green, or red, and covered with spines; three elliptical, glossy, black white, or mottled seeds per capsule.	Entire plant, especially the seeds.	Cultivated as an ornamental or oilseed crop primarily in the southern part of the United States and Hawaii.	Seeds, pressed cake, and leaves poisonous when chewed; contain the phytotoxin ricin.	Burning of the mouth and throat, nausea, vomiting, severe stomach pains, bloody diarrhea, excessive thirst, prostration, dullness of vision, and convulsions; kidney failure and death 1–12 days.	Fatal dose for a child is one to three seeds, and for an adult two to eight seeds; the oil extracted from the seeds is an important commercial product; it is not poisonous and it is used as a medicine (castor oil), for soap, and as a lubricant.
Chinaberry	Melia azedarach	Deciduous tree 20–40 ft (6–12 m) tall; twice, pinnately divided leaves and toothed or lobed leaflets, purple flowers borne in clusters; yellow, wrinkled, rounded berries that persist throughout the winter.	Berries, bark, flowers, and leaves.	A native of Asia introduced as an ornamental in the United States; common in the southern United States and lower altitudes in Hawaii; has become naturalized in old fields, pastures, around buildings, and along fence rows.	Most result from eating pulp of berries; toxic principle is a resinoid with narcotic effects.	Nausea, vomiting, diarrhea, irregular breathing, and respiratory distress.	Six to eight berries can cause the death of a child The berries have been used to make insecticide and flea powder.
Death camas	Zigadenus paniculatus	Perennial herb resembling wild onions but the onion odor lacking; long, slender leaves with parallel veins; pale yellow to pink flowers in clusters on slender seed stalks; fruit, a three-celled capsule.	Entire plant, especially the bulb.	Various species occur throughout the United States and Canada; all are more or less poisonous.	Due to the alkaloids zygadenine, veratrine, and others.	Excessive salivation, muscular weakness, slow heart rate, low blood pressure, subnormal temperature, nausea, vomiting, diarrhea, prostration, coma, and sometimes death.	The members of Lewis and Clark Expedition made four from the bulbs and suffered the symptoms of poisoning. Later some pioneers were killed when they mistook death camas for wild onions or garlic.
Dogbane (Indian hemp)	Apocynum cannabinum	Perennial herbs with milky juice and somewhat woody stems; simple, smooth, and oppositely paired leaves; bell-shaped, small, white to pink flowers borne in clusters at ends of axillary stems; paired, long, slender seed pods.	Entire plant.	Various species growing throughout North America in fields and forests, and along streams and roadsides.	Only suspect since it contains the toxic glycoside cymarin, and is poisonous to animals.	In animals, increased temperature and pulse, cold extremities, dilation of the pupils, discoloration of the mouth and nose, sore mouth, sweating, loss of appetite, and death.	Compounds extracted from roots of dogbane have been used to make a heart stimulant.

Common name	Scientific name	Description	Poisonous parts	Distribution	Cause	Symptoms	Remarks
Foxglove	*Digitalis purpurea*	Biennial herb with alternate, simple, toothed leaves; terminal, showy raceme of flowers, purple, pink, rose, yellow, or white; dry capsule fruit.	Entire plant, especially leaves, flowers, and seeds.	Native of Europe commonly planted in gardens of the United States; naturalized and abundant in some parts of the western United States.	Due to digitalis component.	Nausea, vomiting, dizziness, irregular heartbeat, tremors, convulsions, and possible death.	Foxglove has long been known as a source of digitalis and steroid glycosides; it is an important medicinal plant when used correctly.
Henbane	*Hyoscyamus niger*	Erect annual or biennial herb with coarse, hairy stems 1–5 ft (30–152 cm) high; simple, oblong, alternate leaves with a few coarse teeth, not stalked; greenish-yellow or yellowish with purple vein flowers; fruit, a rounded capsule.	Entire plant.	Along roads, in waste places across southern Canada and northern United States, particularly common in the Rocky Mountains.	Caused by the alkaloids hyoscyamine, hyoscine, and atropine.	Increased salivation, headache, nausea, rapid pulse, convulsions, coma, and death.	A gastric lavage of 4% tannic acid solution may be used to treat the poisoning.
Iris (Rocky Mountain iris)	*Iris missouriensis*	Lily-like perennial plants often in dense patches; long, narrow leaves; flowers blue-purple; fruit, a three-celled capsule.	Leaves, but especially the root stalk.	Wet land of meadows, marshes, and along streams from North Dakota to British Columbia, Canada; south to New Mexico, Arizona, and California; scattered over entire Rocky Mountain area; cultivated species also common.	An irritating resinous substance, irisin.	Burning, congestion, and severe pain in the digestive tract; nausea and diarrhea	Rootstalks have such an acrid taste that they are unlikely to be eaten.
Jasmine	*Gelsemium sempervirens*	A woody, trailing, or climbing evergreen vine; opposite, simple, lance-shaped, glossy leaves; fragrant, yellow flowers; flattened two-celled, beaked capsule fruits.	Entire plant, but especially the root and flowers.	Native to the southeastern United States; commonly grown in the Southwest as an ornamental.	Alkaloids, gelsemine, gelseminine, and gelsemoidine found throughout the plant.	Profuse sweating, muscular weakness, convulsions, respiratory depression, paralysis, and death possible.	Jasmine has been used as a medicinal herb, but overdoses are dangerous. Children have been poisoned by chewing on the leaves.
Jimmy weed (rayless goldenrod)	*Haplopappus heterophyllus*	Small, bushy, half-shrub with erect stems arising from the woody crown to a height of 2–4 ft (61–122 cm); narrow, alternate, sticky leaves; clusters of small, yellow flower heads at tips of stems.	Entire plant.	Common in fields or ranges around watering sites and along streams from Kansas, Oklahoma, and Texas to Colorado, New Mexico, and Arizona.	Contains higher alcohol, tremetol, which accumulates in the milk of cows and causes human poisoning known as "milk sickness."		Other species of *Haplopappus* probably are equally dangerous. White snakeroot also contains tremetol and causes "milk sickness."

(Continued)

TABLE 41 (Continued)
Some Important Poisonous Plants of North America

Common Name	Scientific Name	Description	Toxic Parts	Geographical Distribution	Poisoning	Symptoms	Remarks
Jimson weed (thorn apple)	*Datura stramonium*	Coarse, weedy plant with stout stems and foul-smelling foliage; large, oval leaves with wavy margins; fragrant, large, tubular, white to purple flowers; round, nodding, or erect prickly capsule.	Entire plant, particularly the seeds and leaves.	Naturalized throughout North America; common weed of fields, gardens, roadsides, and pastures.	Due to the alkaloids, hyoscyamine, atropine, and hyoscine (scopolamine).	Dry mouth, thirst, red skin, disturbed vision, pupil dilation, nausea, vomiting, headache, hallucination, rapid pulse, delirium, incoherent speech, convulsion, high blood pressure, coma, and possibly death.	Sleeping near the fragrant flowers can cause headache, nausea, dizziness, and weakness. Children pretending the flowers were trumpets have been poisoned.
Lantana (red sage)	*Lantana camara*	Perennial shrub with square twigs and a few spines; simple, opposite or whorled oval-shaped leaves with tooth margins; white, yellow, orange, red, or blue flowers occurring in flat-topped clusters; berry-like fruit with a hard, blue-black seed.	All parts, especially the green berries.	Native of the dry woods in the southeastern United States; cultivated as an ornamental shrub in pots in the northern United States and Canada; or a lawn shrub in the southeastern coastal plains, Texas, California, and Hawaii.	Fruit contains high levels of an alkaloid, lantanin or lantadene A.	Stomach and intestinal irritation, vomiting, bloody diarrhea, muscular weakness, jaundice, and circulatory collapse; death possible but not common.	In Florida, these plants are considered a major cause of human poisoning. The foliage of lantana may also cause dermatitis.
Larkspur	*Delphinium* sp.	Annual or perennial herb 2–4 ft (61–122 cm) high; finely, palmately divided leaves on long stalks; white, pink, rose, blue, or purple flowers each with a spur; fruit, a many-seeded, three-celled capsule.	Entire plant.	Native of rich or dry forest and meadows throughout the United States but common in the West; frequently cultivated in flower gardens.	Contains the alkaloids delphinine, delphinidine, ajacine, and others.	Burning sensation in the mouth and skin, low blood pressure, nervousness, weakness, prickling of the skin, nausea, vomiting, depression, convulsions, and death within 6 hours if eaten in large quantities.	Poisoning potential of larkspur decreases as it ages, but alkaloids still concentrated in the seeds. Seeds are used in some commercial lice remedies.
Laurel (mountain laurel)	*Kalmia latifolia*	Large evergreen shrubs growing to 35 ft (11 m) tall; alternate leaves dark green on top and bright green underneath; white to rose flowers in terminal clusters; fruit in a dry capsule.	Leaves, twigs, flowers, and pollen grains.	Found in moist woods and along streams in eastern Canada southward in the Appalachian Mountains and Piedmont, and sometimes in the eastern coastal plain.	Contains the toxic resinoid andromedotoxin.	Increased salivation, watering of eyes and nose, loss of energy, slow pulse, vomiting, low blood pressure, lack of coordination, convulsions, and progressive paralysis until eventual death.	The mountain laurel is the state flower of Connecticut and Pennsylvania. By making "tea" from the leaves or by sucking on the flowers, children have been poisoned.

Common name	Scientific name	Description	Part poisonous	Distribution	Toxic principle	Symptoms	Remarks
Locoweed (crazyweed)	*Oxytropis* sp.	Perennial herb with erect or spreading stems; pea-like flowers and stems—only smaller.		Common throughout the southwestern United States.	Contains alkaloid-like substances—a serious threat to livestock.	In animals, loss of weight, irregular gait, loss of sense of direction, nervousness, weakness, and loss of muscular control.	Locoweeds are seldom eaten by humans; hence, they are not a serious problem. There are more than 100 species of locoweeds.
Lupine (bluebonnet)	*Lupinus* sp.	Annual or perennial herbs; digitately divided, alternate leaves; peak-shaped blue, white, red, or yellow flowers borne in clusters at ends of stems; seeds in flattened pods.	Entire plant, particularly the seeds.	Wide distribution but most common in western North America; many cultivated as ornamentals.	Contains lupinine and related toxic alkaloids.	Weak pulse, slowed respiration, convulsions, and paralysis.	Rarely have cultivated varieties poisoned children. Not all lupines are poisonous.
Marijuana (hashish, Mary Jane, pot, grass)		A tall coarse, annual herb; palmately divided and long stalked leaves; small, green flowers clustered in the leaf axils.	Entire plant, especially the leaves, flowers, sap and resinous secretions.	Widely naturalized weed in temperate North America; cultivated in warmer areas.	Various narcotic resins but mainly tetrahydrocannabinol (THC) and related compounds.	Exhilaration, hallucinations, delusions, mental confusion, dilated pupils, blurred vision, poor coordination, weakness, and stupor; coma and death in large doses.	Poisoning results from drinking the extract, chewing the plant parts, or smoking a so-called "reefer" (joint). The hallucinogenic and narcotic effects of marijuana have been known for more than 2000 years. Laws in the United States and Canada restrict the possession of living or dried parts of marijuana.
Mescal bean (frijolito)	*Sophora secundiflora*	Evergreen shrub or small tree growing to 40 ft (12 m) tall; stalked, alternate leaves 4–6 in. (10–15 cm) long, which are pinnately divided and shiny, yellow-green above and silky below when young; violet-blue, pea-like flowers; bright red seeds.	Entire plant, particularly the seed.	Native to southwestern Texas and southern New Mexico; cultivated as ornamentals in the southwestern United States.	Contains cytisine and other poisonous alkaloids.	Nausea, vomiting, diarrhea, excitement, delirium, hallucinations, coma, and death; deep sleep lasting 2–3 days in nonlethal doses.	One seed, if sufficiently chewed, is enough to cause the death of a young child. The Indians of Mexico and the Southwest have used the seeds in medicine as a narcotic and as a hallucinatory drug. Many necklaces have been made from the seeds.

(Continued)

TABLE 41   (Continued)
Some Important Poisonous Plants of North America

Common Name	Scientific Name	Description	Toxic Parts	Geographical Distribution	Poisoning	Symptoms	Remarks
Mistletoes	*Phoradendron serotinum*	Parasitic evergreen plants that grow on trees and shrubs; oblong, simple, opposite leaves, which are leathery; small, white berries.	All parts, especially the berries.	Common on the branches of various trees from New Jersey and southern Indiana southward to Florida and Texas; other species throughout North America.	Contains the toxic amines β-phenylethylamine and tyrosamine.	Gastrointestinal pain, diarrhea, slow pulse, and collapse; possibly nausea, vomiting, nervousness, difficult breathing, delirium, pupil dilation, and abortion; in sufficient amounts, death within a few hours.	Mistletoe is a favorite Christmas decoration. It is the state flower of Oklahoma. Poisonings have occurred when people eat the berries or make "tea" from the berries. Indians chewed the leaves to relieve toothache. Small amounts can be lethal.
Monkshood (wolfsbane)	*Aconitum columbianum*	Perennial herb about 2–5 ft (61–152 cm) high; alternate, petioled leaves which are palmately divided into segments with pointed tips; generally dark blue flowers with a prominent hood; seed in a short-beaked capsule.	Entire plant, especially roots and seeds.	Rich, moist soil in meadows and along streams from western Canada south to California and New Mexico.	Due to several alkaloids, including aconine and aconitine.	Burning sensation of the mouth and skin; nausea, vomiting, diarrhea, muscular weakness, and spasms, weak, irregular pulse, paralysis of respiration, dimmed vision, convulsions, and death within a few hours.	Death in humans reported from eating the plant or extracts made from it. It has been mistaken for horseradish.
Mushrooms (toadstools)	*Amanita muscaria, Amanita verna, Chlorophyllum molybdites*	Common types with central stalk, and cap; flat plates (gills) underneath cap; some with deeply ridged, cylindrical top rather than cap.	Entire fungus.	Various types throughout North America.	Depending on type of mushroom; complex polypeptides such as amanitin and possibly phalloidin; a toxic protein in some; the poisons ibotenic acid, muscimol, and related compounds in others.	Vary with type of mushroom but include death-like sleep, manic behavior, delirium, seeing colored visions, feeling of elation, explosive diarrhea, vomiting, severe headache, loss of muscular coordination, abdominal cramps, and coma and death from some types; permanent liver, kidney, and heart damage from other types.	Wild mushrooms are extremely difficult to identify and are best avoided. There is no simple rule of thumb for distinguishing between poisonous and nonpoisonous mushrooms—only myths and nonsense. Only one or two bites are necessary for death from some species; during the month of December 1981, three people were killed and two hospitalized in California after eating poisonous mushrooms.

Nightshade	*Solanum nigrum, Solanum elaeagnifolium*	Annual herbs or shrub-like plants with simple alternate leaves; small, white, blue, or violet flowers; black berries or yellow to yellow-orange berries depending on species.	Primarily the unripe berries.	Contains the alkaloid solanine; possibly saponin, atropine, and perhaps high levels of nitrate.	Headache, stomach pain, vomiting, diarrhea, dilated pupils, subnormal temperature, shock, circulatory and respiratory depression, and possible death.	Some individuals use the completely ripe berries in pies and jellies.
Oleander	Nerium oleander	An evergreen shrub or small tree growing to 25 ft (8 m) tall; short-stalked, narrow, leathery leaves, opposite or in whorls of three; white to pink to red flowers at tips of twigs.	Entire plant, especially the leaves.	Contains the poisonous glycosides oleandrin and nerioside, which act similar to digitalis.	Nausea, severe vomiting, stomach pain, bloody diarrhea, cold feet and hands, irregular heartbeat, dilation of pupils, drowsiness, unconsciousness, paralysis of respiration, convulsions, coma, and death within a day.	One leaf of an oleander is said to contain enough poison to kill an adult. In Florida, severe poisoning resulted when oleander branches were used as skewers. Honey made from oleander flower nectar is poisonous.
Peyote (mescal buttons)	*Lophophora williamsii*	Hemispherical, spineless member of the cactus family growing from carrot-shaped roots; low, rounded sections with a tuft of yellow-white hairs on top; flower from the center of the plant, white to rose-pink; pink berry when ripe; black seeds.	Entire plant, especially the buttons.	Contains mescaline, lophophorine, and other alkaloids.	Illusions and hallucinations with vivid color, anxiety, muscular tremors and twitching, vomiting, diarrhea, blurred vision, wakefulness, forgetfulness, muscular relaxation, and dizziness.	The effects of chewing fresh or dried "buttons" of peyote are similar to those produced by LSD, only milder. In some states, peyote is recognized as a drug. Peyote has long been used by the Indians and Mexicans in religious ceremonies.

(Continued)

TABLE 41 (Continued)
Some Important Poisonous Plants of North America

Common Name	Scientific Name	Description	Toxic Parts	Geographical Distribution	Poisoning	Symptoms	Remarks
Poison hemlock (poison parsley)	Conium maculatum	Biennial herb with a hairless purple-spotted or lined, hollow stem growing up to 8 ft (2.4 m) tall; turnip-like, long, solid taproot; large, alternate, pinnately divided leaves; small, white flowers in umbrella-shaped clusters; dry; ribbed, two-part capsule fruit.	Entire plant, primarily seeds and root.	A native of Eurasia, now a weed in meadows and along roads and ditches throughout the United States and southern Canada where moisture is sufficient.	The poisonous alkaloid coniine and other related alkaloids.	Burning sensation in the mouth and throat, nervousness, unco-ordination, dilated pupils, muscular weakness, weakened and slowed heartbeat, convulsions, coma, and death.	Poisoning occurs when the leaves are mistaken for parsley, the roots for turnips, or the seeds for anise. Toxic quantities seldom consumed because the plant has such an unpleasant odor and taste. Assumed by some to be the poison drunk by Socrates.
Poison ivy (poison oak)	Toxicodendron radicans	A trailing or climbing vine, shrub, or small tree; alternate leaves with three leaflets; flowers and fruits hanging in clusters; white to yellowish fruit (drupes).	Roots, stems, leaves, pollen, flowers, and fruits.	An extremely variable native weed throughout southern Canada and the United States with the exception of the west coast; found on flood plains, along lake shores, edges of woods, stream banks, fences, and around buildings.	Skin irritation due to an oil-resin-containing urushiol.	Contact with skin causes itching, burning, redness, and small blisters; severe gastric disturbance and even death by eating leaves or fruit.	Almost half of all persons are allergic to poison ivy. Skin irritation may also result from indirect contact such as animals (including dogs and cats), clothing, tools, or sports equipment.
Pokeweed (pokeberry)	Phytolacca americana	Shrub-like herb with a large fleshy taproot; large, entire, oblong leaves that are pointed; white to purplish flowers in clusters at ends of branches; mature fruit, a dark purple berry with red juice.	Rootstalk, leaves, and stems.	Native to the eastern United States and southeastern Canada.	Highest concentration of poison mainly in roots; contains the bitter glycoside saponin, and a glycoprotein.	Burning and bitter taste in mouth, stomach cramps, nausea, vomiting, diarrhea, drowsiness, slowed breathing, weakness, tremors, convulsions, spasms, coma, and death if eaten in large amounts.	Young tender leaves and stems of pokeweed are often cooked as greens. Cooked berries are used for pies without harm. It is one of the most dangerous poisonous plants because people prepare it improperly.

Common name	Scientific name	Description	Distribution	Part toxic	Toxic principle	Symptoms	Remarks
Poppy (common poppy)	*Papaver somniferum*	An erect, annual herb with milky juice; simple, coarsely toothed, or lobed leaves; showy red, white, pink, or purple flowers; fruit an oval, crowned capsule; tiny seeds in capsule.	Introduced from Eurasia and widely grown in the United States until cultivation without a license became unlawful.	Unripe fruits of their juice.	Crude resin from unripe seed capsule source of narcotic opium alkaloids.	From unripe fruit, stupor, coma, shallow and slow breathing, and depression of the central nervous system; possibly nausea and severe retching (straining to vomit).	The use of poppy extracts is a double-edged sword—addictive narcotics and valuable medicines. Poppy seeds that are used as toppings on breads are harmless.
Rhododendron; azaleas	*Rhododendron* sp.	Usually evergreen shrubs; mostly entire, simple, leathery leaves in whorls or alternate; showy white to pink flowers in terminal clusters; fruit, a wood capsule.	Throughout the temperate parts of the United States as a native and as an introduced ornamental.	Entire plant.	Contains the toxic resinoid andromedotoxin.	Watering eyes and mouth, nasal discharge, nausea, severe abdominal pain, vomiting, convulsions, lowered blood pressure, lack of coordination and loss of energy; progressive paralysis of arms and legs until death, in severe cases.	Cases of poisoning are rare in this country but rhododendrons should be suspected of possible danger.
Rosary pea (precatory pea)	*Abrus precatorius*	A twining, more or less, woody perennial vine; alternate and divided leaves with small leaflets; red to purple or white flowers; fruit, a short pod containing ovoid seeds that are glossy, bright scarlet over three-fourths of their surface, and jet black over the remaining one-fourth.	Native to the tropics, but naturalized in Florida and the Keys.	Seeds.	Contains the phytotoxin abrin and tetanic glycoside, abric acid.	Severe stomach pain, in 1–3 days, nausea, vomiting, severe diarrhea, weakness, cold sweat, drowsiness, weak, fast pulse, coma, circulatory collapse, and death.	The beans are made into rosaries, necklaces, bracelets, leis, and various toys, which receive wide distribution. Seeds must be chewed and swallowed to cause poisoning. Whole seeds pass through the digestive tract without causing symptoms; one thoroughly chewed seed is said to be potent enough to kill an adult or child.

(Continued)

TABLE 41 (Continued)
Some Important Poisonous Plants of North America

Common Name	Scientific Name	Description	Toxic Parts	Geographical Distribution	Poisoning	Symptoms	Remarks
Snow-on-the-mountain	*Euphorbia marginata*	A tall annual herb, growing up to 4 ft (122 cm) high; smooth, lance-shaped leaves with conspicuously white margins; whorls of white petal-like leaves border flowers; fruit, a three-celled, three-lobed capsule.	Leaves, stems, and milky sap.	Native to the western, dry plains and valleys from Montana to Mexico; sometimes escapes in the eastern United States.	Toxins causing dermatitis and severe irritation of the digestive tract.	Blistering of the skin, nausea, abdominal pain, fainting, diarrhea, and possibly death in severe cases.	Milky juice of this plant is very caustic. Outwardly, snow-on-the-mountain resembles a poinsettia.
Skunk cabbage	*Veratrum californicum*	Tall, broad-leaved herbs of the lily family, growing to 6 ft (183 cm) high; large, alternate pleated, clasping, and parallel-veined leaves; numerous whitish to greenish flowers in large terminal clusters; three-lobed, capsule fruit.	Entire plant.	Various species throughout North America in wet meadows, forests, and along streams.	Contains such alkaloids as veratridine and veratrine.	Nausea, vomiting, diarrhea, stomach pains, lowered blood pressure, slow pulse, reduced body temperature, shallow breathing, salivation, weakness, nervousness, convulsions, paralysis, and possibly death.	These plants have been used for centuries as a source of drugs and as a source of insecticide. Since the leaves resemble cabbage, they are often collected as an edible wild plant but with unpleasant results.
Tansy	*Tanacetum vulgare*	Tall, aromatic herb with simple stems to 3 ft (91 cm) high; alternate, pinnately divided, narrow leaves; flower heads in flat-topped clusters with numerous small, yellow flowers.	Leaves, stems, and flowers.	Introduced from Eurasia; widely naturalized in North America; sometimes found escaped along roadsides, in pastures, or other wet places; grown for medicinal purposes.	Contains an oil, tanacetum, or oil of tansy.	Nausea, vomiting, diarrhea, convulsions, violent spasms, dilated pupils, rapid and feeble pulse, and possibly death.	Tansy and oil of tansy are employed as an herbal remedy for nervousness, intestinal worms, to promote menstruation, and to induce abortion. Some poisonings have resulted from the use of tansy as a home remedy.

Common name	Scientific name	Description	Poisonous part	Distribution	Toxin	Symptoms	Remarks
Water hemlock	*Cicuta* sp.	A perennial with parsley-like leaves; hollow, jointed stems and hollow, pithy roots; flowers in umbrella clusters; stems streaked with purple ridges; 2–6 ft (61–183 cm) high.	Entire plant, primarily the roots and young growth.	Wet meadows, pastures, and flood plains of western and eastern United States, generally absent in the plains states.	Contains the toxic resin-like higher alcohol cicutoxin.	Frothing at the mouth, spasms, dilated pupils, diarrhea, convulsions, vomiting, delirium, respiratory failure, paralysis, and death.	One mouthful of the water hemlock root is reported to contain sufficient poison to kill a man. Children making whistles and peashooters from the hollow stems have been poisoned. The water hemlock is often mistaken for the edible wild artichoke or parsnip; however, it is considered to be one of the most poisonous plants of the North Temperate Zone.
White snakeroot	Eupatorium rugosum	Erect perennial with stems 1–5 feet (30–152 cm) tall; opposite oval leaves with pointed tips and sharply toothed edges, and dull on the upper surface but shiny on the lower surface; showy, snow white flowers in terminal clusters.	Entire plant.	From eastern Canada to Saskatchewan and south to Texas, Louisiana, Georgia, and Virginia.	Contains the higher alcohol tremetol and some glycosides.	Weakness, nausea, loss of appetite, vomiting, tremors, labored breathing, constipation, dizziness, delirium, convulsions, coma, and death.	Recovery from a nonlethal dose is a slow process, due to liver and kidney damage. Poison may be in the milk of cows that have eaten white snakeroot—"milk sickness."

Source: From Ensminger et al. 1994. *Foods and Nutrition Encyclopedia.* 2nd ed. 1776–85. Boca Raton, FL.: CRC Press.

POLAR

A characteristic of a molecule possessing a positive or negative charge.

POLYADENYLATION

The addition of a sequence of polyadenylic acid to the 5′ end of a eukaryotic RNA after its transcription.

POLYCHLORINATED DIBENZODIOXINS

See Contamination with Organic Chemicals under Contamination of Food.

POLYCHLORINATED DIBENZOFURANS

See Contamination with Organic Chemicals under Contamination of Food.

POLYMERASE CHAIN REACTION (PCR)

An enzymatic method for the repeated copying, and thus amplification of two strands of DNA that make up a particular gene sequence.

POLYNEURITIS

Inflammation of many nerve endings.

POLYPEPTIDE

A string of amino acids in excess of eight. See Protein Structure.

POLYPHENOLS

Compounds with a phenol structure that serve as antioxidants. Found in a variety of foods such as grapes, cranberries, and cherries. Polyphenols stimulate AMP-activated protein kinase, lower blood lipids, and inhibit accelerated atherosclerosis in diabetic LDL-receptor-deficient individuals. Polyphenols improve endothelial function and inhibit platelet aggregation.

POLYSACCHARIDE

A string of monosaccharides joined together. If the linkage is an α-1,4 or α-1,6, mammalian enzymes can break the bond. If the linkage is a β-linkage, mammalian saccharidases cannot sever it.

POLYUNSATURATED FATTY ACID

A fatty acid having more than one double bond.

POLYURIA

Excessive urination.

POMPE'S DISEASE

A rare genetic disease due to a mutation in the gene for the enzyme α-1,– glucosidase; characterized by excess glycogen stores in the muscle. Also called Type II glycogen storage disease.

PONDERAL INDEX

An expression of leanness: height (inches) divided by the cube root of weight in pounds.

PORK

Meat from a pig.

PORPHYRIN

An iron-containing ring structure that is a part of hemoglobin.

PORTAL HYPERTENSION

Increased pressure in the portal vein resulting from an obstruction of blood flow through the liver.

PORTAL VEIN

The vein that carries the absorbed nutrients from the intestinal tract to the liver.

POSTERIOR PITUITARY HORMONES

Oxytocin, vasopressin (antidiuretic hormone, ADH).

POSTPRANDIAL

After a meal.

POTASSIUM (K^+)

An essential mineral. Main intracellular cation; plays an important role in the Na^+K^+ pump, and in the maintenance of cell volume, acid-base balance, muscle contraction, nerve conductance, and protein synthesis.

POTASSIUM^{40} (K^{40})

Naturally occurring nonradioactive isotope of potassium.

PPC10

The concentration at which in 10% of the population the critical organ is affected.

PRADER-WILLI SYNDROME

Obesity caused by a chromosome deletion and characterized by persistent food-seeking behavior.

PRAVASTATIN SODIUM (EPTASTATIN)

A member of the statin family of drugs that act as HMG CoA inhibitors and thus inhibit cholesterol synthesis in the body. Trade name: Pravachol.

PRAZOSIN HYDROCHLORIDE

A drug that is an α-blocker and serves as an antihypertensive drug. Trade name: Minipress.

PREALBUMIN

A blood protein smaller than albumin, which migrates ahead of it when a sample of blood proteins are separated by electrophoresis.

PREBIOTICS

Nondigestible carbohydrates that beneficially affect the host by selectively stimulating the growth and/or activity of one or a limited number of bacteria in the colon and thus improve host health.

PRECISION

No random errors in the measurements; also referred to as reproducibility. The reproducibility of a measurement is high if there is good concordance between repeated measurements.

PRECURSOR

A predecessor molecule.

PREDNISOLONE (PREDNISONE)

Synthetic glucocorticoid used as an anti-inflammatory drug.

PRE-ECLAMPSIA

Toxemia of pregnancy characterized by hypertension, albuminuria, edema of the lower extremities, and headaches that must be corrected to avoid true eclampsia.

PREGNANCY-INDUCED ANEMIA

Dilution of the red cell number due to the increase in blood volume associated with pregnancy.

PREGNANCY-INDUCED HYPERGLYCEMIA

Abnormal glucose tolerance that occurs during gestation (gestational diabetes) but not before or after.

PREGNANCY-INDUCED HYPERTENSION

An increase in blood pressure due to pregnancy. If markedly elevated, it is a sign of pending toxemia.

PREGNENOLONE

A steroid produced from cholesterol that is a precursor to cortisol and progesterone.

PREKALLIKREINS

Precursor of the kallikreins that are a group of serine proteases. These act on plasma a2-globulins to release kinins such as bradykinin, a potent vasodilator.

PREMATURE BABIES

Infants born before prenatal development is complete; infants born prior to 37 weeks of gestation.

PREPROOPIOMELANOCORTINS

Precursor molecule formed in the pituitary cells, neurons, and other tissues for ACTH, γ-MSH, β-LPH, α-MSH, CL IP, γ-LPH, β-endorphin, and met-enkephalin.

PREPROOXYTOCIN

Precursor molecule formed in the posterior pituitary for oxytocin.

PREPROVASOPRESSIN

Precursor molecule formed in the posterior pituitary for vasopressin.

PRESERVATIVES

See Additives, Table 4.

PRESSURE SORES

Ulceration of tissue, usually located over a bony prominence thinly covered with flesh such as the spine, heels, elbows, shoulder blades, or hip, resulting from impaired blood circulation or pressure from prolonged confinement in bed.

PREVALENCE

The number of existing cases of X in a given population at a given time.

PRIMIGRAVIDA

A woman during her first pregnancy.

PRIMIPARA

A woman who is experiencing her first pregnancy.

PRIMOSOME

The mobile complex of helicase and primase that is involved in DNA replication.

PROBE

A molecule used to detect the presence of a specific fragment of DNA or RNA, for instance, in a bacterial colony that is formed from a genetic library or during analysis by blot transfer techniques; common probes are cDNA molecules, synthetic oligodeoxynucleotides, or defined sequence or antibodies to specific proteins.

PROBLEM-ORIENTED MEDICAL RECORD (POMR)

Method of charting in a patient's medical record, which identifies the problems, usually in order of importance, and plans for intervention.

PROENKEPHALIN

Precursor molecule produced by the adrenal medulla for enkephalin.

PROGESTERONE

Female steroid hormone produced by the ovaries and the corpus luteum that serves to prepare the uterus for implantation of the fertilized egg (blastocyte). It also serves to stimulate the development of the mammary alveolar system.

PROGESTINS

A general term that covers the female steroid hormones related to progesterone.

PROINSULIN

Precursor molecule for insulin. It consists of an A chain, a B chain, and a C chain. The C chain is split off when the proinsulin is converted to insulin.

PROKARYOTES

Single-cell organisms.

PROLACTIN

Hormone that stimulates milk production by the mammary cell.

PROLINE

A nonessential amino acid. (See Table 5, Amino Acids.)

PROMOTER

A region of DNA involved in binding RNA polymerase and various regulatory transcription factors to initiate transcription.

PROOPIOMELANOCORTIN

Precursor molecule for ACTH, β-endorphin, β-lipotropin, and three forms of dynorphin.

PROPAFENONE HYDROCHLORIDE

A sodium channel blocker that can be used to help regulate heart rhythm. Trade name: Rythmol.

PROPYLTHIOURACIL (PTU)

A drug that is a thyroid hormone antagonist. Trade name: Propyl-Thyracil.

PRORENIN

Precursor molecule for rennin.

PROSTACYCLIN

See Eicosanoids.

PROSTAGLANDINS

See Eicosanoids.

PROSTATE GLAND

A muscular organ containing 30–50 tubuloalveolar glands that encompass the junction of the ejaculatory duct with the male urethra.

PROSTHETIC GROUP

A nonprotein component of an enzyme (or other body protein) that is necessary to the activity of that enzyme or protein.

PROTEASE

An enzyme that catalyzes the degradation of protein.

PROTEASE INHIBITORS

Compounds that inhibit the protein degradative action of the protease enzymes.

PROTECTIVE FOODS

Foods that are rich in essential nutrients, so called because they protect the body against deficiency diseases.

PROTEINS

A large group of complex molecules that are polymers of amino acids. They are classified as simple proteins or conjugated proteins. Simple proteins have no prosthetic group attached. Examples include albumins, globulins, glutelins, scleroproteins, prolamines, and protamines. Conjugated proteins are characterized by the type of prosthetic group attached to the protein. The prosthetic group can be a carbohydrate (glycoprotein), a lipid (lipoprotein), or other material. The metalloproteins, mucoproteins, nucleoproteins, hemoproteins, and flavoproteins are conjugated proteins.

CLASSIFICATION BY NUTRITIVE VALUE

Nutritionists are interested in food proteins as sources of needed amino acids. Those proteins that contain the essential amino acids in the proportions needed by the body are referred to as complete proteins. They are primarily of animal origin. Eggs, milk, meat, and fish are sources of complete protein. Proteins lacking in one or more essential amino acids or that have a poor balance of amino acids relative to the body's needs are incomplete or imbalanced proteins. These proteins are usually of plant origin, although some animal proteins are incomplete. The connective tissue protein called collagen, from which gelatin is isolated, lacks tryptophan; zein, the protein in corn, is low in lysine as well as tryptophan. When food selection is limited by the availability of protein-rich foods, incomplete proteins can be combined so that all of the essential amino acids are provided. For example, corn or wheat and soy or peanut proteins can be combined in the same meal so that all of the essential amino acids are provided. When these proteins are combined, they will provide sufficient amounts of the needed amino acids. The combination of incomplete proteins needed to provide all the needed amino acids must be consumed within a relatively short time interval (less than 4 hours) to obtain the appropriate and needed amounts of amino acids. Maximum benefit is obtained when the combination is consumed at the same time. Supplementation of incomplete proteins with missing amino acids has been suggested for populations consuming diets having a single dietary item as its main protein source. This supplementation is not very practical over a long period of time due to the cost of the pure amino acid supplement. Such populations are also likely to develop other nutritional disorders when their food supply is so limited. With judicious use of a variety of foods available to these populations, amino acid deficiencies or imbalances can be overcome.

In addition to the amino acid content, protein quality, or rather the quality of the food containing the protein, is classed according to its total protein content. Potatoes, for example, contain a very good distribution of essential and nonessential amino acids, yet, because the potato contains very little protein (1.7%), it is not considered a good protein source. One would have to consume a lot of potatoes (3.18 kg or approximately 7 lbs) to meet one's daily amino acid and total nitrogen requirements. Total protein content can be determined rather easily, but analysis of a food to establish the individual amino acid content can be tedious and difficult.

PROTEIN DENATURATION

One of the most striking characteristics of proteins is the response to heat, alcohol, and other treatments, which affect their quaternary, tertiary, and secondary structures. This characteristic response is called denaturation. Denaturation results in the unfolding of a protein molecule, thus breaking its hydrogen bonds and the associations between functional groups; as a result, the three-dimensional structure is lost. Denaturation affects many of the properties of the protein molecule. Its physical shape is changed, its solubility in water is decreased, and its reactivity with other proteins may be lost. When denatured, the protein loses its biological activity.

PROTEIN ABSORPTION

See Amino Acid Absorption.

PROTEIN ANALYSIS (FOOD)

Total protein content is estimated from the total nitrogen content of the test sample as determined by the classical Kjeldahl method. This method also determines nonprotein nitrogen, however, the amount of error in the method due to the inclusion of these compounds is very small. Most proteins contain 16% nitrogen. To convert the nitrogen content to protein, one uses the following formula:

$$P_G = N_G \times 100 / 16 = N_G \times 6.25$$

where P_G = grams of protein in 100 grams of food and N_G = grams of nitrogen in 100 grams of food.

The 6.25 conversion factor is an average factor. If one wishes more exact figures, established conversion factors for each food category are available. For example, cereals generally have less protein nitrogen and more nonprotein nitrogen, thus the conversion factor of 5.7 is used for cereal foods. On the other hand, milk has more protein nitrogen and the conversion factor of 6.4 may be used. Generally speaking, because humans usually consume a mixed diet, the lower and higher factors tend to average out and the value of 6.25 is correct to use when the protein intake of a day's food intake is chemically determined.

The amino acid determination of a protein has two phases: qualitative identification and quantitative estimation of the residues. The peptide bond that connects the residues is cleaved by acid, base, or enzyme-catalyzed hydrolysis to give a mixture of separated amino acids. The free amino acids are separated from one another and identified using chromatographic and/or electrophoretic techniques. Once separated and identified, each amino acid present can be determined quantitatively. Several amino acid–specific reactions are available. These assays do not establish the sequence of the amino acids or the primary structure of the proteins, but merely tell how much of each amino acid is present. The sequence of amino acids can be determined by cleaving, one by one, the amino acids from the protein and analyzing the individual amino acids. High performance liquid chromatography (HPLC) can be used for this analysis.

PROTEIN CONTENT IN FOODS

Foods vary in their protein content. A complete list of foods and their nutrient content can be found in the USDA website at http://www.nal.usda.gov/fnic/foodcomp/Data.

PROTEIN DIGESTION

The degradation of food protein into its component amino acids and dipeptides. The purpose of protein digestion is to liberate the amino acids contained by the food proteins. Protein digestion does not begin until the protein reaches the stomach and the food is acidified with the gastric hydrochloric acid. Hydrochloric acid denatures the food proteins, thus making them more vulnerable to attack by pepsin, an endopeptidase. Actually, pepsin is not a single enzyme. It consists of pepsin A, which attacks peptide bonds involving phenylalanine or tyrosine, and several other enzymes that have specific attack points. The pepsins are released into the stomach as pepsinogen. Food entering the stomach stimulates HCl release, the pH of the gastric contents fall below 2, and the pepsinogen loses a 44-amino-acid sequence. The activation of the pepsins from pepsinogen occurs by one of two processes. The first, called autoactivation, occurs when the pH drops below 5. At low pH, the bond between the 44th and 45th amino acid residue falls apart and the 44-amino-acid residue (from the amino terminus) is liberated. The liberated residue acts as an inhibitor of pepsin by binding to the catalytic site until pH 2 is achieved. The inhibition is relieved when this fragment is degraded, as happens at pH 2 or below or when it is attacked by pepsin. Since the fragment binds at the catalytic site of pepsin, this can happen. The other process is called autocatalysis and occurs when already active pepsin attacks the precursor pepsinogen. This is a self-repeating process and serves to ensure ongoing catalyses of the resident protein. The cleavage of the 44-amino-acid residue, in addition to providing activated pepsin, has another purpose. That is, it serves as a signal peptide for cholecystokinin release in the duodenum. This then sets the stage for the subsequent pancreatic phase of protein digestion.

As described in the units on lipids and carbohydrates, cholecystokinin stimulates both the exocrine pancreas and the intestinal mucosal epithelial cell to release its digestive enzymes. The intestinal cell releases an enzyme, enteropeptidase or enterokinase, which serves to activate the protease trypsin, released as trypsinogen by the exocrine pancreas. This trypsin not only acts on food proteins, but also acts on other preproteases, released by the exocrine pancreas, activating them. Thus, trypsin acts as an endoprotease, on chymotrypsinogen, releasing chymotrypsin, on proelastase, releasing elastase, and on procarboxypeptidase, releasing carboxypeptidase. Trypsin, chymotrypsin, and elastase are all endoproteases, each having specificity for particular peptide bonds. Each of these three proteases have serine as part of their catalytic site so any compound that ties up the serine will inhibit the activity of these proteases. Inhibitors such as diisopropylphosphofluoridate react with this serine and halt protein digestion.

The daily protein intake of about 100 g plus the protein that appears in the gut as enzymes, sloughed epithelial gut cells, and mucins, is almost completely digested and absorbed. This is a very efficient process that ensures a continuous supply of amino acids to the whole-body amino acid pool. Less than 1% of the total protein that passes through the gastrointestinal tract appears in the feces. If the food contributes between 70 and 100 g of protein and the endogenous protein contributes another 100 g (range: 35–200 g) then one might expect to see about 1–2 g of nitrogen in the feces. This is equivalent to 6–12 g of protein. Of the dietary protein, the fecal protein might include the hard to chew or digest tough fibrous connective tissue of meat, nitrogen-containing indigestible kernel coats of grains, or particles of nuts that are not attacked by the digestive enzymes. The enzymes that are responsible for protein digestion are listed in Table 42.

The protein hydrolases, called peptidases, fall into two categories: those that attack internal peptide bonds and liberate large peptide fragments for subsequent attack by other enzymes are called the endopeptidases, and those that attack the terminal peptide bonds and liberate single amino acids from the protein structure are called exopeptidases. The exopeptidases are further subdivided according to whether they attack at the carboxy end of the amino acid chain (carboxypeptidases) or the amino end of the chain (aminopeptidases). The initial attack on an intact protein is catalyzed by endopeptidases, while the final digestive action is catalyzed by the exopeptidases. The final products of digestion are free amino acids and some di- and tripeptides that are absorbed by the intestinal epithelial cells.

PROTEIN EVALUATION (BIOLOGICAL VALUE OF PROTEIN)

Methods for determining how well the food protein meets the biological need for protein by the consumer. Biological value (BV) is high when the protein is rich in all the amino acids in the right amounts needed by the consumer. Several techniques have been developed for this assessment. The nitrogen N balance technique for evaluating protein quality assumes that a given protein, when fed at maintenance levels, will completely replace the protein being catabolized during the normal course of metabolic events in the body. It also assumes that all nitrogen gains and losses can be measured. Thus, for good quality proteins, nitrogen balance (intake versus excretion) should be zero for an adult individual, and for poor quality proteins, nitrogen balance will be negative. For growing individuals, good quality proteins result in high nitrogen retentions, while poor quality proteins result in low nitrogen retention. The amount of protein retained can be determined by analyzing the total nitrogen content of the food, the feces, and the urine.

The BV was conceived as a ratio of the nitrogen absorbed to that retained multiplied by 100. In the original method, animals were fed a nitrogen-free diet for 7–10 days, then fed a diet containing the test protein at a level commensurate with their protein maintenance requirements for the same time interval. During each of these periods, the urine and feces were collected and analyzed

TABLE 42
Digestive Enzymes and Their Target Linkages

Enzyme	Location	Target
Pepsin	Stomach	Peptide bonds involving the aromatic amino acids
Trypsin	Small intestine	Peptide bonds involving arginine and lysine
Chymotrypsin	Small intestine	Peptide bonds involving tyrosine, tryptophan, phenylalanine, methionine, and leucine
Elastase	Small intestine	Peptide bonds involving alanine, serine, and glycine
Carboxypeptidase A	Small intestine	Peptide bonds involving valine, leucine, isoleucine, and alanine
Carboxypeptidase B	Small intestine	Peptide bonds involving lysine and arginine
Endopeptidase Aminopeptidase Dipeptidase	Cells of brush border	Di- and tripeptides that enter the brush border of the absorptive cells

for total nitrogen. Knowing the nitrogen intake and the nitrogen excretion during both the nitrogen-free and test periods, the BV was calculated as follows:

$$BV = 100 \times N_{absorbed} / N_{retained} = 100 \times N_I - (N_{FT} - N_{FF}) - (N_{UT} - N_{UF}) / N_I - (N_{FT} - N_{FF})$$

where BV = biological value, N_I = nitrogen intake, N_{FT} = fecal nitrogen during test period, N_{FF} = fecal nitrogen during nitrogen-free period, N_{UT} = urinary nitrogen during test period, and N_{UF} = urinary nitrogen during nitrogen-free period.

This method is noninvasive and very useful for calculating BV in humans. However, nitrogen can be lost via routes other than urine and feces. In hot climates or in physically active subjects, significant nitrogen losses can occur through the sweat. On an adequate protein intake, it has been estimated that up to 1 g N/dL can be lost. On an inadequate or low-protein diet, sweat losses can amount of 0.5 g N/dL. Hair, nail, and menstrual losses can also contribute error to the nitrogen balance technique. Usually sweat, hair, skin, and nail losses are ignored since they are minor in comparison to the urine and fecal losses. Other errors in the method include the possibility of daily cumulative errors in the collection and analysis of the food, urine, and feces, and the effects of poor nutritional status on the responses of the subject to this procedure. Good subject cooperation is essential to insure quantitative ingestion of the food and the quantitative collection of the urine and feces.

The main disadvantage of this method is theoretical in character. The basic assumption of the "replaceability" of body protein by a food protein is valid only when comparing good-quality proteins. When poor-quality proteins such as zein, gelatin, or gluten are evaluated, unrealistically high values result. This overestimation results from the failure of the method to account for the mobilization of body protein to meet particular amino acid needs. If there is a deficiency of one or more of the essential amino acids in the test protein, the animal will catabolize body proteins in an effort to provide the missing amino acid so as to support the synthesis of vital or needed proteins. There appears to be a hierarchy of body proteins—those which are most essential to the survival of the animal are synthesized in preference to those which are not as essential, such as muscle protein. In any event, when the body proteins are mobilized, the needed amino acids they contain are utilized and the remaining ones are deaminated and used for energy. The amino group is then converted to urea and excreted, contributing to the urinary nitrogen level. The nitrogen balance technique does not differentiate the source of the nitrogen in the excreta and, because of this, is not as valid as a technique to evaluate incomplete proteins.

The nitrogen balance index (NBI) relates the absorbed nitrogen to the nitrogen excretion of a separate but concurrent group of individuals fed a nitrogen-free diet. This technique requires less time than the Thomas-Mitchell method but is subject to many of the same kinds of errors. Both methods suffer from the inaccuracies contributed by the methodological measure of the so-called endogenous nitrogen loss. Both methods assume that this loss is represented by the nitrogen excreted by the animal during the nitrogen-free period.

One must consider the dynamic state of the body proteins, that is, the constant need to synthesize proteins having a short half-life. This synthesis must be accommodated by the catabolism of tissue protein; it is a catabolic process unlikely to occur extensively if good-quality proteins are consumed. Because this overestimation of endogenous loss is more serious with proteins of poor quality, inconsistent BVs are obtained. This is particularly true when unrefined proteins or food mixtures are evaluated.

A more accurate method for the evaluation of protein quality is one which actually measures the retention of nitrogen in the carcass from the ingested protein nitrogen. This is called the NPU-BV or NPU method. Using this method, which calculates BV from the change in carcass protein, groups of animals, usually rats, are fed diets containing graded amounts of the test protein or a nitrogen-free diet. After a period of 7–10 days, the animals are killed and the nitrogen content of the carcasses determined. Obviously, proteins of high quality will evoke a greater retention of nitrogen in the carcass than proteins of poor quality. Using this technique, BV can be calculated as follows:

$$NPU\ BV = (B_f - B_k + I_k) / I_f \times 100$$

where B_f = carcass nitrogen of animals fed test-protein diet, B_k = carcass nitrogen of animals fed nitrogen-free diet, I_k = absorbed nitrogen of animals fed nitrogen-free diet, and I_f = absorbed nitrogen of animals fed test-protein diet.

While this method has the obvious advantage of actually measuring nitrogen retention, its disadvantages are also obvious. This method is inappropriate for large animals because of the technical difficulties associated with the determination of body composition and because of the excessive cost. Obviously, too, human studies would not be possible. However, conceptually, the method has merit, and several investigators have devised variations that are useful in a variety of species.

One variation that is useful in man is to measure the changes in body composition indirectly. Using a stable isotope of nitrogen, ^{15}N, the rates of total body protein synthesis and breakdown as a response to variation in amounts of dietary protein can be determined. Constant infusions of ^{15}N-glycine allows the assessment of the value of given proteins in the homeostatic situation where there is constant protein synthesis and breakdown. While a very useful technique, it is also very expensive and requires sophisticated techniques and equipment to make the appropriate measurements.

Another variation of the carcass retention method, which uses a radioactive isotope, measures the change in ^{40}K concentration in the body as a result of consuming a given protein for a period of 7–10 days. This method is based on the constancy of potassium as an intracellular ion. The concentration of potassium in the body can be directly related to the number of cells in the body and indirectly related to the protein in the body. Since a set percentage of this potassium exists as the naturally occurring radioactive isotope ^{40}K, measuring ^{40}K levels is a direct measure of body cell number and an indirect measure of body protein. Again, while this method has the advantage of its applicability to the human, its disadvantage is one of cost and availability of the whole body counters needed to determine the presence of the isotope.

By far the easiest variation of the carcass retention method is the protein efficiency ratio (PER). In this method, carcass composition is not determined. It makes the assumption that the gain in body weight of a given animal is related to the quality of the protein fed. Thus, young growing animals are fed test protein–containing diets for a period of 28 days. The weight gain is computed and divided by the total protein intake:

$$PER = \text{Weight gain in grams} / \text{protein intake in grams}$$

This formula is easy to use, and the method requires no specialized expensive equipment. This is the method used for protein quality evaluation by most food companies and has been adopted by the regulatory agencies of the United States and Canada as their method of choice in evaluating the nutritional quality of foods. However, the ease and simplicity of the method should not lull the reader into thinking that it is a "choice" method. PER can vary from species to species, and, within a given species, from strain to strain. Variation can be introduced if levels of protein intake are higher or lower than 10% by weight. In addition, the methods make no allowance for the maintenance requirement of the animal. Values obtained from a variety of food proteins are nonlinear. That is, a protein having a PER of 2 may not have twice the nutritional value of a protein having a PER of 1.

A modification of the PER is the net protein ratio. This method attempts to account for the maintenance needs of the animals. In this method, two groups of animals are used. One is fed a nitrogen-free diet, the other the test diet. This modification is accompanied by all the pitfalls of using the nitrogen-free diets that have been discussed.

Attempts to circumvent the time and expense of whole animal work have resulted in a number of useful techniques. One method, the amino acid score or chemical score, is a nonbiological method and requires the amino acid analysis of the test protein. The amount of the most limiting amino acid (only the essential amino acids are considered) is related to the content of that same amino acid in a reference protein. In most cases, this reference is egg protein; however, a theoretical protein based on the amino acid requirements of the species in question could also be used.

Thus,

$$\text{Chemical score} = \frac{\text{mg of limiting amino acid / gram protein}}{\text{mg of amino acid / gram ideal protein}} \times 100$$

While this method is quick and does not use animals, it does not make any allowance for the digestibility or availability of the constituent amino acids. This is a rather important aspect of protein nutrition. Some amino acids form sugar-amino acid complexes that render the amino acids less available to the body. This occurs with the browning of baked goods such as bread; while bread is not considered a prime protein source, evaluation of its protein quality using the amino acid score would be in error due to the browning reaction.

A variation on this chemical method tries to account for digestibility. In this method, test proteins are first digested in vitro using conditions resembling those in the gastrointestinal tract. The amino acid score is then determined on the products of this digestion. This is a promising approach to evaluating protein quality. It will require work to validate it, but at present, it represents an innovative approach to the problems associated with assessing protein quality.

PROTEIN STRUCTURE

Proteins are complex molecules having characteristic primary, secondary, tertiary, and quaternary structures. The primary structure is determined genetically as the particular sequence of amino acids in a given protein. Under normal pH and temperature conditions, a protein is characterized not only by its amino acid sequence but also by its three-dimensional structure, that is, how the chain of amino acids twists and turns and what shape this long chain of amino acids assumes. This three-dimensional shape, unique to each protein's particular amino acid sequence, is known as the native conformation of the protein. This assumption of shape may be spontaneous or may be catalyzed by enzymes and reflects the lowest energy state of the protein in its native environment. Protein conformation is usually divided into two categories: secondary and tertiary. The secondary and tertiary structures of a protein result from interactions between the reactive groups on the amino acids in the protein.

Secondary structure is the local conformation of the protein molecule. It is due to the formation of hydrogen bonds, disulfide bridges, and ionic bonds (in the case of the polar amino acids) between adjacent or nearby amino acids in an amino acid chain. As a result of these bonds, there is a regular recurring arrangement in space of the amino acids within the chain, which can extend over the entire chain or only in small segments of it. Two kinds of periodic structures are found in proteins: the helix and the pleated sheet. In the helix, the amino acid chain can be viewed as wrapping itself around a long cylinder. The most common helical arrays are the α-helix and triple helix. The other periodic shape is the pleated sheet. It is essentially a linear array of the amino acid chain. All of these structures are stabilized by hydrogen bonding and sulfide bridges.

The tertiary structure is the regional conformation a protein molecule possesses; it develops after the secondary structure is established. Tertiary structure refers to how the amino acid chain bends or folds in three dimensions to form a compact or tightly folded protein. Tertiary structure results from hydrogen bonding, disulfide cross-linkages, ionic bonds between polar amino acids, and interactions between hydrophobic R groups. This last feature tends to locate the hydrophobic

R groups internally in the protein structure, away from the aqueous environment. A protein that clearly demonstrates tertiary structure is hemoglobin. Some parts of the amino acid chains in this molecule can form helices; others cannot. This gives the molecule the fluidity to assume different three-dimensional shapes along the chain—it will bend back upon itself to accomplish the maximum number of hydrogen bonds and disulfide bridges.

As a result of the various bonds that can form within a protein molecule, essentially two kinds of proteins exist: fibrous protein and globular protein. Fibrous proteins resemble long ribbons or hairs. They tend to be insoluble in most solvents and include such tough, resilient protein structures as collagen and elastin. Fibrous protein can have either the helical or pleated sheet structure. Collagen is an example of the triple helix; silk, a pleated sheet structure. The fibrous proteins appear to have a long "stringy" shape, whereas globular proteins are roughly spherical or elliptical. Many enzymes and antibodies have a globular structure.

The quaternary structure refers to how groups of individual amino acid chains are arranged in relation to each other within a given protein. It is the structure that results when two or more polypeptide chains combine. The chains (subunits) may be different or identical, yet each subunit still possesses its own primary, secondary, and tertiary structure. The number of subunits in a protein may vary; some proteins have only two subunits while others have as many as 2130 subunits. The protein, hemoglobin, for example, consists of four subunits and is one of the few proteins whose primary, secondary, tertiary, and quaternary structures are known. It contains four separate peptide chains: two α chains that contain 141 amino acid residues and two β chains that contain 146 amino acid residues. To each of these is bound a heme (iron) residue in a non-covalent linkage.

PROTEIN SYNTHESIS

Protein synthesis is dependent upon the simultaneous presence of all the amino acids necessary for the protein being synthesized and upon the provision of energy. If there is an insufficient supply of either, protein biosynthesis will not proceed at its normal pace. Chemically, the polymerization of amino acids into protein is a series of dehydration reactions between two amino acids.

DNA

The process whereby proteins are synthesized provides the basis for understanding genetic differences. It is also the basis for understanding how the unique properties of each cell type are maintained, since the properties that make cells unique are usually conferred by the proteins within them. Some of these proteins are the structural elements of the cell. Others are enzymes that catalyze specific reactions and processes that characterize the cell in question. Still other proteins confer a particular biochemical function on the cell. The amino acid sequence of a particular protein is genetically controlled. This control is exerted through the polynucleotide, DNA. DNA is found in both the nucleus and the mitochondria. It is composed of four bases: adenine, guanine, thymine, and cytosine. These bases are condensed to form the DNA chain in a process analogous to the condensation of amino acids that comprise the primary structure of a protein. Species vary in the percent distribution of these bases in their DNA. In mammals, the adenine-thymine content varies from 45% to 53%. Small amounts of the base, 5-methyl cytosine, as well as methylated derivatives of the other bases, can also be found.

The chain of nucleotides that comprise DNA is formed by joining adenine, guanine, thymine, and cytosine through phosphodiester bonds. The phosphodiester linkage is between the 5′ phosphate group of one nucleotide and the 3′ OH group of the adjacent nucleotide. This provides a direction (5′ to 3′) to the chain. A typical segment of the chain is illustrated in Figure 38.

The hydrophobic properties of the bases plus the strong charges of the polar groups within each of the component units are responsible for the helical conformation of the DNA chain. The bases

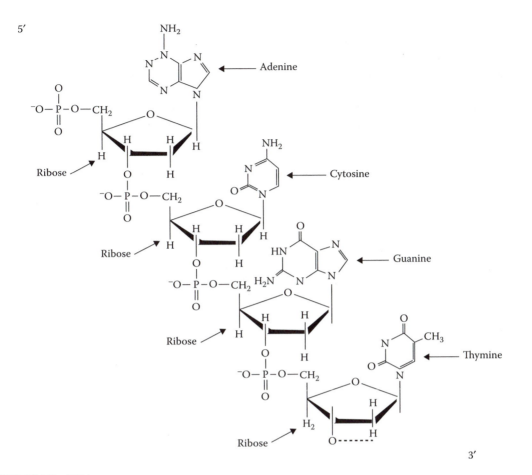

5'

Adenine

Cytosine

Guanine

Thymine

Ribose

Ribose

Ribose

Ribose

3'

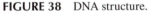

FIGURE 38 DNA structure.

themselves interact such that in the nucleus, the two chains are intertwined. Hence, the term double helix applies to DNA. In the mitochondria, the DNA is circular with connections between the light and heavy strands. Hydrogen bonds between the bases stabilize this conformation. Other factors as well serve to stabilize the structure of the DNA. Unwinding a small portion of the DNA, a necessary step in the initiation of transcription, occurs when these stabilizing factors are perturbed and signals are sent to the nucleus that transcription should begin. Unwinding exposes a small (~17 kb) segment of the DNA (the gene) allowing its base sequence to be available for complementary base pairing as happens when mRNA is synthesized (transcription). The segment that is exposed contains not only the 600 to 1800 nucleotide-structural gene but also a sequence called the promoter region. The promoter region precedes the start site of the structural gene, and this is said to be upstream of the structural gene. Those bases following the start site are downstream. The nucleotides that code for a specific protein may not be adjacent to each other on the DNA strand but may be located nearby as the DNA exists in a doubly coiled chain of bases, the double helix.

The DNA base sequence is unique for every protein that is synthesized in the body. While only a few bases are used for the DNA, the combinations and sequences of the combinations provide a specific code for each and every protein and peptide. Thus, the function of DNA is to determine the properties of the cell through the provision of a code that directs protein synthesis. It also functions to transmit genetic information from one generation to the next in a given species. Thus, DNA has a broad spectrum of functions—it ensures the identity of both specific cell types and specific species.

The sequence of amino acids in each protein synthesized by the body is determined from a subunit of the DNA molecule known as the gene. It consists of several thousand bases (abbreviated as kb). The gene, through the sequence of bases that are found in its constituent nucleotides, codes for a polypeptide. The DNA in the nucleus is very stable with respect to the base sequence and content. It can be damaged by certain chemicals, free radicals, X-rays, and other agents. Nuclear DNA can self-repair; mitochondrial DNA has very limited repair capability. If a change in the base sequence of either genome does occur and is not repaired, a mutation is said to have occurred. Base substitution, duplication, and base deletion can occur as mutations. This mutation will then become part of the genetic information transmitted to the next generation.

Some of the base substitutions have no effect on the gene product. This is because some amino acids have more than one combination of bases (codons) that stipulate a particular amino acid in the gene product (see Table 43). In addition, some mutations occur that have little effect on the functional or conformational characteristics of the resultant protein. For example, a mutation could occur that would result in an amino acid substitution of one neutral amino acid for another. This substitution might occur in a region outside of the active site(s) of the protein and with little effect on that protein's size and shape. Actually, such mutations and resultant amino acid substitutions are not mutations per se but polymorphisms. The resultant gene product retains its premutation function yet has a slightly different amino acid sequence. However, such polymorphisms are useful tools because they allow population geneticists to track mutation and evolutionary events through related family members.

TABLE 43
Codons for the Amino Acids

		Second Base			
		U	C	A	G
First Base	U	UUU ⎫ Phe UUC ⎭ UUA ⎫ Leu UUG ⎭	CUU ⎫ CUC ⎬ Leu CUA ⎭ CUG	AUU ⎫ Ile AUC ⎭ AUA AUG[a] MET	GUU ⎫ GUC ⎬ Val GUA ⎭ GUG
	C	UCU ⎫ UCC ⎬ Ser UCA ⎭ UCG	CCU ⎫ CCC ⎬ Pro CCA ⎭ CCG	ACU ⎫ ACC ⎬ Thr ACA ⎭ ACG	GCU ⎫ GCC ⎬ Ala GCA ⎭ GCG

	A	UAU ⎫ Tyr
		UAC ⎭
		UAA
		   STOP
		UAG
		   STOP
			CAU ⎫ His
			CAC ⎭
			CAA ⎫ Gln
			CAG ⎭
				AAU ⎫ Asn
				AAC ⎭
				AAA ⎫ Lys
				AAG ⎭
					GAU ⎫ Asp
					GAC ⎭
					GAA ⎫ Glu
					GAG ⎭

	G	UGU ⎫ Cys
		UGC ⎭
		UGA
		   STOP
		UGG
		   Trp
			CGU ⎫
			CGC ⎬ Arg
			CGA ⎭
			CGG
				AGU ⎫ Ser
				AGC ⎭
				AGA ⎫ Arg
				AGG ⎭
					GGU ⎫
					GGC ⎬ Gly
					GGA ⎭
					GGG

[a] AUG also serves as a start codon.

In the nucleus, the DNA is found in the chromosomal chromatin. Chromatin contains very long double strands of DNA and a nearly equal mass of histone and nonhistone proteins. Histones are highly basic proteins varying in molecular weight from ~11,000 to ~21,000. As a result of their high content of basic amino acids, histones serve to interact with the polyanionic phosphate backbone of the DNA so as to produce uncharged nucleoproteins. The histones also serve to keep the DNA in a very compact form and serve to protect this DNA from free-radical attack. In mammals, the mitochondrial DNA does not have this protective histone coat. It is "naked" and much more vulnerable to damage. This damage can be quite severe, yet because there are so many copies of the mitochondrial DNA and so many mitochondria in a cell, the effects of this damage might not be apparent.

During cell division, the nuclear DNA, as soon as its replication is completed, becomes highly condensed into distinct chromosomes of characteristic shapes. These chromosomes exist as pairs and are numbered. There are 46 chromosomes in the human. Included in this number are the sex chromosomes, the X and Y chromosomes. If the individual has one X and one Y sex chromosome, the individual is a male; if two X sex chromosomes are present, the individual is a female. The chromosomes are the result of a mixing of the nuclear DNA of the egg and sperm. Approximately half of each pair comes from each parent. If identical codes for a given protein are inherited from each parent, the resultant progeny will be a homozygote for that protein. If nonidentical codes are inherited, the progeny will be a heterozygote. Within the heterozygote population, there may be certain codes that are dominant, for example, eye color or hair color. These are dominant traits and are expressed despite the fact that the individual has inherited two different codes for this trait. A mutation in a code that is not expressed is a recessive trait. If by chance two identical mutated genes are present that encode a certain protein, the expression of this mutated code will be observed. This is the basis for genetic diseases of the autosomal recessive or dominant type. Autosomal means a mutation in any of the chromosomal DNA except that which is in the X or Y chromosome. A mutation of the DNA in this chromosome is called a sex-linked mutation. If it results in a disease, it is called a sex-linked genetic disease. There is another inheritance pattern based on the mitochondrial genome. Because this genome is primarily of maternal origin, certain of the characteristics of the OXPHOS system will be inherited via maternal inheritance. A number of mitochondrial mutations result in a number of degenerative diseases.

Having the codes in the nucleus for the synthesis of protein in the cytoplasm implies communication between the cytoplasm and the nucleus and between the nucleus and the cytoplasm. Signals are sent to the nucleus, which "inform" this organelle of the need to synthesize certain proteins. We do not know what all these signals are. Some are substrates for the needed proteins, some are nutrients, some are hormones, and some are signaling compounds that have yet to be identified. The communication between the nucleus and the cytoplasm is carried out by mRNA.

TRANSCRIPTION

mRNA is used to carry genetic information from the DNA of the chromosomes to the surface of the ribosomes. It is synthesized as a single strand in the nucleus by a process known as transcription. Chemically, RNA is similar to DNA. It is an unbranched linear polymer in which the monomeric subunits are the ribonucleoside 5'-monophosphates. The bases are the purines, adenine, and guanine, and the prymidines, uracil, and cytosine. Note that thymine is not used in RNA and uracil is not present in DNA. RNA is single stranded rather than double stranded. It is held together by molecular base pairing and will contract if in a solution of high ionic strength. RNA, particularly the mRNA, is a much smaller molecule than DNA and is far less stable. It has a very short half-life (from minutes to hours) compared to that of nuclear DNA (years). Because it has a short half-life, the bases that constitute it must be continually resynthesized. This synthesis requires a number of micronutrients as well as energy. This explains some of the symptoms of malnutrition. Among these symptoms are skin lesions. This is because the epithelial cells are among the shortest lived cells and must be constantly renewed. This renewal depends on both an adequate energy and amino acid supply and on the micronutrients that are involved in mRNA synthesis as well cell renewal. The synthesis of mRNA from DNA is called transcription (Figure 39).

The basic mechanism is known and involves three steps: initiation, elongation, and termination. Initiation is the process whereby basal transcription factors recognize and bind the start point for transcription on DNA and form a complex with RNA polymerase II. Most gene expressions can be defined as trans-acting factors binding cis-acting elements. Upstream of the transcription start site on DNA is a region called the promoter (Figure 40).

Within the promoter, approximately 25 base pairs upstream of the start site, is a consensus sequence called the TATA box, which contains A-T base pairs. One of the basal transcription factors, the TATA binding protein (TBP), recognizes this sequence of DNA and binds there. This begins the process of transcription initiation as the trans-acting TBP binds the cis-acting TATA box and a large complex of basal transcription factors, RNA polymerase II, and DNA is formed. Elongation is the actual process of RNA formation through the use of a DNA template in the 5′ to 3′ direction. Shortly after elongation begins, the 5′ end of mRNA is capped by 7-methylguanosine triphosphate. This cap stabilizes the mRNA and is necessary for processing and translation. The third step is the termination of the chain.

FIGURE 39   Transcription.

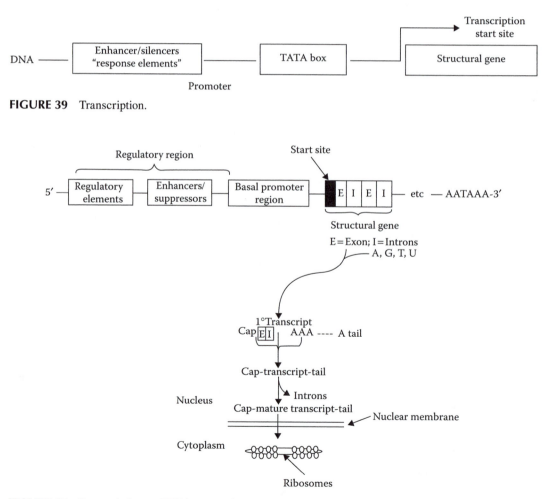

FIGURE 40   Transcription and RNA processing.

The regulation of transcription occurs at the initiation step. The promoter region contains many cis-acting elements, each named for the factor that controls them. In general, these regions are called enhancers, silencers, or more recently named response elements. Examples include the retinoic acid response element (RARE), heat shock element (HSE), and cAMP response element (CRE). The trans-acting factors that bind these elements are in general called transcription factors. They are proteins with at least two domains: DNA binding and transcription activation. Recently it has been shown that coactivators are needed to bind transcription factors and increase transcription by both interacting with basal transcription factors and altering chromatin structure. Corepressors act to decrease transcription both at the level of basal transcription factors and chromatin structure. Coactivators and corepressors are proteins.

The true regulation of transcription occurs by the regulation of transcription factors. Transcription factors can be regulated by their rates of synthesis or degradation, phosphorylation or dephosphorylation, ligand binding, cleavage of a protranscription segment, or release of an inhibitor. One class of transcription factors important for nutrition is the nuclear hormone receptor superfamily, which is regulated by ligand binding. Ligands for these transcription factors include retinoic acid, fatty acids, vitamin D, thyroid hormone, and steroid hormones. All members of this superfamily contain two zinc fingers in their DNA binding domains. Zinc is bound to histidine- and cysteine-rich regions of the protein that envelops the DNA in a shape that looks like a finger. The zinc ion plays an enormous role in gene expression because of its central use in the zinc finger. The nuclear hormone receptor superfamily is divided into four groups according to their dimerization potential, their site specificity, and their localization (Table 44). Group I receptors bind to the steroid hormones and to the

TABLE 44
Members of the Nuclear Hormone Receptor Superfamily

Receptor Group[a]	Consensus Half Site	Binding Site	
		Group 1	
GR, ER, PR, MR, AR	AGAACA or AGGTCA	→(3)←	Homodimers
		Group 2	
RXR, RAR, TR, VDR,	AGGTCA	→(0–5)→	Heterodimerize with RXR
PPAR, MB67, RLD-1,		→(0)←	
ECR, USP, ARP-1, COUP-TF			
		Group 3	
NGF1-B, FTZ-F1	(A,T)AAGGTCA	→	Monomers or heterodimerize with RXR
(ELP, SF-1) ROR,			
Rev-erb, BD73			
		Group 4	
HNF-4	AGGTCA	→(1)→	Homodimers

[a] It may appear that the names of these receptors are in nonsense code. For ease in identifying specific proteins ligand complexes, letter acronyms have been developed. Some of these codes are readily understood but others appear more arcane. For example, TR means thyroid hormone–binding receptor protein; RXR, a protein that binds 9-cis retinoic acid; VDR, a receptor that binds vitamin D (1,25(OH)$_2$ vitamin D); and so forth. Arrows indicate direction of consensus sequence, for example →(3)←, is an inverted repeat with three nucleotide spaces in between.

DNA as homodimers. Group I response elements are palindromes of either AGAACA or AGGTCA spaced by three nucleotides. The specificity occurs by interactions between the specific nucleotide sequence and the protein sequence of the first zinc finger. The retenoid X receptor ($RXR\alpha,\beta,\gamma$) that binds 9-cis retinoic acid binds to either the DR-1 or the IR-O response element. The DR1 response element also binds the PPAR $\alpha\beta$ receptor that in turn binds fatty acids and the PPARγ that binds prostaglandin E_2. All three of these receptors bind to the same element. If only one were to bind, the process would be called homodimerization. If more than one receptor binds to the same element, we would have heterodimerization.

Group II receptors, also called the retinoid/thyroid subfamily, bind nutrients and metabolites such as retinoic acid, vitamin D, and fatty acids. All of these receptors form heterodimers with the retinoid X receptor (RXR). 9-cis retinoic acid binds RXR and has a synergistic effect on transcription when dimerized with most receptors in this group. Generally, these receptors bind to direct repeats of degenerative AGGTCA sequences spaced by one (RXR, LXR, PPAR), two (alternative RAR, TR), three (VDR), four (TR, LXR), or five (RAR) nucleotides. Specificity occurs due to the spacing between the consensus sequence half sites. In the case of the retinoic acid receptor (RAR) and thyroid receptor (TR) unliganded receptor can bind DNA and repress transcription.

There are numerous proteins aside from those of the steroid receptor superfamily that bind to specific base sequences in the promoter region. Some of these bind minerals, some bind other hormones, and some are by themselves, transcription factors that have control properties.

In addition to the receptor proteins that bind to certain base sequences in the promoter region, we also have smaller molecules that similarly serve to stimulate or suppress transcription. One such is the glucose molecule. It serves to stimulate the transcription of glucokinase that has a glucose-sensitive promoter region. Only the β cell and the hepatocyte DNA have this region exposed and only these cell types express the glucokinase gene. Other cells have the gene but do not express it, probably because their glucose promoter site is unexposed. Instead, these other cell types express a similar (but different) gene called hexokinase. There are a number of instances in the nutrition science literature where specific nutrients influence the transcription of genes that encode enzymes, receptors, or carriers that are important to the use of that nutrient. Table 45 shows the examples of these influences. All of the above serve to control transcription, a vital step in controlling gene expression.

Once the bases are joined together in the nucleus to form mRNA, the nucleus must edit and process it. Processing includes capping, nucleolytic and ligation reactions that shorten it, terminal additions of nucleosides, and nucleoside modifications (Figure 40). Through this processing, less than 25% of the original RNA migrates from the nucleus to the ribosomes where it attaches prior

TABLE 45
Some Examples of Nutrient Effects on Transcription

Nutrient	Gene	Effect
Retinoic acid	Many genes	Increases transcription through its binding to RXR or RAR, which in turn bind to the AGGTCA sequence in the promoter region
Vitamin B_6	Steroid hormone receptor	Suppresses transcription
Vitamin D	Many genes	Increases transcription of genes for calcium-binding proteins
Glucose	Glucokinase	Increases transcription in pancreas and liver
Potassium	Aldosterone synthetase	Increases transcription in adrenal cortex
Fatty acids	Fatty acid synthetase	Suppresses transcription in liver
Selenium	Glutathione peroxidase, 5′-deiodinase	Increases transcription
Sodium	Endothelin 1	Increases transcription
Zinc	Zinc transporters	Increases transcription

to translation. The editing and processing are needed because immature RNA contains all those bases corresponding to the DNA introns. Introns are those groups of bases that are not part of the structural gene. Introns are intervening sequences that separate the exons or coding sequences of the structural gene. The removal of these segments is a cut-and-splice process whereby the intron is cut at its 5′ end, pulled out of the way, and cut again at its 3′ end. At the same time, the two exons are joined. This cut-and-splice routine is continued until all the introns are removed and the exons joined. Some editing of the RNA also occurs with base substitutions made as appropriate. Finally, there is a 3′ terminal poly A tail added.

The editing and processing steps are now complete. This mature mRNA now leaves the nucleus and moves to the cytoplasm for translation. The nucleotides that have been removed during editing and processing are either reused or totally degraded. Of note is the fact that editing and processing also are mechanisms used to degrade the whole message unit. This serves to control the amount and half life of this RNA. The endonucleases and exonucleases used in the cut-and-splice processing also come into play in the regulation of mRNA stability. Some mRNA's have very short half lives (minutes) while other have longer half lives (hours). This is important because some gene products are needed for only a short time. Hormones and cell signals must be short lived and therefore the body needs to control or counterbalance their synthesis and action. One of the ways to do this is by regulating the amount of mRNA (number of copies of mRNA for each gene product) that leaves the nucleus. Thus, this regulation is a key step in metabolic control.

TRANSLATION

Following transcription is translation (Figure 41). Translation is the synthesis of the protein using the order of the assemblage of constituent amino acids as dictated by the mRNA. This process is also influenced by specific nutrients. The translation of the ferritin gene, for example, is influenced by the amount of iron available in the cell. In iron deficiency, the mRNA, the start site for ferritin translation, is covered up by an iron responsive protein. This protein binds the 3′UTR and inhibits

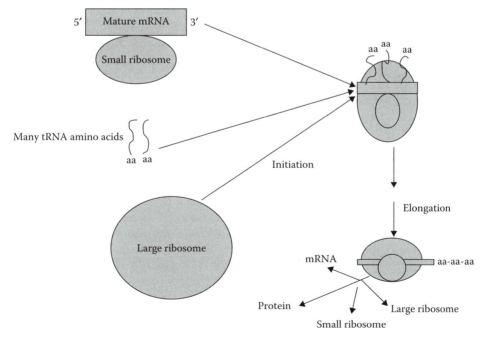

FIGURE 41 Translation.

the movement of the 40S ribosome from the cap to the translation start site. When iron status is improved, the start site is uncovered and translation can proceed. The actual site of translation is on the ribosomes; some ribosomes are located on the membrane of the endoplasmic reticulum and some are free in the cell matrix. Ribosomes consist almost entirely of ribosomal RNA and ribosomal protein. RNA is synthesized via RNA polymerase I in the cell nucleus as a large molecule; there, this RNA molecule is cleaved and leaves the nucleus as two subunits, a large one and a small one. The ribosome is reformed in the cytoplasm by the reassociation of the two subunits; however, the subunits are not necessarily derived from the same precursor.

Ribosomal RNA makes up a large fraction of total cellular RNA. It serves as the "docking" point for the activated amino acids bound to the transfer RNA and the mRNA, which dictates the amino acid polymerization sequence. Transfer RNA (tRNA) is used to bring an amino acid to the polysome (ribosome), the site of protein synthesis. Each amino acid has a specific tRNA. Each tRNA molecule is believed to have a cloverleaf arrangement of nucleotides. With this arrangement of nucleotides, there is the opportunity for the maximum number of hydrogen bonds to form between base pairs. A molecule that has many hydrogen bonds is very stable. Transfer RNA also contains a triplet of bases known, in this instance, as the anticodon. The amino acid carried by tRNA is identified by the codon of mRNA through its anticodon; the amino acid itself is not involved in this identification.

A few general statements can be made about the distribution of ribosomes in cells that have different capacities for the synthesis of proteins: cells that synthesize large numbers of proteins have numerous ribosomes; conversely, cells that synthesize small numbers of proteins contain few ribosomes; of the proteins synthesized by a cell to be secreted from that cell for use elsewhere, most of the ribosomes are attached to the endoplasmic reticulum; and those cells that synthesize protein primarily for intracellular use have relatively few ribosomes attached to the endoplasmic reticulum membrane. Small groups of ribosomes called polysomes are involved in protein synthesis; under physiologic conditions, polysomes are bound to the endoplasmic reticulum. The ribosome is bound to the membrane through its large subunit; the small subunit is involved in the binding of mRNA to the ribosome. The ribosomes have two binding sites used in protein synthesis: the aminoacyl site and the peptidyl site. These two sites have specific functions in protein synthesis.

Translation takes place in four stages. Each stage requires specific cofactors and enzymes. In the first stage, which occurs in the cytosol, the amino acids are activated by esterifying each one to its specific tRNA. This requires a molecule of ATP. In addition to a specific tRNA, each amino acid requires a specific enzyme for this reaction.

During the second stage, the initiation of the synthesis of the polypeptide chain occurs. Initiation requires that mRNA binds to the ribosome. An initiation complex is formed by the binding of mRNA cap and the first activated amino acid-tRNA complex to the small ribosomal subunit. The ribosome finds the correct reading frame on the mRNA by "scanning" for an AUG codon. The large ribosomal unit then attaches, thus forming a functional ribosome. A number of specific protein initiation factors (eIFs) are involved in this step.

In the third stage of protein synthesis, the peptide chain is elongated by the sequential addition of amino acids from the tRNA complexes. The amino acid is recognized by base pairing of the codon of mRNA to the bases found in the anticodon of tRNA and a peptide bond is formed between the peptide chain and the newly arrived amino acid. The ribosome then moves along the mRNA; this brings the next codon in the proper position for attachment of the next activated aminoacyl-tRNA complex. The mRNA and nascent polypeptide appear to "track" through a groove in the ribosomal subunits. This protects them from attack by enzymes in the surrounding environment.

The final stage of protein synthesis is the termination of the chain. The termination is signaled by one of three special codons (stop codons) in the mRNA. After the carboxy terminal amino acid is attached to the peptide chain, it is still covalently attached to tRNA, which is, in turn, bonded to the ribosome. A protein release factor promotes the hydrolysis of the ester link between the tRNA and the amino acid. Once the polypeptide chain is generated and free of the ribosome, it assumes its characteristic three-dimensional structure.

If, during the course of synthesis, there is any interference in the continuity of a supply of the needed amino acids, synthesis is stopped. Here lies the basis for the time factor of protein synthesis, a feature that nutritionists have recognized for several decades. It was established on the basis of animal feeding experiments that protein synthesis would not occur if all the needed amino acids were not provided at the same time. In addition, since protein biosynthesis is very costly in terms of its energy requirement, synthesis is severely inhibited by starvation or energy restriction. In experimental animals, it has been shown that starvation inhibits the polymerization of mRNA units, thus significantly reducing the activity of the transcription process. Other studies have shown that animals starved and then refed "overcompensate" for this period of reduced mRNA synthesis by markedly increasing mRNA synthesis above normal during the period of realimentation after the starvation period. This starved-refed-induced increase in mRNA is manifested as an increase in the synthesis of enzymes necessary for the metabolism of the various ingredients in the diet used for realimentation. The signal(s) for the release of the starvation-induced inhibition of mRNA and enzyme synthesis include the macronutrients in the diet as well as the hormones glucocorticoid, thyroxine, insulin, and others.

If there is a mutation in the sequence of bases that comprise the genetic code for a given protein, the amino acid sequence generated in a protein will be incorrect. Whether this substitution of one amino acid for another in the protein being generated affects the functionality of the protein being generated depends entirely on the amino acid in question. Some amino acids can be replaced without affecting the secondary, tertiary, or quaternary structures of the protein (and hence, its chemical and physical properties), whereas others cannot. In addition, genetic errors in amino acid sequence may pose no threat to the individual if the protein in question is of little importance in the maintenance of health and well being, or it can have large effects on health if the protein is a critical one. In the synthesis of the important protein, hemoglobin, if the genetic code calls for the use of valine instead of the usual glutamic acid in the synthesis of the β chain in the hemoglobin molecule, the resulting protein is less able to carry oxygen. This amino acid substitution not only affects the oxygen carrying capacity of the red blood cell but also affects the solubility of the hemoglobin in the red blood cell cytosol. This, in turn, affects the shape of the red blood cell, changing it from a "dumbbell-shaped" donut to a shape resembling a sickle, hence the name sickle-cell anemia. The decreased solubility of the hemoglobin can be understood if one remembers the relative polarity of the glutamic acid and valine molecules. The glutamic acid side chain is more ionic and thus contributes more to the solubility of the protein than the nonpolar carbon chain of valine. This change in pH decreases its solubility in water, and, of course, a change in solubility leads to an increased viscosity of the blood as the red cells rupture spilling their contents into the blood stream.

The amino acid sequence within a given species for a given protein is usually similar. However, some individual variation does occur. An example of an "acceptable" amino acid substitution would be some of the ones that account for the species differences in the hormone insulin. As a hormone, it serves a variety of important functions in the regulation of carbohydrate, lipid, and protein metabolism. Yet, even though there are species differences in the amino acid sequence of this protein, insulin from one species can be given to another species and be functionally active. Obviously, the species differences in the amino acid sequence of this protein are not at locations in the chains, which determine its biological function in promoting glucose use.

After translation is complete, the primary structure is complete. At this point, some posttranslational modification can occur and again specific nutrients can influence the process. For example, after the translation of osteocalcin and prothrombin, two proteins that have glutamic acid–rich regions, these glutamate residues are carboxylated. This posttranslational carboxylation requires vitamin K. Should vitamin K be in short supply, this carboxylation will not occur (or will occur in only a limited way), and these proteins will not be able to bind calcium. Both must bind calcium in order to function; osteocalcin in bone can bind neither calcium nor can canprothrombin. Hence, bone will be more fragile and blood will not clot as needed.

PROTEIN KINASE

There are four major kinases (A, C, C_E, and G) that catalyze the phosphorylation of specific proteins within the membrane-to-cytosol signaling systems.

PROTEIN TURNOVER

Protein turnover consists of two processes: synthesis and degradation. Synthesis is described in the preceding section. The proteins synthesized by the body have a finite existence. They are subject to a variety of insults and modifications. Some of these modifications have been listed, for example, a prohormone is converted to an active hormone; an enzyme is activated or inactivated with the addition or removal of a substituent and so forth. Thus, it is that a dynamic state within the body exists with respect to its full complement of peptides and proteins. Some proteins have very short lifetimes and very rapid turnover times; other proteins are quite stable and long lived. Their turnover time is quite long. The estimate of the life of a protein, that is, how long it will exist in the body, is its half-life. A half-life is the time interval that occurs when half of the amount of a compound synthesized at time X will have been degraded.

PROTEINURIA

Protein in the urine.

PROTEOLYSIS

Breakdown of proteins or peptides.

PROTEOMICS

A technique for studying a whole body response to an experimental treatment by monitoring the changes in the amounts and kinds of body proteins.

PROTHROMBIN

Precursor of thrombin. The conversion of thrombin is an essential step in the clotting process.

PROTHROMBIN TIME

A laboratory test performed to identify the time that is needed for clotting after thromboplastin and calcium are added to decalcified plasma.

PROTOCOLLAGEN

Protein in the bone matrix onto which minerals are deposited. It is synthesized by the osteoblast cells and polymerized to form a triple helix. The many proline and lysine residues are hydroxylated and then glycosylated to form procollagen that is then secreted around the osteoblast cells. It is then converted to tropocollagen, which with further processing then binds the bone minerals.

PROTON

A particle in the nucleus of an atom that has a positive charge.

PROTO-ONCOGENE

Normal cellular analogs of oncogenes. These analogs contain codes for transcription factors important to the conversion of normal cells to cancer cells.

PROTOPORPHYRIN

A compound found in hemoglobin, myoglobin, and the cytochromes.

PROXIMAL

Toward the center of the body.

PROXIMATE COMPOSITION

The composition of a diet or of an animal in crude (not exact) percentage figures.

P/S RATIO

The ratio of polyunsaturated fatty acids to saturated fatty acids.

PSEUDOGENE

An inactive segment of DNA arising by mutation of a parental active gene.

PSEUDOHYPOPARATHYROIDISM

A rare genetic disorder involving bone and mineral metabolism. Probably inherited as a sex-linked disorder and is characterized by a resistance to parathyroid hormone and an elevated blood level of PTH. Victims are short, have a round face, and have brachydactylia as a result of early epiphyseal closure. In some cases, there is ectopic soft tissue calcification.

PSEUDOVITAMINS

Compounds without vitamin activity.

PSYLLIUM

A food component that has laxative qualities.

PTH

Parathyroid hormone; essential to the regulation of blood calcium levels.

PTOMAINES

Very poisonous organic compounds produced by microorganisms in spoiled foods.

PUBERTY

The period of life when the individual undergoes a physical change from childhood to adulthood. The process is orchestrated by the sex hormones.

PUFA

Polyunsaturated fatty acids.

PUFFERFISH POISONING

Intoxication by tetrodotoxin, which is formed by bacteria (*Shewanella putrefaciens*) in the intestines of the pufferfish. The symptoms include tingling of the lips, vomiting, paralysis of the chest muscles, and death. Consumption of this extremely toxic substance results in a mortality of about 60%.

PULMONARY EDEMA

Accumulation of fluids in the lung.

PULMONARY EMBOLISM

Occlusion of one or more of the pulmonary arteries by a thrombus, which almost always originates in the leg veins from blood stasis, vessel injury, or changes in clotting factors.

PULMONARY FUNCTION TESTS

Tests used to assess the status of individuals with chronic obstructive pulmonary disease. These which include measurements of vital capacity, residual volume, and total lung capacity.

PULSES

Throbbing of blood in response to the heart beat; a family of foods, primarily beans, peas, and lentils, that are the seeds of their respective plants.

PURINE

A nitrogenous base that is an essential structural unit of DNA and RNA; it includes adenine and guanine.

PURINE-RESTRICTED DIET

Therapeutic diet used as an adjunctive therapy to medication for the treatment and control of gout. Foods highest in purines are limited and total protein intake is moderate.

PUTRESCINE

A polyamine derived from arginine.

PVN

Paraventricular nucleus in the hypothalamus; releases hormones that affect food intake.

PYELONEPHRITIS

Inflammation of the kidney; a common renal disease from acute bacterial infection.

PYLORUS

The connection between the stomach and small intestine.

PYRIDOXAL PHOSPHATE

Coenzyme form of the vitamin pyridoxine.

PYRIDOXINE, PYRIDOXAMINE, PYRIDOXIC ACID

Vitamin B_6; an essential nutrient that serves as a coenzyme involved in transamination reactions. Vitamin B_6 occurs in nature in three different forms that are interconvertible. It can be an aldehyde (pyridoxal), an alcohol (pyridoxine), or an amine (pyridoxamine). These three forms are shown in Figure 42. Vitamin B_6 is the generic descriptor for all 2-methyl-3,5-dihydroxymethyl pyridine derivatives. For vitamin activity, it must be a pyridine derivative, phosphorylatable at the 5-hydroxymethyl group, and the substituent at carbon 4 must be convertible to the aldehyde form.

Pyridoxine hydrochloride is the commercially available vitamin form. Pyridoxine HCl is stable to light and heat in acid solutions. In neutral or alkaline solutions, it is unstable to light and heat.The aldehyde form (pyridoxal) is much less stable. Its instability to heat is a major concern in food processing since foods that are rich in the vitamin are neutral to slightly alkaline. When heat treated, as is necessaryto kill food-borne pathogens and prevent spoilage, vitamin activity may be lost. This is particularly true for foods that are autoclaved (i.e., infant formulas).

SOURCES

Pyridoxine, pyridoxal, and pyridoxamine are widely distributed throughout foods from the plant and animal kingdoms. Meats, cereals, legumes, lentils, nuts, fruits, and vegetables all contain the vitamin.

ABSORPTION AND METABOLISM

Pyridoxine uptake is by passive diffusion rather than by active transport (Figure 43).

Once absorbed it is carried by the erythrocyte to all cells in the body. Significant amounts of the vitamin may be found in liver, brain, spleen, kidney, and heart, but like the other water soluble vitamins, there is no appreciable store and this vitamin must be present in the daily diet. It is carried in the blood tightly bound to proteins, primarily hemoglobin and albumin. The vitamin binds via the amino group of the N-terminal valine residue of the hemoglobin α chain, and this binding has twice the strength of its binding to albumin. Pyridoxal is converted via a saturable process to pyridoxal phosphate (PPS). The reaction shown in Figure 44 is catalyzed by pyridoxal kinase, an enzyme present in the cytoplasm of the mucosal cell.

When pyridoxal is phosphorylated, transmural absorption decreases, whereas uptake is unaffected. Phosphorylation thus serves as a means of control of the cellular PP level. Pyridoxal phosphate is essential to the absorption of other nutrients. A major metabolite is 4-pyridoxic acid. It accounts for 50% of B_6 excreted in the urine. Other metabolites have been found in the urine in addition to the three forms of the vitamin. Amphetamines, chlorpromazine, oral con-

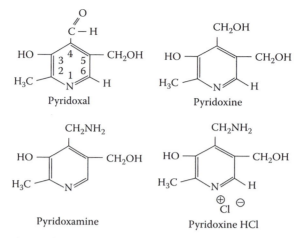

FIGURE 42   Structures of naturally occurring vitamin B_6.

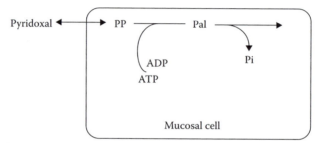

FIGURE 43   Absorption of pyridoxal.

traceptives, and reserpine all increase B_6 loss. Oral contraceptives increase tryptophan use and thus increase B_6 use.

FUNCTION

Pyridoxal phosphate serves as a coenzyme in reactions whose substrates contain nitrogen. Well over 100 reactions are known that involve pyridoxal phosphate. About 50% of these are transaminase reactions. Reactions such as transamination, racemization, decarboxylation, cleavage, synthesis, dehydration, and desulfhydration have been shown to be dependent on pyridoxal phosphate. Intransamination, the α-amino group of amino acids, such as alanine, arginine, asparagine, aspartic acid, cysteine, isoleucine, lysine, phenylalanine, tryptophan, tyrosine, and valine, is removed and transferred to a carbon chain such as α-ketoglutarate, which in turn can transfer the amino group to the urea cycle for urea synthesis. Pyridoxal phosphate functions in transaminations in a Schiff base mechanism, as shown in Figure 45. The binding of pyridoxal phosphate to its apoenzyme is shown in Figure 46. The active coenzyme forms of the vitamin B_6 are pyridoxal phosphate and pyridoxamine phosphate.

Our present understanding of the role of these coenzymes is that pyridoxal will react nonenzymatically at 100°C with glutamic acid to yield pyridoxamine and α-ketoglutaric acid. Pyridoxal phosphate functions as a coenzyme by virtue of the ability of its aldehyde group to react with the α-amino group to yield a Schiff base between the enzyme-bound pyridoxal phosphate and the amino acid, converting it to the α-keto acid; the resulting bound pyridoxamine phosphate enzyme then reacts with another α-keto acid, called an amino acid acceptor, in a

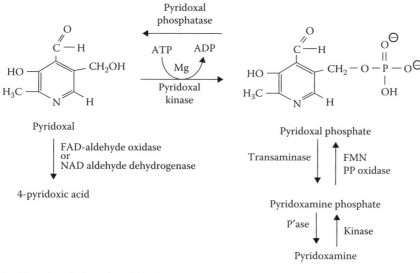

FIGURE 44 Phosphorylation of pyridoxal.

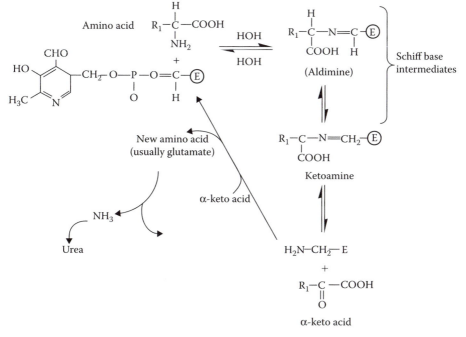

FIGURE 45 Schiff base mechanism for pyridoxal phosphate.

reverse reaction to yield a new amino acid and pyridoxal phosphate. The linkage of pyridoxal phosphate to the enzyme is a noncovalent bonding, presumably through the charged ring containing the nitrogen atom and the lysyl residues of the transaminase enzyme proteins. In transamination, the unprotonated amino group of the amino donor is covalently bound to the carbon atom of the aldehyde group of enzyme-bound pyridoxal phosphate, with the elimination of water, to form an aldimine that tautomerizes to the corresponding ketamine. The step involves the movement of an electron pair from the amino acid to the pyridine ring of the prosthetic

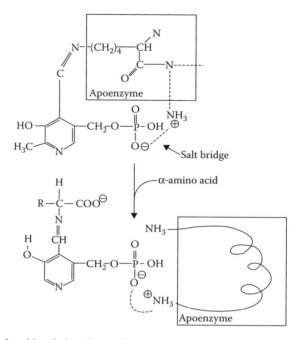

FIGURE 46   Binding of pyridoxal phosphate to its apoenzyme.

group followed by tautomerization to the ketomine. Addition of water leads to the formation of a free α-keto acid and Enz-PP complex. By oscillating between the aldehyde and amino groups, the PP acts as an amino acid carrier. Thus, the transamination reaction is an example of a double displacement reaction.

Pyridoxal phosphate (P'al P) also acts with cystathionine lyase to catalyze the cleavage of cystathionine to yield free enzyme, free cysteine with α-ketobutyrate and NH_3 as other products. Pyridoxal phosphate is important for the synthesis of the neurotransmitters γ aminobutyric acid (GABA), serotonin, dopamine, norepinephrine, and epinephrine. These reactions are outlined in Figure 47.

This role of vitamin B_6 explains the CNS symptoms associated with the deficient state. Convulsions are a common symptom together with other derangements in metabolism and anemia. The symptom of anemia arises from the role of pyridoxal phosphate in hemoglobin synthesis, which is outlined in Figure 48.

More recently we have come to understand a role of vitamin B_6 in steroid hormone-induced protein synthesis. Studies have shown that B_6 has an important role as a physiological mediator of steroid hormone function. In this role, B_6 binds to a steroid hormone receptor and in so doing inhibits the binding of the steroid hormone–receptor complex to specific DNA sites. In this way, B_6 acts as a negative control of steroid hormone action. Progesterone, glucocorticoids, estrogen, and testosterone effects on RNA polymerase II and RNA transcription have been shown to be inhibited by the presence of pyridoxal phosphate. In each of these instances, the pyridoxal phosphate binds to the receptor protein and in so doing has a negative effect on hormone-receptor binding to DNA. This role for B_6 is in addition to its role as a coenzyme in a wide variety of enzymes involved in cell growth and cell division. One of these is ornithine decarboxylase, an enzyme that plays an important role in cell division. In rapidly growing tumor cells, B_6 levels are much lower than in normal cells, and some of the major chemotherapies for cancer are based on the need for B_6 by these cells. Antivitamin B_6 compounds are important chemotherapeutic agents in this setting.

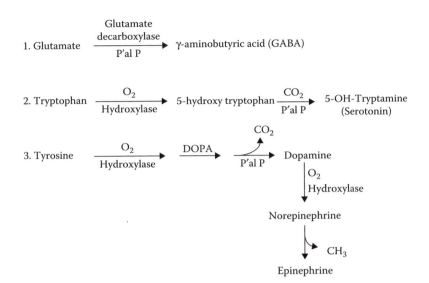

FIGURE 47 B_6 and the synthesis of neurotransmitters.

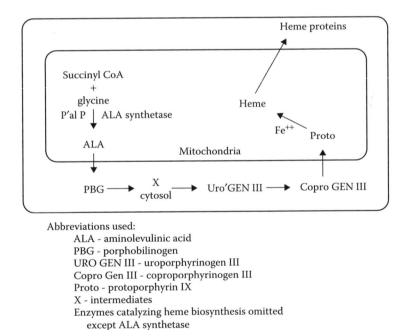

FIGURE 48   Role of pyridoxal phosphate in heme biosynthesis.

Lastly, B_6 status has been associated with chronic inflammatory conditions such as obesity, diabetes, and cardiovascular disease. Individuals whose B_6 status is marginal are more at risk to develop these conditions than individuals whose B_6 intake is excellent.

DEFICIENCY

In humans, the deficiency syndrome is ill defined. It is characterized by weakness, irritability and nervousness, insomnia, and difficulty in walking. Cheilosis (cracks at the corners of the mouth) is not responsive to biotin or riboflavin. Infants consuming B_6-deficient milk formula have convulsive seizures that can be corrected almost immediately with intravenously administered vitamin. There is a deranged tryptophan metabolism and evidence of increased excretion of xanthurenic acid. In B_6 deficiency, the conversion of tryptophan to niacin is impaired and thus skin lesions develop that resemble those of pellagra and riboflavin deficiency. Behavioral changes have been described and include depression and irritability. In the elderly, diet supplementation with a mixture of folacin, vitamin B_{12}, and pyridoxine has been shown to improve mental status and reduce symptoms of confusion and mental disability. Marginal intakes of pyridoxine result in a reduced red-cell glutathione synthesis without affecting red-cell glutathionie concentrations.

Hypochromic sideroblastic anemia is a common finding and is due to the role B_6 in hemoglobin synthesis. While B_6 is found in a wide variety of foods, B_6 deficiency can be observed when antivitamin drugs are used. For example, isoniazid, a drug used in the treatment of tuberculosis, results in excessive B_6 loss. Penicillamine, a drug used in the treatment of Wilson's disease, has antivitamin activity. Lastly, higher than normal doses of B_6 have been prescribed for the treatment of skin disease and for neuromuscular and neurological diseases. Whether this prescription has a positive effect on the pathophysiology of these diseases remains under discussion.

There are several congenital diseases of importance to B_6 status. Homocysteinuria due to a defect in the enzyme cystathionine β-synthase is characterized by dislocation of the lenses in the eyes, thromboses, malformation of skeletal and connective tissues, and mental retardation. Hyperhomocysteinemia is associated with an increased risk of atherosclerosis and is also associated with a proinflammatory state. Pyridoxal phosphate is a coenzyme for this synthase. Cystathionuria due to a defect in cystathionine γ-lyase is characterized by mental retardation, also drives up the need for B_6. GABA deficiency due to mutation in glutamate decarboxylase is manifested by a variety of neuropathies and sideroblastic anemia due to a mutation in δ-aminolevulinate synthetase is characterized by anemia, cystathionuria, and xanthurenic aciduria. All of these genetic disorders can be ameliorated somewhat by massive doses of the vitamin. Why this works is not known, but patients with these disorders do not have any symptoms of B_6 deficiency. The need for B_6 depends on the composition of the diet and on the age and gender of the individual.

PYRIMIDINE GLYCOSIDES

Nonnutritive natural food components of important toxicological relevance. Favism, a disease caused by the ingestion of fava beans, is characterized by acute hemolysis, in serious cases accompanied by jaundice and hemoglobinuria. It is mainly found in Mediterranean populations with a congenital deficiency of NADPH-dependent glucose-6-phosphate dehydrogenase (G6PD). Fava beans contain two pyrimidine glycosides that have been shown to induce hemolysis: vicine and convicine. The aglycons are divicine and isouramil. Divicine and isouramil are powerful reducing agents. In red cells, they are readily oxidized by oxyhemoglobin to form methemoglobin, H_2O_2, and Heinz bodies (thought to consist of denatured hemoglobin). The oxidation products undergo reduction by glutathione, and H_2O_2 is reduced by glutathione peroxidase. The oxidized glutathione produced by these reactions is reduced by NADPH, generated from glucose-6-phosphate and G6PD. The defect leading to hemolysis lies in the red cells that have insufficient G6PD, that is, diminished levels of reduced glutathione, to protect them against oxidative attack.

PYRIMIDINES

A group of nitrogenous bases needed for DNA and RNA structures; includes cytosine, thymine, and uracil.

PYROLYSIS

Decomposition of a compound into smaller, more reactive structures by the action of heat alone. The fragmentation is usually followed by combination of the smaller structures to more stable compounds, provided the conditions do not allow the conversion to CO and CO_2. Pyrolysis products may occur in all three of the macronutrient categories. The formation of pyrolysis products depends on the type of parent compound and the temperature. In the case of food, hazardous compounds are formed from about 300°C. Well-known types of pyrolysis products in foods include polycyclic aromatic hydrocarbons (PAHs) and heterocyclic pyrolysis products from amino acids. PAHs are likely to be formed from degradation products consisting of two- or four-carbon units, such as ethylene and butadiene radicals. The most potent carcinogenic PAH is benz[a]pyrene, which has been identified in the charred crusts of biscuits and bread, in broiled and barbecued meat, in broiled mackerel, and in industrially roasted coffees. Fat is an important precursor for the formation of PAHs (in meat and fish). Furthermore, PAHs are abundantly found in smoked food, originating from the combustion of wood and other fuels. Heterocyclic pyrolysis products from amino acids include 3-amino-1,4-dimethyl-5H-pyrido(4-β)indole (precursor—tryptophan), 3-amino-1-methyl-5H-pyrido (4,3-b)indole (precursor—tryptophan), and 2-amino-5-phenylpyridine (precursor—phenylalanine). These mutagens and several structurally related substances have been isolated from the surface of protein-containing food cooking at 250°C and higher. Other mutagens, such as 2-amino-3-methylimidazo(4,5-f)quinoline and 2-amino-3,8-dimethylimidazole(4,5-f) quinoxaline, have also been isolated from different types of protein-rich foods heated at about 200°C.

PYRROLOQUINOLINE QUINONE

Also called ethoxatin; cofactor for the copper-dependent lysyl oxidase in the cross-linking of collagen and elastin.

PYRUVATE

The end product of glycolysis.

Q

Q CYCLE

A part of the electron transport chain; shuttles reducing equivalents back and forth through the inner mitochondrial membrane.

QUADRIPLEGIA

Paralysis of the limbs due to damage to the spinal cord in the cervical region.

QUANTITATIVE COMPUTED TOMOGRAPHY

An imaging technique consisting of an array of X-ray sources and radiation detectors aligned opposite each other. As X-ray beams pass through the subjects, they are weakened or attenuated by the tissues and picked up by the detectors. The signals are then compared using a computer, which can construct a cross section of the body using sophisticated modeling techniques.

QUICK BREADS

Baked flour products made without yeast using baking powder or baking soda as the leavening agent.

QUINAPRIL HHYDROCHLORIDE

Ace inhibitor, antihypertensive drug. Trade name: Accupril.

QUININE

A compound useful in malaria treatment.

R

RABBIT FEVER

Tularemia. Caused by the microorganism *Fracisella tularensis*. Symptoms include ulcerous lesions of skin, headache, chills, and fever. Organism frequently is carried by wild game.

RABEPRAZOLE SODIUM

Proton pump inhibitor; antiulcerative drug. Trade name: Aciphex.

RADIOACTIVE ISOTOPES

An unstable atom with particles, which when they are released by the atom also results in the release of energy as α, β, or γ rays.

RAFFINOSE

A trisaccharide that is difficult to digest but can be digested by gut flora to result in gas (flatulence) and short-chain fatty acids.

RALOXIFENE HYDROCHLORIDE

This drug is a selective estrogen receptor modulator and acts as an antiosteoporotic drug. Trade name: Evista.

RAMIPRIL

ACE inhibitor and an antihypertensive drug. Trade name: Altace.

RANCIDITY

Deterioration of fats and oils in foods. It is characterized by an unpleasant odor and taste. Two types of rancidity can be defined as follows: (1) hydrolytic rancidity, and (2) oxidative rancidity.

RANDOM MISCLASSIFICATION

Errors in the necessary information (e.g., in exposure measurement) that are not related to the state of disease. This is the case if equal proportions of subjects in the groups, which are compared, are classified incorrectly with respect to exposure or disease. Also known as nondifferential misclassification. This type of misclassification dilutes the true difference and therefore always changes the observed effect toward the null hypothesis (i.e., no relationship between exposure and disease).

RANITIDINE HYDROCHLORIDE

H_2-receptor antagonist that serves as an antiulcerative drug. Trade names: Apo-Ranitidine, Zantac, Zantac-C, Zantac EFFERdose, Zantac 75.

RAPESEED

A seed oil plant. A subspecies of rapeseed is the canola seed, which has no erucic acid in its oil.

RAPID FREEZING

A food processing technique affecting the oxidation of dietary fats and oils. Rapid freezing of raw plant material may be accompanied by lipoxygenase-mediated oxidation, depending on the extent of tissue damage and on the storage temperature and time.

RATE DIFFERENCE

The difference in incidence rate between exposed and unexposed populations, expressed in absolute terms. It is calculated by subtracting the incidence rate in the unexposed group (I0) from the incidence rate in the exposed group (I1). I0 can be interpreted as the baseline incidence rate, and only the incidence rate exceeding this figure is due to exposure. Therefore, the rate difference is also known as attributable rate. A difference in incidence rate of 0 means that the disease is not related to exposure (I1 = I0).

RBC

Red blood cell; erythrocyte.

RBP

Retinol-binding protein. A protein synthesized in the liver and used to transport retinol in the blood or in the cell.

REACTIVE HYPOGLYCEMIA

Blood levels that fall below 80 mg/dL after a glucose challenge; can be life threatening. May be due to an overdose of insulin.

READING FRAME

One of three possible ways of reading a nucleotide sequence as a series of triplets.

RECALL BIAS

A type of information bias that is of importance in case-control studies. It means that cases differ from controls in the recollection of exposure.

24-HOUR RECALL METHOD

A method used to estimate the food intake of subjects by asking them to recall what they ate over the last 24 hours.

RECEPTOR

This is a general term applied to any protein in any part of the cell that binds to a specific compound and allows that compound to do its job in the cell. Most hormones and many nutrients have specific receptors, without which these hormones or nutrients would be ineffective. The term also refers to proteins in the nucleus and mitochondria that have a specific role in binding nutrients, hormones, or metabolites to specific base sequences in the DNA in these compartments. There are both plasma and intracellular membrane receptors. Plasma membrane receptors typically bind peptides or proteins (see Figure 49). These are called ligands.

In many instances, these compounds are hormones or growth factors. Upon binding, one of two processes occurs. In one, the binding of the peptide or protein (ligand) to its cognate receptor is followed by an internalization of this ligand-receptor complex. In the other, the receptor is not internalized but when ligand is bound, it generates a signal that alters cell metabolism and function. Internalization allows for the entry of the ligand or its activated fragment into the cell, where it may target specific intracellular components. The ligand can either transfer to another receptor or move to its target site in the cell by itself as it dissociates from its plasma membrane receptor. The receptor in turn is either recycled back to the plasma membrane or it is degraded. There are actually four types of membrane-spanning receptors: (1) simple receptors that have a single membrane-spanning unit; (2) receptors with a single membrane-spanning unit that also involves a tyrosine kinase component on the interior aspect of the plasma membrane; (3) receptors with several membrane-spanning helical segments of their protein structures that are coupled to a separate G-protein on the interior aspect of the plasma membrane; and (4) receptors that not only have membrane-spanning units but also have a membrane-spanning ion channel. Examples of each of these are shown in Table 46.

Immunoglobulins typically are moved into the cell via the single membrane-spanning receptor; so too are nerve growth factor and several other growth factors. The receptors for these proteins are usually rich in cysteine. The cysteine-rich region projects out from the plasma membrane and is important for the binding of its ligand through disulfide bonds. Insulin and thyroid-stimulating hormone are moved into the cell via a single membrane-spanning unit that contains tyrosine kinase activity. There is considerable homology between the first type and this type of receptor in the portion of the receptor that binds the ligand. Where the receptors differ is in the portion that extends

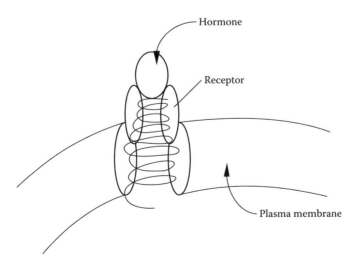

FIGURE 49   Schematic of a hormone bound to its cognate receptor located in the plasma membrane.

TABLE 46
Types of Plasma Membrane Receptors and Examples of Ligands

a) Single membrane-spanning unit, no tyrosine kinase
    Ligands
        Immunoglobulins
        T-cell antibodies
        Insulin-like growth factor (IGF)
        Nerve growth factor (NGF)
        Growth hormone (GH)

b) Single membrane-spanning unit with tyrosine kinase activity
    Ligands
        Thyroid-stimulating hormone (TSH)
        Insulin
        Platelet-derived growth factor (PDGF)

c) Multiple membrane-spanning unit coupled with G-protein
    Ligands
        Calcitonin
        Parathormone
        Luteinizing hormone
        Rhodopsin
        Acetylcholine
        Thyrotropin-releasing hormone

d) Multiple membrane-spanning unit coupled with G-protein and an ion channel
    Ligand
        γ-aminobutyric acid (GABA)

into and projects through the interior aspect of the plasma membrane. On the interior aspect of these single membrane-spanning receptors is a tyrosine kinase domain.

The tyrosine kinase portion of the receptor is involved in the intracellular signaling systems. These can be very complex cascades. There can be an ion (Ca+) channel as part of the two major intracellular signaling systems, the phosphatidylinositol (PIP) and the adenylatecyclase signaling systems.

Once the ligand has entered the cell, one of two events occurs. If the ligand is a hormone that has its primary effect at the plasma membrane, then its "job" is done. It will then be taken into the cell and degraded via the enzymes of the lysosomes. If the ligand has an intracellular function, it will move to its target within the cell. One of these targets may be DNA. The ligand may be transferred to an intracellular transport protein, to another receptor protein that has DNA-binding capacity, or may bind directly to the DNA affecting its transcription. The receptor has several distinct regions; each has a role in receptor activity, as shown in Figure 50. These binding proteins comprise another group of receptor proteins, the intracellular receptors. These intracellular receptors function in the movement of ligands from the plasma membrane to their respective targets. In this instance, the ligands may be lipid-soluble materials, minerals, or vitamins, as well as carbohydrates, peptides, and proteins. There is no evidence that these receptors participate in the intracellular signaling cascades except as recipients of their ligands.

Intracellular receptors bind such compounds as the retinoids, vitamin D, certain minerals, steroid hormones, thyroxine, and some of the small amino acid derivatives that regulate metabolism. As such they serve to move these materials from their site of entry to their site of action. In many instances, these receptors bind DNA and thereby function in the mode of action of their ligand. For example, each steroid receptor binds a specific steroid. These receptor proteins are grouped together and

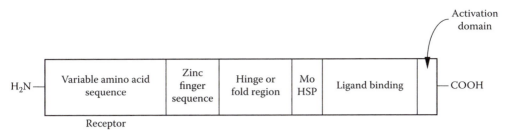

FIGURE 50   Generic structure of a receptor.

referred to as the steroid hormone super family of receptors. This is somewhat of a misnomer because not all of the ring-structured compounds they bind are steroids or steroid hormones. For example, these receptors bind thyroxine, retinoic acid, and the peroxisome proliferator–activated receptors (PPARs). In some instances, the receptor protein binds the DNA and more than one of these ring structures at the same time. Figure 50 illustrates a generic steroid hormone receptor. In this receptor, there are six basic domains that have functional importance with respect to its action in transcription. Of interest is the homology that exists among the various members of this super family of receptors: 60%–95% of the amino acid sequence of the zinc finger domain is homologous, 65%–75% of the heat shock domain (HSP) is homologous, and 30%–60% of the ligand-binding domain is homologous.

The regions where nonhomology exists determine which of the many ligands will be bound. The first hypervariable region allows researchers to separate these receptors based on their immunoreactivity. This has use in the study of gene expression, especially in the area where investigators are trying to understand how specific nutrients affect the expression of specific genes. Other members of the receptor class of cellular components bind specific ligands and in turn may also bind to DNA at specific base sequences called elements. There are specific proteins that bind copper or zinc; one or more of the vitamins; or one of the many amino acids, fatty acids, carbohydrates, or metabolites. In addition, there are intracellular receptors that bind one or more of these substances but do not bind to DNA. Instead, these binding proteins serve as transporters of their ligands from their point of entry to their point of use. Altogether, the family of proteins called receptors is an important structural component of living cells.

RECOMBINANT DNA

DNA isolated and/or synthesized in the laboratory.

RECOMMENDED DIETARY ALLOWANCES (RDA, THE UNITED STATES)

Recommended daily allowance, not to be confused with requirement, and which has been replaced by DRIs. It is a figure for each nutrient that should adequately nourish the average individual in the specified age or gender group. Complete information on the DRIs can be found at http://www.nap.edu.

RECOMMENDED NUTRIENT INTAKES (RDI, CANADA)

Similar to the U.S. RDA.

RECORD METHOD

A method for estimating food intake. It is used to obtain detailed information on food intake during a limited number of days, usually 1–7. During that period, the subjects write down everything they eat and estimate the quantities. A problem with this method is that people tend to forget to write things down or change their eating habits due to the fact that they have to write down everything they eat.

A record method for 2 days cannot be used to obtain information on the usual diet of the study subjects. Due to the large day-to-day variability in the intake of foods, a 2-day period is too short to obtain a valid estimate of the usual food intake. If information on food consumption at an individual level is needed, the record method has to be repeated several times during a certain period of time. However, the 2-day record method can give a good estimate of food consumption at group level because then a large number of 2-day records is averaged to estimate the mean intake by the group.

RECUMBENT

Lying down.

REDOX STATE

Ratio of oxidized to reduced forms of coenzymes that has three forms: NAD/NADH, FAD/FADH, NADP/NADPH.

REDUCING EQUIVALENTS

Hydrogen ions.

REFSUM'S DISEASE

Rare genetic disease characterized by defective oxidation of fatty acids. Symptoms include defective night vision, tremors, and other neurologic symptoms caused by an accumulation of phytanic acid, a metabolite of chlorophyll.

REGISTERED DIETITIAN

See Dietitian.

REGRESSION EQUATION

A statistical method for calculating the relationship between an independent variable such as age with a dependent variable such as metabolic activity.

RELAPSE

Return of disease symptoms.

RELATIVE RISK (RR)

The difference in incidence rate between exposed and unexposed populations, expressed in relative terms. It can be calculated as the incidence rate in the exposed group (I1) divided by the incidence rate in the unexposed group (I0). Also known as rate ratio. A relative risk of 1 indicates that the disease is not related to exposure (I1 = I0).

RELAXIN

A small peptide hormone produced by the corpus luteum of the ovary during the first and second trimesters of pregnancy. It is structurally similar to insulin with two peptide chains (A and B). The role of this hormone is unclear; it has been noticed to increase just prior to parturition (birth).

REMODELING

Reshaping or degrading and rebuilding a body structure.

RENAL FAILURE

See Chronic Renal Failure.

RENAL SOLUTE LOAD

Amount of solute that must be excreted by the kidney.

RENAL THRESHOLD

Concentration of a substance in plasma at which it is excreted in urine.

RENIN

An enzyme that initiates the cascade that generates angiotensin II and III.

RENIN-ANGIOTENSIN-ALDOSTERONE SYSTEM

Hormone system that regulates blood pressure, water balance, and renal function.

REPAGLINIDE

An antidiabetic drug useful in managing type 2 diabetes mellitus. Trade name: Prandin.

REPLICATION

Duplication of the genetic code.

REPORTER GENE

A coding unit whose product is easily assayed. It may be connected to any promoter of interest so that the expression of that gene can be monitored.

RER

Rough endoplasmic reticulum.

RESERPINE

A drug that has catecholamine-depleting activity with respect to the adrenal chromaffin cells.

RESIDUE

Indigestible content of food.

RESISTIN

A 108-residue hormone that blocks insulin action in fat cells.

RESPIRATORY ACIDOSIS

Acid-base imbalance of carbon dioxide retention associated with respiratory failure, sedative overdose, chronic obstructive pulmonary disease, chest wall trauma, acute abdominal distention, and obesity; it is characterized by a rapid respiratory rate that usually provides inadequate ventilation, rapid heart rate, pale and dry skin, diaphoresis, headache, and coma.

RESPIRATORY ALKALOSIS

Acid-base imbalance of decreased carbon dioxide associated with hyperventilation, anxiety, fever, pain, and mechanical over ventilation; it is characterized by increased heart rate, increased rate and depth of respirations, paresthesia, anxiety, irritability, dizziness, and agitation.

RESPIRATORY CHAIN

See Oxidative Phosphorylation.

RESPIRATORY FAILURE

Inability of the lungs to perform their ventilatory function.

RESPIRATORY QUOTIENT (RQ)

The ratio of carbon dioxide exhaled to oxygen consumed.

RESTING ENERGY EXPENDITURE

See Basal Energy.

RESTENOSIS

Recurrent narrowing of an opening.

RESTRICTION ENZYME

An endonuclease enzyme that causes cleavage of both strands of DNA at highly specific sites dictated by the base sequence.

RESTRICTION FRAGMENT LENGTH POLYMORPHISM (RFLP)

Inherited differences in sites for restriction enzymes.

RETICULOCYTE

An immature red blood cell with a network of precipitated basophilic substance and occurring during the process of active blood regeneration.

RETINA

The inner neural bilayer of the eye consisting of an outer pigment layer attached to the inner surface of the choroid, ciliary body, and iris and an inner layer formed by the expansion of the optic nerve.

RETINOIDS

A group of compounds having vitamin A activity.

RETINOL EQUIVALENT

The activity of one mole of all-trans-retinol. Not all retinoids have the same biological activity.

RETINOL-BINDING PROTEIN (RBP)

A protein required for the transport of vitamin A in the blood. A separate but similar carrier protein is located within the cells. Another protein in located within the mitochondrial and nuclear compartments that binds retinoic acid and DNA. It is called the retinoic acid receptor rather than retinol-binding protein.

RETINYL PALMITATE

A palmitoyl ester of retinol.

RETROSPECTIVE COHORT STUDIES

See Follow-Up Studies.

REVERSE TRANSCRIPTION

RNA-directed synthesis of DNA catalyzed by reverse transcriptase.

RHEUMATOID ARTHRITIS

An inflammatory disease of the joints resulting in a progressive destruction of articular and peri-articular structures. Thought to be an autoimmune disease.

RHODOPSIN

The visual pigment in the red cells of the eye. Consists of the protein opsin and 11-cis retinal. When light enters the eye, the 11-cis retinal changes to 11-trans retinal, which then separates from opsin. Recombination is then needed to restore the rhodopsin. This combination requires more retinol (which is changed to retinal) and the niacin-containing coenzyme NAD.

RIA

Radioimmunoassay. Technique useful for determining small quantities of biologically important substances such as hormones.

RIBOFLAVIN

An essential vitamin of the B family. Serves as a coenzyme (FAD, FMN) in reactions where hydrogen ions are transferred. Riboflavin (Figure 51) is a yellow-orange crystalline substance frequently associated with flavoproteins. As a solid it is red-orange in color. In solution the color changes to a greenish yellow. In solution it is quite labile. Milk loses 33% of its riboflavin activity in 1 hour of sunlight. In solution, riboflavin is easily destroyed by light and must be protected at all times from exposure. Riboflavin fluoresces due to a shifting of bonds in the isoalloxazine ring. The fluorescence is due to the presence of a free 3-imino group. If substitutions are made for this group, there is no fluorescence. Fluorescence is pH-dependent and is best between pH 4–8 max at 556 mU.

The oxidized forms of different flavoenzymes are intensely colored. They are characteristically yellow, red, or green due to strong absorption bands in the visible range. Upon reduction, they undergo bleaching with a characteristic change in the absorption spectrum.

In order to have vitamin activity, positions 8 and 7 must be substituted with more than just a hydrogen and the amine group in position 3 must be unattached. There must be a ribityl group on position 10. If the ribityl group is lost, then vitamin activity is lost. There are some antivitamins that interfere with riboflavin's usefulness. These compounds compete for the prosthetic groups or competitively inhibit its phosphorylation to form the coenzymes flavin mononucleotide (FMN) or flavin adenine nucleotide (FAD). The structures of these coenzymes are shown in Figure 52.

Sources

The best sources are foods of animal origin: milk, meat, and eggs. Wheat germ is also a good source.

Absorption, Metabolism

Absorption occurs by way of an active carrier and is energy and sodium dependent. Maximum absorption occurs in the proximal segment (the jejunum) of the small intestine, with significant uptake by the duodenum and ileum.

After a load dose, peak values in the plasma appear within two hours. The phosphorylated forms (coenzyme forms) are dephosphorylated prior to absorption through the action of nonspecific hydrolases from the brush border membrane of the duodenum and jejunum. There is a pyrophosphatase that cleaves FAD and FMN and an alkaline phosphatase that liberates the vitamin from its coenzyme form. Bile salts appear to facilitate uptake, and a small amount of the vitamin circulates via the

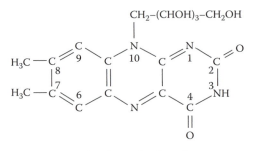

7,8-dimethyl 10 (1′ D-ribityl) isoalloxazine
or
6,7-dimethyl 9 (D-1′ ribityl) isoalloxazine
if only the carbons are numbered.

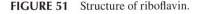

FIGURE 51   Structure of riboflavin.

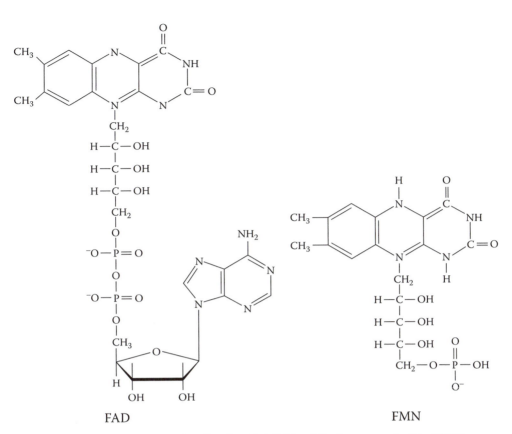

FIGURE 52   Structures of flavin adenine dinucleotide (FAD) and flavin mononucleotide (FMN).

enterohepatic system. Prior to entry into the portal blood, some of the vitamin is rephosphorylated to reform FAD and FMN. After absorption, the vitamin circulates in the blood bound to plasma proteins, notably albumin. Specific riboflavin binding proteins have been isolated and identified in several species. These proteins are of hepatic origin. There is active uptake of the free vitamin by all of the vital organs. For example, isolated liver cells will accumulate up to five times the amount of the vitamin in the fluids that surround them. Although cells will accumulate the vitamin against a concentration gradient, these cells also use the vitamin quite rapidly, so there is little net storage. The usual blood levels of riboflavin are in the range of 20–50 μg/dL, while 500–900 μg/day are excreted in the urine. Excretion products include 7- and 8-hydroxymethyl riboflavin 8-α-sulfonyl riboflavin, riboflavin peptide esters, 10-hydroxyethylflavin, lumiflavin, 10-formylmethylflavin, 10-carboxymethylflavin, lumichrome, and of course free riboflavin. Very small amounts of riboflavin and its metabolites can be found in the feces. Upon entry into the cell, riboflavin is reconverted to FMN and FAD as shown in Figure 53.

The initial phosphorylation reaction is zinc dependent. FMN and FAD synthesis is responsive to thyroid status. Hyperthyroidism is associated with increased synthesis, whereas hypothyroidism is associated with decreased synthesis. FAD is linked to a variety of proteins via hydrogen bonding and also with purines, phenols, and indoles. Covalent bonding with certain enzymes also occurs and involves the riboflavin 8-methyl group, which forms a methylene bridge to the peptide histidyl imidazole function or to the thioether function of a former cysteinyl residue. When bound to these proteins, these coenzymes are protected from degradation. However, flavins in excess of that which are protein bound are rapidly degraded and excreted in the urine. Degradation begins with hydroxylation at positions 7 and 8 of the isoalloxazine ring by hepatic microsomal cytochrome

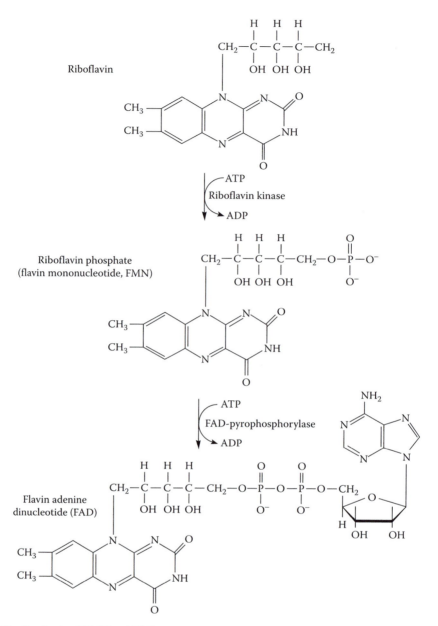

FIGURE 53 Synthesis of FMN and FAD.

P450 enzymes. The methyl groups at these positions are removed and the compound loses its activity as a vitamin. Because degradation and excretion occur at a fairly rapid rate, the rate of riboflavin degradation determines the requirement for the vitamin rather than the need for the vitamin in its function as a coenzyme, that is, the rate of FMN and FAD synthesis.

FUNCTION

FAD and its precursor FMN are coenzymes for reactions that involve oxidation-reduction. Thus, riboflavin is an important component of intermediary metabolism. The respiratory chain in the mitochondria and reactions in numerous pathways, which utilize either FAD or FMN as coenzymes,

---

TABLE 47
Reactions Using FAD or FMN

FAD-Linked Enzymes

Ubiquinone reductase
Monoamine oxidase
NADH-cytochrome P450 reductase
D-amino acid oxidase
Acyl CoA dehydrogenase
Dihydrolipoyl dehydrogenase (component of PDH and α-KGDH)
Xanthine oxidase
Cytochrome reductase
Succinate dehydrogenase
α-glycerohosphate dehydrogenase
Enzymes of the electron transport respiratory chain
Glutathione reductase

FMN-Linked Enzymes

NADH dehydrogenase (respiratory chain)
Lactate dehydrogenase
L-amino acid oxidase
NADH-cytochrome P450 reductase

PDH = Pyruvate dehydogenase; α-KGDH = α-ketoglutarate dehydrogenase.

---

require riboflavin. Table 47 shows a list of some of these enzymes. They include reactions in which reducing equivalents are transferred between cellular compartments as part of a shuttle arrangement as well as reactions that are in a mitochondrial or cytosolic sequence.

In most glutathione reductase flavoenzymes, the flavin nucleotide is tightly but noncovalently bound to the protein; an exception is succinate dehydrogenase, in which the flavin nucleotide, FAD, is covalently bound to a histidine residue of the polypeptide chain. The metalloflavoproteins contain one or more metals as additional cofactors. Flavin nucleotides undergo reversible reduction of the isolloxazine ring in the catalytic cycle of flavoproteins to yield the reduced nucleotides $FMNH_2$ and $FADH_2$. The enzymes that have a riboflavin-containing coenzyme are of three general types:

1. Enzymes whose substrates are a reduced pyridine nucleotide and the acceptor is either a member of the cytochrome or another acceptor
2. Enzymes that accept electrons directly from the substrate and can pass them to one of the cytochromes or directly to oxygen
3. Enzymes that accept electrons from substrate and pass them directly to oxygen (true oxidases)

The mechanism of action is shown in Figure 54.

Each of the steps in this sequence is fully reversible, allowing the flavoprotein to accept or donate reducing equivalents, which in turn can be joined to oxygen. Many of the flavoproteins, proteins linked with FAD or FMN also contain a metal such as iron, molybdenum or zinc and the combination of these metals and the flavin structure allows for its easy and rapid transition between single and double electron donors. Note in Table 47 that a number of enzymes are members of the oxidase family of enzymes. The oxidases transfer hydrogen directly to oxygen to form hydrogen peroxide. Xanthine oxidase uses a variety of purines as its substrate, converting hypoxanthine to

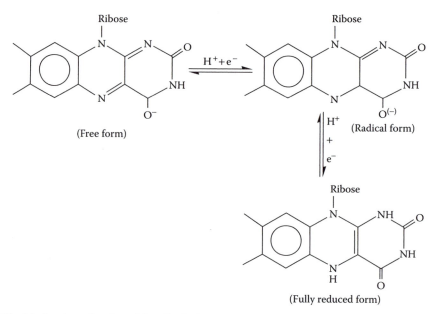

FIGURE 54   Mechanism of action of the riboflavin portion of the coenzyme.

xanthine, which is then converted to uric acid. Xanthine oxidase also catalyzes the conversion of retinal to retinoic acid. Among the important enzymes shown in Table 47 are those that are essential to mitochondrial respiration and ATP synthesis as well as the mitochondrial citric acid cycle. Succinate dehydrogenase is one of these and its activity has been used as a biomarker of riboflavin intake sufficiency. The acyl CoA dehydrogenases catalyze another of the essential pathways, fatty acid oxidation. These are FAD linked. Fatty acid synthesis requires the presence of FMN linked enzymes. While the list of enzymes shown in Table 47 is by no means complete, it gives evidence of the intimate and essential need for riboflavin in the regulation of metabolism. In its absence, profound impairments can be expected and death should follow in a short time once all of the FAD and FMN is used up. In man, clinical signs of deficiency appear in less than 6 weeks on intakes of less than 0.6 mg/day.

DEFICIENCY

Despite our knowledge about riboflavin's function as a coenzyme, there are a few symptoms that are specific to riboflavin deficiency. Poor growth, poor appetite, and certain skin lesions (cracks at the corners of the mouth, dermatitis on the scrotum) have been observed. However, these symptoms can also occur for reasons apart from inadequate riboflavin intake. This lack of direct correlation of symptoms to intake is due to the almost universal need for FAD and FMN as coenzymes in such a wide variety of the reactions of intermediary metabolism. Thus, it is impossible to pinpoint a specific deficiency symptom. Nutrition assessment of adequate riboflavin intake relies upon a few reactions in readily available cells (i.e., blood cells) that can predict intake adequacy. Erythrocyte FAD-linked glutathione reductase is one of these. Low enzyme activity is associated with inadequate intakes. Succinate dehydrogenase is another enzyme frequently used in nutrition assessment.

RIBONUCLEASE

An enzyme that catalyzes the destruction of RNA.

RIBONUCLEIC ACID (RNA)

A single strand of nucleosides having ribose instead of deoxyribose and uracil in place of thymine. There are three types of RNA: mRNA, tRNA, and ribosomal RNA. mRNA serves as the template for the order of amino acids of the particular protein being synthesized, tRNA carries these amino acids, and ribosomal RNA serves as the docking place on the ribosome for the messenger RNA.

RIBOSE

A five-carbon sugar produced by the hexose monophosphate shunt. When a single oxygen is removed, it is deoxyribose and is part of DNA. RNA contains ribose.

RIBOSOME

The organelle of the cell where protein synthesis occurs.

RICKETS

Bone malformation usually due to inadequate intake of vitamins and minerals; some forms of this disease are due to renal disease, while other forms may be due to certain toxins.

RIGOR MORTIS

Stiff rigid muscles characteristic of death.

RISEDRONATE SODIUM

Drug that reduces bone mineral loss. Trade name: Actonel.

ROSIGLITAZONE MALEATE

A thiazolidinedione that is an antidiabetic drug. Useful in managing type 2 diabetes mellitus. Trade name: Avandia. It is also available mixed with metformin hydrochloride with the trade name of Avandamet.

ROTENONE

A compound that inhibits electron transport from complex I to complex III.

ROUX-EN-Y GASTRIC BYPASS

A surgical procedure designed to help obese patients lose weight. It is a modification of the original loop gastric bypass designed to limit oral intake and create a "physiological dumping" effect to discourage patients from consuming high-sugar foods. Iron absorption and iron status are reduced in these patients as is vitamin A and D absorption. The loss of intrinsic factor needed for vitamin B_{12} absorption also means that B_{12} status is compromised unless injections of this vitamin are provided. Bone density decreases as mineral absorption is impaired.

RUMINANTS

Animals with a four-chambered stomach, one of which is called the rumen. It is a large fermentation vat populated by bacteria that can digest the complex carbohydrates of grasses and grains.

S

SACCHARIN

Nonnutritive sweetener that has 300 times the sweetness of sucrose.

SAFROLE

A methylenedioxyphenyl substance. Safrole is one of the natural and synthetic flavoring agents. Sassafras, containing high levels of safrole, used to be added to sarsaparilla root beer. Safrole is still present in the diet as a (minor) component of various herbs and spices, for example, cloves. Safrole and related substances have been shown to be carcinogenic. Biotransformation data suggest that the 1′-hydroxysulfate ester of safrole is the ultimate carcinogenic species capable of binding to DNA.

SALICYLATES

Salts of salicylic acid; anti-inflammatory agent in the amide form. Salicylic acid has been used as a food preservative.

SALIVA

A clear tasteless secretion of the salivary gland containing a lipase, amylase, and mucin. Its function is to lubricate the food, making it easier to swallow.

SALIVARY AMYLASE

An enzyme that initiates starch digestion in the mouth.

SALMONELLA

A genus of bacteria that causes one of the most common food-borne illnesses.

SALT

An inorganic compound having a negative and a positive ion that dissociate in solution. Table salt is sodium chloride.

SAM

S-adenosylmethionine. A principle methyl donor.

SARCOIDOSIS

Disease of unknown etiology characterized by tumor-like lesions that affect any tissue or organ of the body.

SARCOPENIA

Loss of skeletal muscle mass with aging, accompanied by fatty infiltration of the muscle.

SATIETIN

A blood-borne factor that serves as an appetite suppressant.

SATIETY

Feeling of fullness from consuming food.

SATURATED FATTY ACIDS (SFAS)

Fatty acids with no double bonds. The chain length can vary from 4 to 20 C atoms in mammals. Well-known examples are palmitic acid (C16:0) and stearic acid (C18:0).

SAUERKRAUT

A cabbage product made of thinly sliced cabbage and salt and allowed to ferment.

SCLERODERMA

A skin disease characterized by increased thickness.

SCRAPPLE

A pork product using corn meal and meat scraps.

SCURVY

A disease due to ascorbic acid deficiency.

SECRETIN

A 27-amino acid peptide hormone secreted by duodenal cells in response to the low pH of the chyme entering the small intestine from the stomach. Its function is to inhibit hydrochloric acid secretion while stimulating the release of a watery alkaline juice from the pancreatic exocrine cells.

SECRETOGOGE

A compound such as glucose that stimulates the β cell to release insulin. This term refers to any compound that stimulates a secreting cell to release its product.

SELECTION BIAS

The fact that the effect measured is perverted due to the selection of the study subjects. This means that the association between exposure and disease in the study population differs from the association in the total population. Case-control studies are especially sensitive to selection bias. If subjects are systematically excluded from or included in the case or control group, the comparison of these groups can give biased results. Since cases are often recruited from hospitals, controls are sometimes also selected from the same hospitals. Since hospitalized persons are likely to differ from the general population, this may influence the study results. Therefore, in the study design, special attention should be paid to the selection of controls. Often, several control groups are used to estimate the consequences of the choice of the source population of controls. Other source populations of controls that are used in addition to hospital controls are neighborhood controls (to control for socioeconomic differences between cases and controls) or a random population sample, in order to compare the exposure in the cases with that in the general population.

SELENIUM

An essential mineral needed for the antioxidant enzyme glutathione peroxidase. This is important to the suppression of oxygen free radicals. Excess selenium intakes are associated with diabetes and elevated blood lipids.

SENESCENCE

Agedness; the final portion of the life cycle.

SENILE DEMENTIA

The gradual, progressive loss with age of cognitive function.

SENSORY PERCEPTION OF FOOD

The perception of the qualities of food using the senses of taste, smell, sound, sight, and the perception of texture. All of these perceptions are in the framework of culturally expected characteristics of the food in question.

SEPSIS

Infection due to identifiable microorganisms or their products in the blood or tissues.

SEPTIC SHOCK

The end result of a process initiated by pathogenic organisms, altered mental status, inadequate tissue perfusion, decreased urine output, and refractory hypotension.

SEPTICEMIA

Systemic disease caused by the multiplication of blood-borne pathogens and their associated toxins.

SER

Smooth endoplasmic reticulum. The portion of the endoplasmic reticulum where certain lipids are synthesized and drugs are detoxified.

SERINE

A three-carbon nonessential amino acid containing a hydroxyl group on its terminal carbon. (See Amino Acids, Table 5.)

SEROTONIN (5HT)

A neurotransmitter synthesized in the CNS from tryptophan. It serves a number of roles in the body, from mood regulation to food intake regulation. In the latter, it serves as a satiety factor.

SERUM

The cell-free fluid that surrounds the red blood cells and the white blood cells.

SET POINT WEIGHT

Weight that an individual maintains for extended periods of time without conscious effort.

SEX-LINKED TRAIT

A genetic characteristic carried on either the X or the Y chromosome.

SFA

Saturated fatty acid.

SGOT

Serum glutamate oxaloacetate transaminase. A vitamin B_6-dependent enzyme whose level in the serum increases after muscle damage, particularly after a heart attack.

SGPT

Serum glutamate pyruvate transaminase. Another vitamin B_6-dependent enzyme. A rise in activity also indicates muscle damage.

SHELLFISH POISONING

A disease resulting from the consumption of shellfish that have ingested toxic algae. Shellfish poisoning manifests itself in two forms: paralytic shellfish poisoning and diarrheic shellfish poisoning.

SHIGELLOSIS

Dysentery caused by food and/or water contaminated by the organism shigella.

SHOCK

Condition in which the peripheral blood flow is inadequate to return blood to the heart; decreased cardiac output causing poor tissue perfusion.

SI UNITS

Standard units for expressing biological values (see Table 48).

TABLE 48
Conversion Factors for Values in Clinical Chemistry (SI Units)[1]

Component	Present Reference Intervals (Examples)	Present Unit	Conversion Factor	SI Reference Intervals	SI Unit Symbol	Significant Digits	Suggested Minimum Increment
Acetaminophen (P), toxic	>5.0	mg/dL	66.16	>330	mmol/L	XXO	10 mmol/L
Acetoacetate (S)	0.3–3.0	mg/dL	97.95	30–300	mmol/L	XXO	10 mmol/L
Acetone (B, S)	0	mg/dL	172.2	0	mmol/L	XXO	10 mmol/L
Acid phosphatase (S)	0–5.5	U/L	16.67	0–90	nkat/L	XX	2 nkat/L
Adrenocorticotropin [ACTH] (P)	20–100	pg/mL	0.2202	4–22	pmol/L	XX	1 pmol/L
Alanine aminotransferase [ALT] (S)	0–35	U/L	0.01667	0–0.58	mkat/L	X.XX	0.02 mkat/L
Albumin (S)	4.0–6.0	g/dL	10.0	40–60	g/L	XX	1 g/L
Aldolase (S)	0–6	U/L	16.67	0–100	nkat/L	XXO	20 nkat/L
Aldosterone (S)							
Normal salt diet	8.1–15.5	ng/dL	27.74	220–430	pmol/L	XXO	10 pmol/L
Restricted salt diet	20.8–44.4	ng/dL	27.74	580–1240	pmol/L	XXO	10 pmol/L
Aldosterone (U)—sodium excretion							
=25 mmol/d	18–85	mg/24 h	2.774	50–235	nmol/d	XXX	5 nmol/d
=75–125 mmol/d	5–26	mg/24 h	2.774	15–70	nmol/d	XXX	5 nmol/d
=200 mmol/d	1.5–12.5	mg/24 h	2.774	5–35	nmol/d	XXX	5 nmol/d
Alkaline phosphatase (S)	0–120	U/L	0.01667	0.5–2.0	mkat/L	X.X	0.1 mkat/L
α1-Antitrypsin (S)	150–350	mg/dL	0.01	1.5–3.5	g/L	X.X	0.1 g/L
α-Fetoprotein (S)	0–20	ng/mL	1.00	0–20	mg/L	XX	1 mg/L
α-Fetoprotein (Amf)	Depends on gestation	mg/dL	10.0	Depends on gestation	mg/L	XX	1 mg/L
α2-Macroglobulin (S)	145–410	mg/dL	0.01	1.5–4.1	g/L	X.X	1 mg/L
Aluminum (S)	0–15	mg/L	37.06	0–560	nmol/L	XXO	10 nmol/L

(Continued)

TABLE 48 (*Continued*)
Conversion Factors for Values in Clinical Chemistry (SI Units)[1]

Component	Present Reference Intervals (Examples)	Present Unit	Conversion Factor	SI Reference Intervals	SI Unit Symbol	Significant Digits	Suggested Minimum Increment
Amino acid fractionation (P)							
Alanine	2.2–4.5	mg/dL	112.2	245–500	mmol/L	XXX	5 mmol/L
α-Aminobutyric acid	0.1–0.2	mg/dL	96.97	10–20	mmol/L	XXX	5 mmol/L
Arginine	0.5–2.5	mg/dL	57.40	30–145	mmol/L	XXX	5 mmol/L
Asparagines	0.5–0.6	mg/dL	75.69	35–45	mmol/L	XXX	5 mmol/L
Citrulline	0.2–1.0	mg/dL	75.13	0–20	mmol/L	XXX	5 mmol/L
Cystine	0.2–2.2	mg/dL	57.08	15–55	mmol/L	XXX	5 mmol/L
Glutamic acid	0.2–2.8	mg/dL	67.97	15–190	mmol/L	XXX	5 mmol/L
Glutamine	6.1–10.2	mg/dL	68.42	420–700	mmol/L	XXX	5 mmol/L
Glycine	0.9–4.2	mg/dL	133.2	120–560	mmol/L	XXX	5 mmol/L
Histidine	0.5–1.7	mg/dL	64.45	30–110	mmol/L	XXX	5 mmol/L
Hydroxyproline	0–trace	mg/dL	76.26	0–trace	mmol/L	XXX	5 mmol/L
Isoleucine	0.5–1.3	mg/dL	76.24	40–100	mmol/L	XXX	5 mmol/L
Leucine	1.2–3.5	mg/dL	76.24	75–175	mmol/L	XXX	5 mmol/L
Lysine	1.2–3.5	mg/dL	68.40	80–240	mmol/L	XXX	5 mmol/L
Methionine	0.1–0.6	mg/dL	67.02	5–40	mmol/L	XXX	5 mmol/L
Ornithine	0.4–1.4	mg/dL	75.67	30–400	mmol/L	XXX	5 mmol/L
Phenylalanine	0.6–1.5	mg/dL	60.54	35–90	mmol/L	XXX	5 mmol/L
Proline	1.2–3.9	mg/dL	86.86	105–340	mmol/L	XXX	5 mmol/L
Serine	0.8–1.8	mg/dL	95.16	75–170	mmol/L	XXX	5 mmol/L
Taurine	0.9–2.5	mg/dL	79.91	25–170	mmol/L	XXX	5 mmol/L
Threonine	0.9–2.5	mg/dL	83.95	75–210	mmol/L	XXX	5 mmol/L
Tryptophan	0.5–2.5	mg/dL	48.97	25–125	mmol/L	XXX	5 mmol/L
Tyrosine	0.4–1.6	mg/dL	55.19	20–90	mmol/L	XXX	5 mmol/L
Valine	1.7–3.7	mg/dL	85.36	145–315	mmol/L	XXX	5 mmol/L
Amino acid nitrogen (P)	4.0–6.0	mg/dL	0.7139	2.9–4.3	mmol/L	X.X	0.1 mmol/L
Amino acid nitrogen (U)	50–200	mg/24 h	0.07139	3.6–14.3	mmol/d	X.X	0.1 mmol/d

Component	Conventional reference range	Conventional unit	Conversion factor	SI reference range	SI unit	Significant digits	Suggested minimum increment
δ-Aminolevulinate (U) [as levulinic acid]	1.0–7.0	mg/24 h	7.626	8–53	mmol/d	XX	1 mmol/d
Amitriptyline (P, S) therapeutic (vP)	50–200	ng/mL	3.605	180–270	nmol/L	XO	10 nmol/L
Ammonia (vP)							
As ammonia [NH_3]	10–80	mg/dL	0.5872	5–50	mmol/L	XXX	5 mmol/L
As ammonium ion [NH_4^+]	10–85	mg/dL	0.5543	5–50	mmol/L	XXX	5 mmol/L
As nitrogen [N]	10–65	mg/dL	0.7139	5–50	mmol/L	XXX	5 mmol/L
Amylase (S)	0–130	U/L	0.01667	0–2.17	mkat/L	XXX	0.01 mkat/L
Androstenedione (S)							
Male > 18 years	0.2–3.0	mg/L	3.492	0.5–10.5	nmol/L	XX.X	0.5 nmol/L
Female > 18 years	0.8–3.0	mg/L	3.492	3.0–10.5	nmol/L	XX.X	0.5 nmol/L
Angiotensin-converting enzyme (S)	<40	nmol/mL/min	16.67	<670	nkat/L	XXO	10 nkat/L
Arsenic (H) [as As]	<1	mg/g (ppm)	13.35	<13	nmol/g	XX.X	0.5 nmol/g
Arsenic (U) [as As]	0–5	mg/24 h	13.35	0–67	nmol/d	XX	1 nmol/d
Arsenic [as As_2O_3]	<25	mg/dL	0.05055	<1.3	mmol/L	XX.X	0.1 mmol/L
Ascorbate [as ascorbic acid] (P)	0.6–2.0	mg/dL	56.78	30–110	mmol/L	XO	10 mmol/L
Aspartate aminotransferase [AST] (S)	0–35	U/L	0.0167	0–0.58	mkat/L	O.XX	0.01 mkat/L
Barbiturate (S)							
Phenobarbital		mg/dL	43.06		mmol/L	XX	5 mmol/L
sodium phenobarbital		mg/dL	39.34		mmol/L	XX	5 mmol/L
Barbitone		mg/dL	54.29		mmol/L	XX	5 mmol/L
Barbiturate (S) therapeutic	—	—	—	—	—	—	—
	—	—	—	—	—	—	—
	—	—	—	—	—	—	—
Bile acids, total (S) [As chenodeoxycholic acid]	Trace–3.3	mg/mL	2.547	Trace–8.4	mmol/L	X.X	0.2 mmol/L
Cholic acid	Trace–1.0	mg/mL	2.448	Trace–2.4	mmol/L	X.X	0.2 mmol/L
Chenodeoxycholic acid	Trace–1.3	mg/mL	2.547	Trace–3.4	mmol/L	X.X	0.2 mmol/L
Deoxycholic acid	Trace–1.0	mg/mL	2.547	Trace–2.6	mmol/L	X.X	0.2 mmol/L
Lithocholic acid	Trace	mg/mL	2.656	Trace	mmol/L	X.X	0.2 mmol/L

(Continued)

TABLE 48 (*Continued*)
Conversion Factors for Values in Clinical Chemistry (SI Units)[1]

Component	Present Reference Intervals (Examples)	Present Unit	Conversion Factor	SI Reference Intervals	SI Unit Symbol	Significant Digits	Suggested Minimum Increment
Bile acids (Df) [after cholecystokinin stimulation]							
total as							
Chenodeoxycholic acid	14.0–58.0	mg/mL	2.547	35–148	mmol/L	XX.X	0.2 mmol/L
Cholic acid	2.4–33.0	mg/mL	2.448	6.8–81.0	mmol/L	XX.X	0.2 mmol/L
Chenodeoxycholic acid	4.0–24.0	mg/mL	2.547	10.0–61.4	mmol/L	XX.X	0.2 mmol/L
Deoxycholic acid	0.8–6.9	mg/mL	2.547	2–18	mmol/L	XX.X	0.2 mmol/L
Lithocholic acid	0.3–0.8	mg/mL	2.656	0.8–2.0	mmol/L	XX.X	0.2 mmol/L
Bilirubin, total (S)	0.1–1.0	mg/dL	17.10	2–18	mmol/L	XX	2 mmol/L
Bilirubin, conjugated (S)	0–0.2	mg/dL	17.10	0–4	mmol/L	XX	2 mmol/L
Bromide (S), toxic							
As bromide ion	>120	mg/dL	0.1252	>15	mmol/L	XX	1 mmol/L
As sodium bromide	>150	mg/dL	0.09719	>15	mmol/L	XX	1 mmol/L
Cadmium (S)	>15	mEq/L	1.00	>15	mmol/L	XX	1 mmol/L
Calcitonin (S)	<3	mg/dL	0.08897	<0.3	mmol/L	X.X	0.1 mmol/L
Calcium (S)	<100	pg/mL	1.00	<100	ng/L	XXX	10 ng/L
Male	8.8–10.3	mg/dL	0.2495	2.20–2.58	mmol/L	X.XX	0.02 mmol/L
Female <50 years	8.8–10.0	mg/dL	0.2495	2.20–2.50	mmol/L	X.XX	0.02 mmol/L
Female >50 years	8.8–10.2	mg/dL	0.2495	2.20–2.56	mmol/L	X.XX	0.02 mmol/L
Calcium ion (S)	4.4–5.1	mEq/L	0.500	2.20–2.56	mmol/L	X.XX	0.02 mmol/L
	2.00–2.30	mEq/L	0.500	1.00–1.15	mmol/L	X.XX	0.01 mmol/L
Calcium (U), normal diet	<250	mg/24 h	0.02495	<6.2	mmol/d	X.X	0.1 mmol/d
Carbamazepine (P), therapeutic	4.0–10.0	mg/L	4.233	17–42	mmol/L	XX	1 mmol/L
Carbon dioxide content (B, P, S) [bicarbonate + CO_2]	22–28	mEq/L	1.00	22–28	mmol/L	X	1 mmol/L

Analyte	Conventional Reference Interval	Conventional Unit	Conversion Factor	SI Reference Interval	SI Unit	Significant Digits	Suggested Minimum Increment
Carbon monoxide (B) [proportion of Hb, which is COHb]	<15	%	0.01	<0.15	1	0.XX	0.01
β-carotenes (S)	50–250	mg/dL	0.01863	0.9–4.6	mmol/L	X.X	0.1 mmol/L
Catecholamines, total (U) [as norepinephrine]	<120	mg/24 h	5.911	<675	nmol/d	XXO	10 mg/d
Ceruloplasmin (S)	20–35	mg/dL	10.0	200–350	mg/L	XXO	10 mg/L
Chlordiazepoxide (P)							
Therapeutic	0.5–5.0	mg/L	3.336	2–17	mmol/L	XX	1 mmol/L
Toxic	>10.0	mg/L	3.336	>33	mmol/L	XX	1 mmol/L
Chloride (S)	95–105	mEq/L	1.00	95–105	mmol/L	XXX	1 mmol/L
Chlorimipramine (P) [includes desmethyl metabolite]	50–400	ng/mL	3.176	150–1270	nmol/L	XXO	10 nmol/L
Chlorpromazine (P)	50–300	ng/mL	3.136	150–950	nmol/L	XXO	10 nmol/L
Chlorpropamide (P), therapeutic	75–250	mg/L	3.613	270–900	mmol/L	XXO	10 nmol/L
Cholestanol (P) [as a fraction of total cholesterol]	1–3	%	0.01	0.01–0.03	1	0.XX	0.01
Cholesterol (P)							
<29 years	<200	mg/dL	0.02586	<5.20	mol/L	X.XX	0.05 mmol/L
30–39 years	<225	mg/dL	0.02586	<5.85	mmol/L	X.XX	0.05 mmol/L
40–49 years	<245	mg/dL	0.02586	<6.35	mmol/L	X.XX	0.05 mmol/L
>50 years	<265	mg/dL	0.02586	<6.85	mmol/L	X.XX	0.05 mmol/L
Cholesterol esters (P) [as a fraction of total cholesterol]	60–75	%	0.01	0.60–0.75	1	O.XX	0.01
Cholinesterase (S)	620–1370	U/L	0.01667	10.3–22.8	mkat/L	XX.X	0.1 mkat/L
Chorionic gonadotropin (P) [β-HCG]	0 if not pregnant	mIU/mL	1.00	0 if not pregnant	IU/L	XX	1 IU/L
Citrate (B) [as citric acid]	1.2–3.0	mg/dL	52.05	60–160	mmol/L	XXX	5 mmol/L
Complement, C3 (S)	70–160	mg/dL	0.01	0.7–1.6	g/L	X.X	0.1 g/L
Complement, C4 (S)	20–40	mg/dL	0.01	0.2–0.4	g/L	X.X	0.1 g/L
Copper (S)	70–140	mg/dL	0.1574	11.0–22.0	mmol/L	XX.X	0.2 mmol/L
Copper (U)	<40	mg/24 h	0.01574	<0.6	mmol/d	X.X	0.2 mmol/d
Coproporphyins (U)	<200	mg/24 h	1.527	<300	nmol/d	XXO	10 nmol/d

(Continued)

TABLE 48 (*Continued*)
Conversion Factors for Values in Clinical Chemistry (SI Units)[1]

Component	Present Reference Intervals (Examples)	Present Unit	Conversion Factor	SI Reference Intervals	SI Unit Symbol	Significant Digits	Suggested Minimum Increment
Cortisol (S)							
800 hour	4–19	mg/dL	27.59	110–520	nmol/L	XXO	10 nmol/L
1600 hour	2–15	mg/dL	27.59	50–410	nmol/L	XXO	10 nmol/L
2400 hour	5	mg/dL	7.59	140	nmol/L	XXO	10 nmol/L
Cortisol, free (U)	10–110	mg/24 h	2.759	30–300	nmol/d	XXO	10 nmol/d
Creatine (S)							
Male	0.17–0.50	mg/dL	76.25	10–40	mmol/L	XO	10 mmol/L
Female	0.35–0.93	mg/dL	76.25	30–70	mmol/L	XO	10 mmol/L
Creatine (U)							
Male	0–40	mg/24 h	7.625	0–300	mmol/d	XXO	10 mmol/d
Female	0–80	mg/24 h	7.625	0–600	mmol/d	XXO	10 mmol/d
Creatine kinase [CK] (S)	0–130	U/L	0.01667	0–2.16	mkat/L	X.XX	0.01 mkat/L
MB fraction	>5 in myocardial infarction	%	0.01	>0.05	1	O.XX	0.01
Creatinine (S)	0.6–1.2	mg/dL	88.40	50–110	mmol/L	XXO	10 mmol/L
Creatinine (U)	Variable	g/24 h	8.840	Variable	mmol/d	XX.X	0.1 mmol/d
Creatinine clearance (S, U)	75–125	mL/min	0.01667	1.24–2.08	mL/s (where A is the body surface area in square meters [m^2])	X.XX	0.02 mL/s
Cyanide (B)—lethal	>0.10	mg/dL	384.3	>40	mmol/L	XXX	5 mmol/L
Cyanocobalamin (S) [vitamin B_{12}]	100–200	pg/mL	0.7378	150–750	pmol/L	XXO	10 pmol/L
cyclic AMP (S)	2.6–6.6	mg/L	3.038	8–20	nmol/L	XXX	1 nmol/L
Cyclic AMP (U)							

Total urinary	2.9–5.6	mmol/g creatinine	113.1	330–630	nmol/mmol creatinine	XXO	10 nmol/mmol creatinine
Renal tubular	<2.5	mmol/g creatinine	113.1	<280	nmol/mmol creatinine	XXO	10 nmol/mmol creatinine
Cyclic GMP (S)	0.6–3.5	mg/L	2.897	1.7–10.1	nmol/L	XX.X	0.1 nmol/L
Cyclic GMP (U)	0.3–1.8	mmol/g creatinine	113.1	30–200	nmol/mmol creatinine	XXO	10 nmol/mmol creatinine
Cystine (U)	10–100	mg/24 h	4.161	40–420	mmol/d	XXO	10 mmol/d
Dehydroepiandrosterone [DHEA] (P, S)							
1–4 years	0.2–0.4	mg/L	3.467	0.6–1.4	nmol/L	XX.X	0.2 nmol/L
4–8 years	0.1–1.9	mg/L	3.467	0.4–6.6	nmol/L	XX.X	0.2 nmol/L
8–10 years	0.2–2.9	mg/L	3.467	0.6–10.0	nmol/L	XX.X	0.2 nmol/L
10–12 years	0.5–9.2	mg/L	3.467	1.8–31.8	nmol/L	XX.X	0.2 nmol/L
12–14 years	0.9–20.0	mg/L	3.467	3.2–69.4	nmol/L	XX.X	0.2 nmol/L
14–16 years	2.5–20.0	mg/L	3.467	8.6–69.4	nmol/L	XX.X	0.2 nmol/L
Premenopausal female	2.0–15.0	mg/L	3.467	7.0–52.0	nmol/L	XX.X	0.2 nmol/L
Male	0.8–10.0	mg/L	3.467	2.8–34.6	nmol/L	XX.X	0.2 nmol/L
Dehydroepiandrosterone (U)	See Steroids	Fractionation	—	—	—	—	—
Dehydroepiandrosterone sulfate [DHEA-S] (P, S)							
Newborn	1670–3640	ng/mL	0.002714	4.5–9.9	mmol/L	XX.X	mmol/L
Prepubertal children	100–600	ng/mL	0.002714	0.3–1.6	mmol/L	XX.X	mmol/L
Male	2000–3500	ng/mL	0.002714	5.4–9.1	mmol/L	XX.X	mmol/L
Female (premenopausal)	820–3380	ng/mL	0.002714	2.2–9.2	mmol/L	XX.X	mmol/L
Female (postmenopausal)	110–610	ng/mL	0.002714	0.3–1.7	mmol/L	XX.X	mmol/L
Pregnancy [term]	0–1170	ng/mL	0.002714	0.6–3.2	mmol/L	XX.X	mmol/L
11-Deoxycortisol (S)	0–2	mg/dL	28.86	0–60	nmol/L	XXO	10 nmol/L
Desipramine (P), therapeutic	50–200	ng/mL	3.754	170–700	nmol/L	XXO	10 nmol/L
Diazepam (P)							
Therapeutic	0.10–0.25	mg/L	3512	350–900	nmol/L	XXO	10 nmol/L
Toxic	>1.0	mg/L	3512	>3510	nmol/L	XXO	10 nmol/L
Dicoumarol (P), therapeutic	8–30	mg/L	2.974	25–90	mmol/L	XX	5 mmol/L

(*Continued*)

TABLE 48 (Continued)
Conversion Factors for Values in Clinical Chemistry (SI Units)[1]

Component	Present Reference Intervals (Examples)	Present Unit	Conversion Factor	SI Reference Intervals	SI Unit Symbol	Significant Digits	Suggested Minimum Increment
Digoxin (P)							
Therapeutic	0.5–2.2	ng/mL	1.281	0.6–2.8	nmol/L	X.X	0.1 nmol/L
Toxic	>2.5	ng/mL	1.281	>3.2	nmol/L	X.X	0.1 nmol/L
Dimethadione (P), therapeutic	<1.00	g/L	7.745	<7.7	mmol/L	X.X	0.1 mmol/L
Disopyramide (P), therapeutic	2.0–6.0	mg/L	2.946	6–18	mmol/L	XX	1 mmol/L
Doxepin (P), therapeutic	50–200	n/mL	3.579	180–720	nmol/L	XO	10 nmol/L
Electrophoresis, protein (S)							
Albumin	60–65	%	0.01	0.60–0.65	1	O.XX	0.01
α1-Globulin	1.7–5.0	%	0.01	0.02–0.05	1	O.XX	0.01
α2-Globulin	6.7–12.5	%	0.01	0.07–0.13	1	O.XX	0.01
β-Globulin	8.3–16.3	%	0.01	0.08–0.16	1	O.XX	0.01
γ-Globulin	10.7–20.0	%	0.01	0.11–0.20	1	O.XX	0.01
Albumin	3.6–5.2	g/dL	10.0	36–52	g/L	XX	1 g/L
α1-Globulin	0.1–0.4	g/dL	10.0	1–4	g/L	XX	1 g/L
α2-Globulin	0.4–1.0	g/dL	10.0	4–10	g/L	XX	1 g/L
β-Globulin	0.5–1.2	g/dL	10.0	5–12	g/L	XX	1 g/L
γ-Globulin	0.6–1.6	g/dL	10.0	6–16	g/L	XX	1 g/L
Epinephrine (P)	31–95 (at rest for 15 min)	pg/mL	5.458	170–520	pmol/L	XXO	10 pmol/L
Epinephrine (U)	<10	mg/24 h	5.458	<55	nmol/d	XX	5 nmol/L
Estradiol (S) male >18 years	15–40	pg/mL	3.671	55–150	pmol/L	XX	1 pmol/L
Estriol (U) [nonpregnant]							
Onset of menstruation	4–25	mg/24 h	3.468	15–85	nmol/d	XXX	5 nmol/d
Ovulation peak	28–99	mg/24 h	3.468	95–345	nmol/d	XXX	5 nmol/d
Luteal peak	22–105	mg/24 h	3.468	75–365	nmol/d	XXX	5 nmol/d
Menopausal woman	1.4–19.6	mg/24 h	3.468	5–70	nmol/d	XXX	5 nmol/d
Male	5–18	mg/24 h	3.468	15–60	nmol/d	XXX	5 nmol/d

Estrogen (S) [as estradiol]							
Female	20–300	pg/mL	3.671	70–1100	pmol/L	XXXO	10 pmol/L
Peak production	200–800	pg/mL	3.671	750–2900	pmol/L	XXXO	10 pmol/L
Male	<50	pg/mL	3.671	<180	pmol/L	XXO	10 pmol/L
Estrogen, placental (U) [as estriol]	Depends on period of gestation	mg/24 h	3.468	Depends on period of gestation	mmol/d	XXX	1 mmol/d
Estrogen receptors (T), negative	0–3	fmol estradiol bound/mg cytosol protein	1.00	0–3	fmol estradiol/mg cytosol protein	XXX	1 fmol/mg protein
Doubtful	4–10	fmol estradiol bound/mg cytosol protein	1.00	4–10	fmol estradiol/mg cytosol protein	XXX	1 fmol/mg protein
Positive	>10	fmol estradiol bound/mg cytosol protein	1.00	>10	fmol estradiol/mg cytosol protein	XXX	1 fmol/mg protein
Estrone (P, S)							
Female, 1–10 days of cycle	43–180	pg/mL	3.699	160–665	pmol/L	XXX	5 pmol/L
Female, 11–20 days of cycle	75–196	pg/mL	3.699	275–725	pmol/L	XXX	5 pmol/L
Female, 20–39 days of cycle	131–201	pg/mL	3.699	485–745	pmol/L	XXX	5 pmol/L
Male	29–75	pg/mL	3.699	105–275	pmol/L	XXX	5 pmol/L
Estrone (U) female	2–25	mg/24 h	3.699	5–90	nmol/d	XXX	5 nmol/d
Ethanol (P)							
Legal limit [driving]	<80	mg/dL	0.2171	<17	mmol/L	XX	1 mmol/L
Toxic	>100	mg/dL	0.2171	>22	mmol/L	XX	1 mmol/L
Ethchlorvynol (P), toxic	>40	mg/L	6.915	>280	mmol/L	XXO	10 mmol/L
Ethosuximide (P), therapeutic	40–110	mg/L	7.084	280–780	mmol/L	XXO	10 mmol/L
Ethylene glycol (P), toxic	>30	mg/dL	0.1611	>5	mmol/L	XX	1 mmol/L
Fat (F) [as stearic acid]	2.0–6.0	g/24 h	3.515	7–21	mmol/d	XXX	1 mmol/d
Fatty acids, nonesterified (P)	8–20	mg/dL	10.00	80–200	mg/L	XXO	10 mg/L
Ferritin (S)	18–300	ng/mL	1.00	18–300	mg/L	XXO	10 mg/L

(Continued)

TABLE 48 (Continued)
Conversion Factors for Values in Clinical Chemistry (SI Units)[1]

Component	Present Reference Intervals (Examples)	Present Unit	Conversion Factor	SI Reference Intervals	SI Unit Symbol	Significant Digits	Suggested Minimum Increment
Fibrinogen (P)	200–400	mg/dL	0.01	2.0–4.0	g/L	X.X	0.1 g/L
Fluoride (U)	<1.0	mg/24 h	52.63	<50	mmol/d	XXO	10 mmol/d
Folate (S) [as pteroylglutamic acid]	2–10	ng/mL	2.266	4–22	nmol/L	XX	2 nmol/L
Folate (Erc)	140–960	mg/dl	22.66		mg/dl		2 nmol/l
		ng/mL	2.266	550–2200	nmol/L	XXO	10 nmol/L
Follicle-stimulating hormone [FSH] (P)							
Female	2.0–15.0	mIU/mL	1.00	2–15	IU/L	XX	1 IU/L
Peak production	20–50	mIU/mL	1.00	20–50	IU/L	XX	1 IU/L
Male	1.0–10.0	mIU/mL	1.00	1–10	IU/L	XX	1 IU/L
Follicle-stimulating hormone [FSH] (U)							
Follicular phase	2–15	IU/24 h	1.00	2–15	IU/d	XXX	1 IU/d
Midcycle	8–40	IU/24 h	1.00	8–40	IU/d	XXX	1 IU/d
Luteal phase	2–10	IU/24 h	1.00	2–10	IU/d	XXX	1 IU/d
Menopausal women	35–100	IU/24 h	1.00	35–100	IU/d	XXX	1 IU/d
Male	2–15	IU/24 h	1.00	2–15	IU/d	XXX	1 IU/d
Fructose (P)	<10	mg/dL	0.05551	<0.6	mmol/L	X.XX	0.1 mmol/L
Galactose (P) [children]	<20	mg/dL	0.05551	<1.1	mmol/L	X.XX	0.1 mmol/L
Gases							
pO$_2$	75–105	mm Hg (=torr)	0.1333	10.0–14.0	kPa	XX.X	0.1 kPa
pCO$_2$	33–44	mm Hg (=torr)	0.1333	4.4–5.9	kPa	X.X	0.1 kPa
γ-glutamyltransferase [GGT] (S)	0–30	U/L	0.01667	0–0.50	mkat/L	X.XX	0.01 mkat/L
Gastrin (S)	0–180	pg/mL	1.00	0–180	ng/L	XXO	10 ng/L
Globulins (S) [see immunoglobulins]	—	—	—	—	—	—	—

Analyte	Conventional Reference Interval	Conventional Unit	Conversion Factor	SI Reference Interval	SI Unit	Significant Digits	Suggested Minimum Increment
Glucagon (S)	50–100	pg/mL	1.00	50–100	ng/L	XXO	10 ng/L
Glucose (P) fasting	70–110	mg/dL	0.05551	3.9–6.1	mmol/L	XX.X	0.1 mmol/L
Glucose (Sf)	50–80	mg/dL	0.05551	2.8–4.4	mmol/L	XX.X	0.1 mmol/L
Glutethimide (P)							
Therapeutic	<10	mg/L	4.603	<46	mmol/L	XX	1 mmol/L
Toxic	>20	mg/L	4.603	>92	mmol/L	XX	1 mmol/L
Glycerol, free (S)	<1.5	mg/dL	0.1086	<0.16	mmol/L	X.XX	0.01 mmol/L
Gold (S), therapeutic	300–800	mg/dL	0.05077	15.0–40.0	mmol/L	XX.X	0.1 mmol/L
Gold (U)	<500	mg/24 h	0.005077	<2.5	mmol/d	X.X	0.1 mmol/d
Palmitic acid (Amf)	Depends on gestation	mmol/L	1000	Depends on gestation	mmol/L	XXX	5 mmol/L
Pentobarbital (P)	20–40	mg/L	4.419	90–170	mmol/L	XX	5 mmol/L
Phenobarbital (P), therapeutic	2–5	mg/L	43.06	85–215	mmol/L	XXX	5 mmol/L
phensuximide (P)	4–8	mg/L	5.285	20–40	mmol/L	XX	5 mmol/L
phenylbutazone (P), therapeutic	<100	mg/L	3.243	<320	mmol/L	XXO	10 mmol/L
Phenytoin (P)							
Therapeutic	10–20	mg/L	3.964	40–80	mmol/L	XX	5 mmol/L
Toxic	>30	mg/L	3.964	>12	mmol/L	XX	5 mmol/L
Phosphate (S) [as phosphorus, inorganic]	2.5–5.0	mg/dL	0.3229	0.80–1.60	mmol/L	X.XX	0.05 mmol/L
Phosphate (U) [as phosphorus, inorganic]	Diet dependent	g/24 h	32.29	Diet dependent	mmol/d	XXX	1 mmol/d
Phospholipid phosphorus, total (P)	5–12	mg/dL	0.3229	1.60–3.90	mmol/L	X.XX	0.05 mmol/L
Phospholipid phosphorus, total (Erc)	1.2–12.0	mg/dL	0.3229	0.40–3.90	mmol/L	X.XX	0.05 mmol/L
Phospholipids (P) substance fraction of total phospholipid							
Phosphatidylcholine	65–70	%/total	0.01	0.65–0.70	1	O.XX	0.01
Phosphatidylethanolamine	4–5	%/total	0.01	0.04–0.05	1	O.XX	0.01
Sphingomyelin	15–20	%/total	0.01	0.15–0.20	1	O.XX	0.01
Lysophosphatidylcholine	3–5	%/total	0.01	0.03–0.05	1	O.XX	0.01

(Continued)

TABLE 48 (*Continued*)
Conversion Factors for Values in Clinical Chemistry (SI Units)[1]

Component	Present Reference Intervals (Examples)	Present Unit	Conversion Factor	SI Reference Intervals	SI Unit Symbol	Significant Digits	Suggested Minimum Increment
Phospholipids (Erc) substance fraction of total phospholipid							
Phosphatidylcholine	28–33	%/total	0.01	0.28–0.33	1	O.XX	0.01
Phosphatidylethanolamine	24–31	%/total	0.01	0.24–0.31	1	O.XX	0.01
Sphingomyelin	22–29	%/total	0.01	0.22–0.29	1	O.XX	0.01
Phosphatidylserine + phosphatidylinositol	12–20	%/total	0.01	0.12–0.20	1	O.XX	0.01
Lysophosphatidylcholine	1–2	%/total	0.01	0.01–0.02	1	O.XX	0.01
Phytanic acid (P)	Trace–0.3	mg/dL	32.00	<10	mmol/L	XX	5 mmol/L
[Human] placental lactogen [HPL] (SO)	>4.0 after 30 wk gestation	mg/mL	46.30	>180	nmol/L	XXO	10 nmol/L
Porphobilinogen (U)	0–2	mg/24 h	4.420	0–9	mmol/d	X.X	0.5 mmol/d
Porphyrins							
Coproporphyrin (U)	45–180	mg/24 h	1.527	68–276	nmol/d	XXX	2 nmol/d
Protoporphyrin (Erc)	15–50	mg/dL	0.0177	0.28–0.90	mmol/L	X.XX	0.02 mmol/L
Uroporphyrin (U)	5–20	mg/24 h	1.204	6–24	nmol/d	XX	2 nmol/d
Uroporphyrinogen							
Synthetase (Erc)	22–42	mmol/mL/h	0.2778	6.0–11.8	mmol/(l.s)	X.X	0.2 mmol/(l.s)
Potassium ion (S)	3.5–5.0	mEq/L	1.00	3.5–5.0	mmol/L	X.X	0.1 mmol/L
		mg/dL	0.2558		mmol/L	X.X	0.1 mmol/L
Potassium ion (U) [diet dependent]	25–100	mEq/24 h	1.00	25–100	mmol/d	XX	1 mmol/d

	Conventional Reference Interval	Conventional Unit	Factor	SI Reference Interval	SI Unit	Significant Digits	Suggested Minimum Increment
Pregnaediol (U)							
Normal	1–6	mg/24 h	3.120	3.0–18.5	mmol/d	XX.X	0.5 mmol/d
Pregnancy	Depends on gestation						
Pregnanetriol (U)	0.5–2.0	mg/24 h	2.972	1.5–6.0	mmol/d	XX.X	0.5 mmol/d
Primidone (P)							
Therapeutic	6–10	mg/L	4.582	25–46	mmol/L	XX	1 mmol/L
Toxic	>10	mg/L	4.582	>46	mmol/L	XX	1 mmol/L
Procainamide (P)							
Therapeutic	4–8	mg/L	4.249	17–34	mmol/L	XX	1 mmol/L
Toxic	>12.0	mg/L	4.249	>50	mmol/L	XX	1 mmol/L
N-acetyl procainamide (P)							
Therapeutic	4–8	mg/L	3.606	14–29	mmol/L	XX	1 mmol/L
Progesterone (P)							
Follicular phase	<2	ng/mL	3.180	<6	nmol/L	XX	2 nmol/L
Luteal phase	2–20	ng/mL	3.180	6–64	nmol/L	XX	2 nmol/L
Progesterone receptors (T)							
Negative	0–3	fmol progesterone bound/mg cytosol protein	1.00	0–3	fmol progesterone bound/mg cytosol protein	XX	1 fmol/mg protein
Doubtful	4–10	fmol progesterone bound/mg cytosol protein	1.00	4–10	fmol progesterone bound/mg cytosol protein	XX	1 fmol/mg protein
Positive	>10	fmol progesterone bound/mg cytosol protein	1.00	>10	fmol progesterone bound/mg cytosol protein	XX	1 fmol/mg protein
Prolactin (P)	<20	ng/mL	1.00	<20	mg/L	XX	1 mg/L
Propoxyphene (P), toxic	>2.0	mg/L	2.946	>5.9	mmol/L	X.X	0.1 mmol/L
Propranolol (P) [Inderal], therapeutic	50–200	ng/mL	3.856	190–770	nmol/L	XXO	10 nmol/L
Protein, total (S)	6.0–8.0	g/dL	10.0	60–80	g/L	XX	1 g/L
Protein, total (Sf)	<40	mg/dL	0.01	<0.40	g/L	X.XX	0.1 g/L
Protein, total (U)	<150	mg/24 h	0.001	<0.15	g/d	X.XX	0.01 g/d
Protriptyline (P)	100–300	ng/mL	3.797	380–1140	nmol/L	XXO	10 nmol/L

(Continued)

TABLE 48 (*Continued*)
Conversion Factors for Values in Clinical Chemistry (SI Units)[1]

Component	Present Reference Intervals (Examples)	Present Unit	Conversion Factor	SI Reference Intervals	SI Unit Symbol	Significant Digits	Suggested Minimum Increment
Pyruvate (B) [as pyruvic acid]	0.30–0.90	mg/dL	113.6	35–100	mmol/L	X.XX	1 mmol/L
Quinidine (P)							
Therapeutic	1.5–3.0	mg/L	3.082	4.6–9.2	mmol/L	X.X	0.1 mmol/L
Toxic	>6.0	mg/L	3.082	>18.5	mmol/L	X.X	0.1 mmol/L
Renin (P) normal sodium diet	1.1–4.1	ng/mL/h	0.2778	0.30–1.14	ng/(l.s)	X.XX	0.2 ng/(l.s)
Restricted sodium diet	6.2–12.4	ng/mL/h	0.2778	1.72–3.44	ng/(l.s)	X.XX	0.02 ng/(l.s)
Salicylate (S) [salicylic acid], toxic	>20	mg/dL	0.07240	>1.45	mmol/L	X.XX	0.05 mmol/L
Serotonin (B) [5-hydroxytryptamine]	8–21	mg/dL	0.05675	0.45–1.20	mmol/L	X.XX	0.05 mmol/L
Sodium ion (S)	135–147	mEq/L	1.00	135–147	mmol/L	XXX	1 mmol/L
Sodium ion (U)	Diet dependent	mEq/24 h	1.00	Diet dependent	mmol/d	XXX	2 mmol/d
Steroids 17-hydroxy-corticosteroids (U) [as cortisol]							
Female	2.0–8.0	mg/24 h	2.759	5–25	mmol/d	XX	1 mmol/d
Male	3–10	mg/24 h	2.759	10–30	mmol/d	XX	1 mmol/d
17-Ketogenic steroids (U) [as dehydroepiandrosterone]							
Female	7–12	mg/24 h	3.467	25–40	mmol/d	XX	1 mmol/d
Male	9–17	mg/24 h	3.467	30–60	mmol/d	XX	1 mmol/d
17-Ketosteroids (U) [as dehydroepiandrosterone]							
Female	6–17	mg/24 h	3.467	20–60	mmol/d	XX	1 mmol/d
Male	6–20	mg/24 h	3.467	20–70	mmol/d	XX	1 mmol/d
Ketosteroid fractions (U) androsterone							
Female	0.5–2.0	mg/24 h	3.443	1–10	mmol/d	XX	1 mmol/d
Male	2.0–5.0	mg/24 h	3.443	7–17	mmol/d	XX	1 mmol/d

Dehydroepiandrosterone							
Female	0.2–1.8	mg/24 h	3.467	1–6	mmol/d	XX	1 mmol/d
Male	0.2–2.0	mg/24 h	3.467	1–7	mmol/d	XX	1 mmol/d
Etiocholanolone							
Female	0.8–4.0	mg/24 h	3.443	2–14	mmol/d	XX	1 mmol/d
Male	1.4–5.0	mg/24 h	3.443	4–17	mmol/d	XX	1 mmol/d
Sulfonamides (B) [as sulfanilamide]							
Therapeutic	10–15	mg/dL	58.07	580–870	mmol/L	XXO	10 mmol/L
testosterone (P)							
Female	0.6	ng/mL	3.467	2.0	nmol/L	XX.X	0.5 nmol/L
Male	4.6–8.0	ng/mL	3.467	14–28	nmol/L	XX.X	0.5 nmol/L
Theophylline (P), therapeutic	10–20	mg/L	5.550	55–110	mmol/L	XX	1 mmol/L
Thiocyanate (P) (nitroprusside toxicity)	10.0	mg/dL	0.1722	1.7	mmol/L	X.XX	0.1 mmol/L
Thiopental (P)	individual	mg/L	4.126	individual	mmol/L	XX	5 mmol/L
Thyroid tests							
Thyroid-stimulating hormone [TSH] (S)	2–11	mU/mL	1.00	2–11	mU/L	XX	1 mU/L
Thyroxine [T4] (S)	4–11	mg/dL	12.87	51–142	nmol/L	XXX	1 nmol/L
Thyroxine-binding globulin [TGB] (S) [as thyroxine]	12–28	mg/dL	12.87	150–360	nmol/L	XXO	1 nmol/L
Thyroxine, free (S)	0.8–2.8	ng/dL	12.87	10–36	pmol/L	XX	1 pmol/L
Triiodothyronine [T3] (S)	75–220	ng/dL	0.01536	1.2–3.4	nmol/L	X.X	0.1 nmol/L
T3 uptake (S)	25–35	%	0.01	0.25–0.35	1	O.XX	0.01
Tolbuamide (P), therapeutic	50–120	mg/L	3.699	180–450	mmol/L	XXO	10 mmol/L
Transferrin (S)	170–370	mg/dL	0.01	1.70–3.70	g/L	X.XX	0.01 g/L
Triglycerides (P) [as triolein]	<160	mg/dL	0.01129	<1.80	mmol/L	X.XX	0.02 mmol/L
Trimethadione (P), therapeutic	<50	mg/L	6.986	<350	mmol/L	XXO	10 mmol/L
Trimipramine (P), therapeutic	50–200	ng/mL	3.397	170–680	nmol/L	XXO	10 nmol/L
Urate (S) [as uric acid]	2–7	mg/dL	59.48	120–420	nmol/L	XXO	10 nmol/L
Urate (U) [as uric acid]	Diet dependent	g/24 h	5.948	Diet dependent	mmol/d	XX	1 mmol/d
Urea nitrogen (S)	8–18	mg/dL	0.3570	3.0–6.5	mmol/L UREA	X.X	0.5 mmol/L
Urea nitrogen (U)	2–20 diet dependent	g/24 h	35.700	450–700	mmol/d UREA	XXO	10 mol/d
Urobilinogen (U)	0–4	mg/24 h	1.693	0.0–6.8	mmol/d	X.X	0.1 mmol/d

(Continued)

TABLE 48 (Continued)
Conversion Factors for Values in Clinical Chemistry (SI Units)[1]

Component	Present Reference Intervals (Examples)	Present Unit	Conversion Factor	SI Reference Intervals	SI Unit Symbol	Significant Digits	Suggested Minimum Increment
Valproic acid (P), therapeutic	50–100	mg/L	6.934	350–700	mmol/L	XO	10 mmol/L
Vanillylmandelic acid [VMA], urine	<6.8	mg/24 h	5.046	<35	mmol/d	XX	1 mmol/d
Vitamin A [retinol] (P,S)	10–50	mg/dL	0.03491	0.35–1.75	mmol/L	X.XX	0.05 mmol/L
Vitamin B$_1$ [thiamine hydrochloride] (U)	60–500	mg/24 h	0.002965	0.18–1.48	mmol/d	ZX.XX	0.01 mmol/d
Vitamin B$_2$ [riboflavin] (S)	2.6–3.7	mg/dL	26.57	70–100	nmol/L	XXX	5 nmol/L
Vitamin B$_6$ [pyridoxal] (B)	20–90	ng/mL	5.982	120–540	nmol/L	XXX	5 nmol/L
Vitamin B$_{12}$ (P,S) [cyanocobalamin]	200–1000	pg/mL	0.7378	150–750	pmol/L	XO	10 pmol/L
Vitamin C [see ascorbate] (B,P,S)	—	—	—	—	—	—	—
Vitamin D$_3$ [cholecalciferol] (P)	24–40	mg/mL	2.599	60–105	nmol/L	XXX	5 nmol/L
25-OH-cholecalciferol	18–36	ng/mL	0.496	45–90	nmol/L	XXX	5 nmol/L
Vitamin E [α-tocopherol] (P,S)	0.78–1.25	mg/dL	23.22	18–29	mmol/L	XX	1 mmol/L
Warfarin (P), therapeutic	1–3	mg/L	3.243	3.3–9.8	mmol/L	XX.X	0.1 mmol/L
Xanthine (U), hypoxanthine	5–30	mg/24 hmg/24 h	6.574 7.347	30–200	mmol/d mmol/d	XXO XXO	10 mmol/d 10 mmol/d
D-xylose (B) [25 g dose]	30–40 (30–60 minutes)	mg/dL	0.06661	0–2.7 (30–60 minutes)	mmol/L	X.X	0.1 mmol/L
D-xylose excretion (U) [25 g dose]	21–31	%	0.01	0.21–0.31 (excreted in 5 h)	1	0.XX	0.01
Zinc (S)	75–120	mg/dL	0.1530	11.5–18.5	mmol/L	XX.X	0.1 mmol/L
Zinc (U)	150–1200	mg/24 h	0.01530	2.3–18.3	mmol/d	XX.X	0.1 mmol/d

Source: From Young, D. S. 1987. *Ann Int Med* 106:20.

[1] Abbreviations used (S), serum; (P), plasma; (B) whole blood; (U) urine; (Erc), erythrocyte; (Amf) amniotic fluid; (Df) digesta fraction; (Sf), serum fraction; (T) cytosol protein; (F) fat; (SO) placental fluid.

SIBUTRAMINE HYDROCHLORIDE

An inhibitor of the reuptake of dopamine and norepinephrine reuptake; can be used as an antiobesity drug. Trade name: Meridia.

SICKLE-CELL ANEMIA

A genetic disease caused by a mutation in the code for one of the subunits of hemoglobin. Because of this mutation, the amino acid sequence of the protein is aberrant, which in turn affects its quatenary structure and its ability to carry oxygen. The name comes from the change in shape of the red blood cell. Instead of being round, it is sickle shaped.

SIDEROSIS (HEMOSIDEROSIS)

Also called hemochromatosis. A nutritional disorder due to a low protein intake together with a high iron intake. The iron is absorbed and accumulates in the liver causing damage.

SIGNAL

The end product observed when a specific sequence of DNA or RNA is detected by autoradiography or by some other method. Hybridization with complimentary radioactive polynucleotide (e.g., by southern or northern blotting) is commonly used to generate the signal. This term also applies to the transmission of intracellular reactions as in signal transduction or signal transmission that occurs when a hormone is bound to its cognate receptor on the exterior surface of the cell.

SIGNAL TRANSDUCTION

The process by which a receptor interacts with a ligand at the surface of the cell and then transmits a signal to trigger a series of reactions within that cell.

SIMPLE SIMILAR ACTION

Combination of substances with common sites of main action and no interaction between the components. The action can be additive. An example is the combined toxic action of mixtures of polychlorinated dibenzodioxins, polychlorinated dibenzofurans, and polychlorinated biphenyls (particularly congeners with planar structures) occurring in, for example, mother's milk. The effects of these substances have been shown to be additive. Usually, the toxicity of such mixtures is expressed in terms of the concentration of 2,3,7,8-tetrachlorodibenzo-p-dioxin (TCDD) by adding the so-called TCDD toxicity equivalent concentrations of the individual components—concentration addition.

SIMPLESSE

A fat substitute derived from egg or milk proteins. It cannot be used in cooked or baked products because it breaks down easily.

SIMVASTATIN

A member of the statin group of drugs that act as HMGCoA reductase inhibitors, thus reducing the endogenous synthesis of cholesterol. Trade name: Zocor.

SINES

Short interspersed repeat sequences.

SKINFOLD THICKNESS

A double fold of skin and underlying tissue that can be used as a measure of the subcutaneous fat store. The general formulas for calculating body fat from these measurements are shown in Table 18.

SMALL FOR GESTATIONAL AGE BABY

A baby whose birth weight is small even though the baby has not been born prematurely.

SNP, SNP$_3$

Single nucleotide polymorphism; variation in the base sequence of a given gene.

SNRNA

Small nuclear RNA. This family of RNAs is best known for its role in splicing and other RNA processing reactions.

SOAP NOTE

Acronym for subjective data, objective information, assessment, and plan; a method of organizing information to be written in a medical record. Subjective data provides pertinent information obtained from the client, objective information includes relevant verifiable facts, assessment is the interpretation of the problems and related facts, and the plan indicates what actions are to be taken to resolve the identified problems.

SOD

Superoxide dismutase. An enzyme important to the suppression of free radicals. See Oxidation.

SODIUM (N$_A$$^+$)

An essential cation in the extracellular fluids. This ion is essential for muscle contraction, active transport of solutes, and the maintenance of fluid balance.

SODIUM BENZOATE

An additive involved in idiosyncratic food intolerance reactions. This preservative is used in foods such as lemonades, margarine, jam, ice cream, fish, sausages, and dressings. Sometimes it is also added to flavorings. Benzoates can elicit asthmatic attacks in asthma patients. Furthermore, they may play a role in patients with urticaria.

SODIUM BICARBONATE

An alkalizer both systemically and in the urinary tract. Trade names: Bell/ans, Citrocarbonate, Soda Mint.

SODIUM PUMP

The energy requiring process by which a high potassium concentration is maintained inside cells and a high sodium level is maintained outside the cells. The energy is provided by ATP.

SODIUM-DEPENDENT ACTIVE TRANSPORT

See Active Transport.

SOFT DIET

Therapeutic diet characterized by soft foods and liquids; the diet is typically reduced in fiber and residue.

SOFT TISSUE

Tissues and organs that are not mineralized.

SOLUTE LOAD

The amount of solutes on one side of a membrane. Usually refers to the filtering function of the convoluted tubule in the kidney.

SOMATOSTATIN

Hormone released by D cells of pancreatic islets and other organs (intestine, brain, etc.); serves as an appetite suppressant.

SOMOGYI EFFECT

Rebound hyperglycemia indicated by change from hypoglycemia to hyperglycemia within one to two hours.

SORBIC ACID

A food additive possessing antimicrobial activity.

SORBITOL

A sugar alcohol derived from the six-carbon sugar sorbose; provides less energy (~2 kcal/g) than glucose.

SORGHUM

A cereal grain; used in both human and animal foods.

SOUTHERN BLOTTING

A method for transferring DNA from an agarose gel to a nitrocellulose filter on which DNA can be detected by a suitable probe.

SOYBEAN HYDROLYSATE

A protein mixture isolated from soybeans and subjected to hydrolysis to improve its digestibility.

SPECIAL COHORTS

See Follow-Up Studies.

SPECIFIC DYNAMIC ACTION

Heat production resulting from the metabolism of food. It is estimated to be about 10% of energy value of the food consumed; also known as thermic effect of food or diet-induced thermogenesis.

SPECIFIC GRAVITY

Ratio of the weight of the body to the weight of an equal volume of water.

SPECIFIC-HEAT

The heat-absorbing capacity of a substance compared to water.

SPERMATOGENESIS

The production of sperm by the testes in the male.

SPERMATOZOA

Reproductive cell of the male.

SPHINCTER

A muscle, surrounding a body opening or vessel, that can contract and close that opening.

SPHINGOMYELIN

A group of phospholipids found in the myelin sheath covering the nerves.

SPHINGOSINE

An alcohol that forms the backbone of sphingomyelin.

SPINA BIFIDA

Congenital defect in the structure of the spinal column characterized by an open area around the nerve trunk leaving it unprotected and subject to infection or injury.

SPIRONOLACTONE

A potassium-sparing diuretic that is an antihypertensive drug. Trade names: Aldactone, Novo-Spiroton.

SPLICEOSOME

A 50S to 60S particle containing snRNPs and pre-mRNA; it carries out the splicing reactions whereby a pre-mRNA is converted to a mature RNA.

SPLICING

The removal of introns from RNA accompanied by the joining of exons to produce a mature transcript.

SPORTS ANEMIA

A decrease in red cell volume from excessive red cell breakdown due to excessive physical activity.

SPRUE

Malabsorption syndrome caused by either sensitivity to gluten or fat intolerance.

SQUELCHING

The inhibition of the activity of a transcription factor by another transcription factor that competes with it for binding to DNA.

STABLE ISOTOPE

An isotope that is nonradioactive. K_{40} is a stable isotope.

STACHYOSE

A nondigestible carbohydrate found in dried beans and peas.

STANDARD OF IDENTITY

A term used by the U.S. Food and Drug Administration to indicate that standard ingredients in standard amounts are used to make a food product. Deviations from these standards must be so labeled.

STARCH

A glucose polymer having α-1,4 and α-1,6 linkages. (See Carbohydrates.)

STARVATION

Involuntary absence of feeding.

STASIS

A slowing or stoppage of normal fluid flow.

STEATORRHEA

Excess fat in feces.

STEATOSIS

Fatty degenerative change in tissues.

STEER

A castrated male bovine.

STEM CELL

A cell from which all other cell types can be generated given the appropriate environment and signaling factors.

STENOSIS

Narrowing of an opening.

STEREOISOMER

Isomers having the same atoms but whose structure has one or two slight differences in the position of these atoms. (See Carbohydrate, Protein.)

STERIGMATOCYSTIN

A carcinogenic mycotoxin that is primarily produced by *Aspergillus versicolor* and *Aspergillus nidulans*, although other molds (e.g., *Aspergillus flavus*, *Aspergillus rugulosus*, *Bipolaris* spp., *Penicillium luteum*) are also capable of producing sterigmatocystin. Sterigmatocystin is structurally related to the aflatoxins and is equally stable. It is a potent hepatotoxin causing bile duct hyperplasia in ducklings and hyperplasia of the hepatocytes with little bile duct proliferation and liver necrosis in rats. Factors involved in fungal growth and toxin production include lactose, fat, and some fat hydrolysis products. Occurrence of sterigmatocystin has been reported in grains and the outer layer of hard cheeses when these have been colonized by *Aspergillus versicolor*.

STEROL

A four-ring structure typical of all steroid molecules.

STICKY-ENDED DNA

Complimentary single strands of DNA that protrude from opposite ends of a DNA duplex or from the ends of different duplex molecules.

STOMATITIS

Inflammation of the mucous membrane of the mouth.

STOOL

Feces.

STREPTOCOCCUS MUTANS

A food-borne pathogen.

STRESS RESPONSE

Whole body response to physiological or psychological trauma. The response is mediated by the hormones listed in Table 49.

STROKE

Blockage or rupture of blood vessel(s) supplying the brain resulting in loss of consciousness, paralysis, and other symptoms. Apoplexy is a common term for stroke.

TABLE 49
Hormones Directly Involved in the Stress Response

Hormone	Origin	Physiological Functions
ACTH	Anterior pituitary	Synthesis and release of hormones from the adrenal cortex, mainly the glucocorticoids.
Aldosterone (mineralocorticoid)	Adrenal cortex	Stimulates kidney to excrete potassium into the urine and to conserve sodium.
Epinephrine (adrenaline), norepinephrine (noradrenaline)	Adrenal medulla	Both hormones alter heart output; dilate or constrict blood vessels; elevate blood pressure; release free fatty acids into the blood; stimulate the brain to increase alertness; increase metabolic rate; cause rapid release of glucose from the liver.
Glucagon	α cells of islets of Langerhans	Mobilizes glucose from liver glycogen; increases gluconeogenesis.
Glucocorticoids (cortisone, corticosterone, and cortisol)	Adrenal cortex	Increases protein catabolism; increases gluconeogenesis.
Growth hormone	Anterior pituitary	Growth of all tissues; protein synthesis; mobilization of fats for energy while conserving glucose by preventing glucose uptake by some tissues.
Prolactin	Anterior pituitary	Growth of all tissues; protein synthesis; mobilization of fats for energy while conserving glucose by preventing glucose uptake by some tissues.
Triiodothyronine (T3), thyroxine (T4)	Thyroid	Both hormones have similar actions; however, triiodothyronine is more potent and its actions are faster. Steps up metabolic rate; increases heart performance; increases nervous system activity; stimulates protein synthesis; increases motility and secretion of gastrointestinal tract; increases absorption of glucose from the intestine.
Vasopressin (ADH)	Posterior pituitary	Acts on the kidneys to reduce urine volume and conserve body water, thus preventing body fluids from becoming too concentrated; urine becomes concentrated and urine volume decreases.

SUBCUTANEOUS FAT

The fat cell layer just beneath the skin.

SUBSTRATE

The substance upon which an enzyme works.

SUBUNIT BACTERIAL TOXINS

Compounds produced by food-borne microorganisms. To this group belong the toxins produced by *Clostridium botulinum*, which are a group of motile, gram-positive, rod-shaped, spore-forming, anaerobic bacteria that are capable of producing neurotoxins. According to the toxin they produce, there are seven types and three subtypes of *Clostridium botulinum*: type A, subtype Af (A toxin); type B (B toxin); type C, subtype Ca (C1, C2, and D toxins), subtype Cb (C2 toxin); type D (C1 and D toxins); type E (E toxin); type F (F toxin); and type G (G toxin). Based on their ability to digest proteins and break down sugars, *Clostridium botulinum* can be divided into four groups: group I, strains that are strongly proteolytic and saccharolytic (all strains of type A, several strains of types B and F); group II, strains that are nonproteolytic but strongly saccharolytic (all strains of type E, several strains of types B and F); group III, strains that are nonproteolytic except that they can digest gelatin (all strains of types C and D); and group IV, strains that are proteolytic but nonsaccharolytic (a single strain of type G). All types can deaminate and decarboxylate amino acids and desulfurize cystine to produce H_2S. Thus, all types can produce NH_3, H_2S, CO_2, and volatile amines from amino acids.

Clostridium botulinum produces an intracellular protoxin consisting of a nontoxic progenitor toxin (a hemagglutinin with a molecular weight of 500,000) and a highly toxic neurotoxin (molecular weight 150,000). The protoxin is released upon lysis of the vegetative bacterial cell. The neurotoxin is formed by proteolytic degradation of the protoxin. This proteolysis is caused by *Clostridium botulinum* proteolytic enzymes or by exogenous proteases (e.g., trypsin) when nonproteolytic strains of *Clostridium botulinum* are involved. Botulinum toxin is heat sensitive (inactivated at 80°C for 10 minutes or 100°C for a few minutes). It is acid resistant and survives the gastric passage. Botulinum toxin is an exotoxin; it is excreted by the cell, but most of it is released upon lysis of the cell after sporulation.

Botulism, caused by the ingestion of food containing the neurotoxin, is the most severe bacterial food-borne intoxication known. Humans are susceptible to types A, B, E, and F neurotoxins, whereas type A is toxic to chickens, types Ca and E to birds, types Cb and D to cattle, type Cb to sheep, types Cb and E to mink, and types A, B, Cb, and D to horses. Dogs, cats, and pigs are quite resistant to ingested toxin. The minimum lethal oral dose for man based on estimates in lethal poisoning is of the order of 1.4 ¥ 10–2 mg/kg, and doses that have caused nonfatal botulism, as judged from accidental cases, range from 0.1 to 1.0 mg. The toxin appears to be transported by way of the lymph as well as the blood. It has a direct action on the nerves, particularly the peripheral nerves, resulting in neuromuscular paralysis. Clinical symptoms of botulinum poisoning usually occur in 12–36 hours, starting with vomiting and dizziness, accompanied or followed by weakness, dryness of the mouth with difficulty in swallowing, paralysis, double vision, and respiratory distress. Death, resulting from respiratory paralysis and/or obstruction of the airways, pulmonary infection, and cardiac arrest, may occur as early as 10 hours after symptoms appear.

Factors affecting growth and toxin production by *Clostridium botulinum* include as follows:

- Type and nutrient composition of substrate (in general, complex organic media provide better support for more efficient toxin production than synthetically defined ones).
- Temperature of growth (optimum temperature: 36–37°C at pH 7.0–7.2 [types A, B, and D], 33°C at pH 7.6 [type C], 30°C at pH 7.0–7.2 [types E and F]).
- Acidity and salt concentration of substrate (in general, the required inhibitory salt concentration and pH increases and decreases, respectively, as the number of viable spores contaminating a product increases).
- Moisture activity (sufficient water activity is required).
- Oxygen concentration (*Clostridium botulinum*, being an obligate anaerobe, is inhibited by oxygen or may be directly poisoned by it).
- Presence of other microorganisms (effects: lowering of redox potential or production of growth factors; lowering or increasing of pH of medium by production or consumption of acids or acid-forming substances; production of proteolytic enzymes that destroy or activate the toxin; and production of antibiotic or antimicrobial substances).
- Other inhibitors (inhibitors of spore germination, e.g., various metals, rancidified unsaturated fatty acids, some flavonoids and spices; and inhibitors of vegetative growth, e.g., antibiotics).

Sources of *Clostridium botulinum* causing botulism include soil, mud, water, and intestinal tract of animals. At particular risk are low-acid foods that are insufficiently heated. Examples are home-canned vegetables contaminated with soil-borne *Clostridium botulinum*, meat and fish contaminated during slaughtering with *Clostridium botulinum* originating from the intestinal tract, and chilled vacuum-packed foods, which usually have had minimal heat treatment, contain no preservatives other than any naturally occurring antimicrobial substances, and are not reheated or only mildly heated prior to consumption. Preventive measures against botulism include the heating and cooking of all foods with high water activity ($a_w > 0.90$) and low acidity (pH > 4) and storage above 3°C. Additionally, sanitary and proper food preservation procedures can minimize botulism.

SUCCINATE

A metabolic intermediate in the citric acid cycle. See Citric Acid Cycle.

SUCCINYL COA

A metabolic intermediate in the citric acid cycle. See Citric Acid Cycle.

SUCRALFATE

Pepsin inhibitor that serves as an antiulcer drug. Trade names: Carafate, Sulcrate.

SUCRASE

Enzyme that catalyzes the cleavage of sucrose to glucose and fructose.

SUCROSE

A disaccharide consisting of one molecule of glucose and one molecule of fructose linked together.

SUCROSE DIGESTION/ABSORPTION

See Carbohydrate Absorption.

SUCROSE POLYESTER (OLESTRA)

A polymer of sucrose and fatty acids that can be used as a fat substitute.

SUCROSE-INDUCED FATTY LIVER

This is due to the fructose-induced increase in fatty acid synthesis. Adaptation can and does occur and the liver returns to its normal fat level. Not observed in humans.

SUCROSE-INDUCED LIPEMIA

When rats and some humans are fed sucrose-rich, low-fat diets, blood lipids, particularly triacylglycerols, increase. This is due to the fact that the fructose of the sucrose is metabolized primarily by the liver, and the product of this metabolism is triacylglyceride, which is then exported to the periphery for storage. In normal individuals, there is adaptation to this diet and the lipemia subsides.

SULFITES

Additives involved in idiosyncratic food intolerance reactions. Sodium and potassium bisulfite and metabisulfite are used in food products to prevent spoilage by microorganisms as well as oxidative discoloration. They are added, among others, to salads, wine, dehydrated fruits, potatoes, seafood, baked goods, and tea mixtures. Symptoms that may occur in sulfite-intolerant persons are airway constriction, flushing, itching, urticaria, angioedema, nausea, and in extreme cases, hypotension.

SULFORAPHANE

A histone deacetylase inhibitor that may have anticancer activity.

SULFUR

An essential element needed for the formation of disulfide bridges. Also important to hold iron in the centers of heme and the cytochromes and as a structural element in mucopolysaccharides and sulfolipids.

SULFUR-CONTAINING AMINO ACIDS

Methionine, cysteine, cystine (see Table 5).

SUPINE

Lying on one's back.

SURFACTANT

A compound that reduces the surface tension of a liquid so that another liquid can be mixed with it.

SWEETENING AGENTS

Compounds that elicit a sweet taste.

SYMPTOMS

Signs or indications of disease.

SYNDROME

A group of signs and symptoms associated with a specific disease.

SYNERGISM

The effect resulting when two substances work together to produce an effect greater than each could produce individually.

T

T CELLS

Cells of the immune system that originated from the thymus gland. These cells recognize antigens and produce antibodies to them.

T3

Triiodothyronine. The active thyroid hormone.

T_4

Thyroxine. The form of thyroid hormone released by the thyroid gland to the blood.

TACHYCARDIA

Rapid heart beat.

TAGASEROD MALEATE

A partial agonist of the 5-HT_4 receptor that is used to treat irritable bowel syndrome. Trade name: Zelhorm.

TALLOW

Beef or sheep fat.

TANDEM

Used to describe multiple copies of the same sequence that lie adjacent to each other in the gene.

TANGIER DISEASE

Familial HDL deficiency. A genetic disease due to a mutation in the gene for the HDL protein. Characterized by very low plasma HDL and cholesterol levels, an accumulation of cholesterol esters in the tissues, and a peculiar yellow orange color to the tonsils.

TANNINS

A heterogeneous group of substances in plants. They include all the plant polyphenolic substances with a molecular weight higher than 500. Two types of tannins are distinguished on the basis of their properties, breakdown products, botanical distribution, and whether they are hydrolyzable or condensed tannins. Hydrolyzable tannins are gallic, digallic, and ellagic acid esters of glucose or quinic acid. One type of hydrolyzable tannins is tannic acid (also known as gallotannic acid, gallotannin, or simply tannin). In tannic acid all the hydroxyl groups of glucose are esterified with gallic or digallic acid. It may cause acute liver injury, that is, liver necrosis and fatty liver. The condensed tannins (also known as flavonols) are polymers of flavonoids and in most cases are leucoanthocyanidins. The monomers are linked through carbon-carbon bonds between positions 4 and 6, or positions 4 and 8. The occurrence of tannins is reported in unripe fruits such as mango, dates, and persimmons. The tannins diminish in amounts as the fruits ripen. Furthermore, tannins are found in variable amounts in coffee (regular coffee: 1.1% tannins; instant coffee: 4.3% tannins; decaffeinated ground coffee: 1.2% tannins; instant decaffeinated coffee: 5.2% tannins), cocoa (unsweetened cocoa: 2.5% tannins; cocoa made by treatment with alkali: 4% tannins), and tea (bulk black tea and green tea: 10.5%–11.8% tannins; tea bags [black and green tea]: 9.1%–13.1% tannins; black instant tea: 14.7% tannins). Green tea may yield more soluble tannins, while black tea contains tannins with a higher molecular mass, as a result of oxidation of phenolic precursors during fermentation. Other food sources of tannins are grapes (condensed tannins, on average 500 mg/kg of grapes), grape juice, wines (red wine: 1.2–4.4 g/L of wine), and some sorghum grain varieties.

TARGETED MUTATION (KNOCKOUT MUTATION)

A specific gene at a specific location that has been altered or deleted.

TASTE BUDS

Sensory cells on the surface of the tongue, soft palate, cheeks, and throat.

TASTE THRESHOLD

The lowest concentration of a food or beverage at which its taste can be determined. Altered taste thresholds are often noted by individuals undergoing chemotherapy.

TAURI'S DISEASE

Glycogen storage disease type VII due to a mutation in the gene for phosphofructokinase. Characterized by excess glycogen stores in muscles.

TAURINE

2-aminoethyl sulfonic acid; synthesized from methionine and excreted via the kidneys; involved in neurotransmission; an end product of taurocholic acid (a bile acid) degradation.

TAUROCHOLATE

A bile acid derived from taurine produced by the liver, stored in the gall bladder, and released into the duodenum to serve as an emulsifier of lipid in the ingesta.

TAY-SACHS DISEASE

A genetic disease due to a mutation in the gene for the enzyme hexo-amidase A that is involved in the normal degradation of brain gangliosides. When these accumulate, the child loses mental function and dies.

TBF

Total body fat.

TBG (THYROID HORMONE BINDING GLOBULIN)

Protein that carries the thyroxine from the thyroid gland to its target tissue.

TBW

Total body water.

TCA CYCLE

See Citric Acid Cycle and Metabolic Maps, Appendix 2.

TDP, TPP

Thiamin-containing coenzyme required for decarboxylation reactions.

TELOMERES

The structures at the ends of the chromosomes.

TERATOGENIC RISK

Risk associated with specific compounds, based on the chance that these compounds will have deleterious effects on the embryo or fetus.

TERAZOSIN HYDROCHLORIDE

A selective α_1-blocking agent used to treat hypertension. Trade name: Hytrin.

TERBINAFINE HYDROCHLORIDE

An antifungal agent. Trade name: Lamisil.

TERBUTALINE SULFATE

A β_2 adrenergic agonist that serves as a bronchodilator or as an inhibitor of premature labor. Trade names: Brethine, Bricanyl.

TERIPARATIDE

Synthetic parathyroid hormone that can be used as a hormone replacement or to combat osteoporosis. Trade name: Forteo.

TERMINAL TRANSFERASE

An enzyme that adds nucleotides of one type to the 3′ end of a DNA strand.

TERPENOIDS

All steroids belong to the class of compounds known as terpenoids. All of these compounds have in common the same two C_5H_8 isoprene precursors employed for their synthesis, namely, isopentenyl pyrophosphate and dimethylallyl pyrophosphate.

TESTOSTERONE

Male hormone (androgen). Synthetic forms are available for therapeutic use. Trade names: Testamone, Depo-Testosterone, Testex, Androderm, Testoderm.

TETANY

A disorder characterized by intermittent tonic muscular contractions accompanied by fibrillary tremors, paresthesia, and muscle pain.

TETRAHYDROFOLATE

A coenzyme form of the vitamin folacin; a carrier of methyl groups. (See Folacin/Folic Acid.)

THALASSEMIA

A genetic disorder characterized by a defect in one of the hemoglobin chains, which reduces its oxygen-carrying capacity.

THEOPHYLLINE

An alkaloid found in tea; acts as a diuretic, vasodilator, and a cardiac stimulant.

THERAPEUTIC DIETS

Diets designed to manage the symptoms of metabolic disorders such as obesity, diabetes, hypertension.

THERMIC EFFECT OF FOOD

Heat-producing response of the body to the ingestion of food.

THERMOGENESIS

Heat production.

THERMOGENIN

Uncoupling protein produced by brown adipose fat cells; when produced/released it serves to dissipate the proton gradient in the mitochondria with the result of a failure to trap some of the energy released by the respiratory chain into the high-energy bond of ATP. Instead, all of this energy is released as heat.

THERMOPHILES

Bacteria that thrive or tolerate temperatures above 55°C.

THIAMIN, THIAMIN HYDROCHLORIDE (VITAMIN B₁)

Vitamin that serves as a coenzyme (thiamin pyrophosphate [TPP]) and is required for oxidative decarboxylation reactions. Thiamin is an essential nutrient and a member of the B family of vitamins. It is a relatively simple compound of a pyrimidine and a thiazole ring (Figure 55).

It exists in cells as TPP, which used to be called cocarboxylase. The name thiamin comes from the fact that the compound contains both a sulfur group (the thiol group) and nitrogen in its structure.

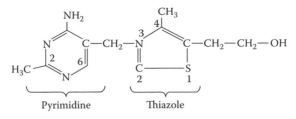

FIGURE 55   Structure of thiamin.

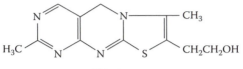

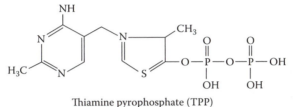

FIGURE 56   Structures of thiochrome and the coenzyme thiamin pyrophosphate.

Its biological function depends on the conjoined pyrimidine and thiazole rings, the presence of an amino group on carbon 4 of the pyrimidine ring, and the presence of a quaternary nitrogen, an open carbon at position 2 and a phosphorylatable alkyl group at carbon 5 of the thiazole ring. In its free form it is unstable. For this reason, it is available commercially as either a hydrochloride or mononitrate salt. It is stable in acids up to 120°C but readily decomposes in alkaline solutions, especially when heated. It can be split by nitrite or sulfite at the bridge between the pyrimidine and thiazole rings. The mononitrate form is a white crystalline substance that is more stable to heat than the hydrochloride form. This form is used more often for food processing than the hydrochloride (HCl) form. Other forms are also available. These include thiamin allyl disulfide, thiamin propyl disulfide, thiamin tetrahydrofurfuryl disulfide, and o-benzoyl thiamin disulfide.

When oxidized the bridge is attacked and thiamin is converted to thiochrome. Thiochrome is biologically inactive. These structures are shown in Figure 56.

THIAMIN ANTAGONISTS

The two most commonly used antagonists to thiamin are oxythiamine and pyrithiamine. A pyridine ring is substituted for the thiazole ring of thiamin in pyrithiamine. A hydroxyl group is substituted for the amino group of the pyrimidine moiety of the thiamin molecule in oxythiamine. It appears that thiamin activity is decreased when the number 2 position of the pyridine ring is changed.

Both the molecules are potent thiamin antagonists but differ in the mechanism by which this is accomplished. Oxythiamine is readily converted to the pyrophosphate and competes with thiamin for its place in the TPP-enzyme systems. Pyrithiamine prevents the conversion of thiamin to TPP by interfering with the activity of thiamin kinase.

Oxythiamine depresses appetite, growth, and weight gain and produces bradycardia, heart enlargement, and an increase in blood pyruvate level, but it does not produce neurological symptoms. Pyrithiamine results in a loss of thiamin from tissues, bradycardia, and heart enlargement but does not produce an increase in blood pyruvate level.

A natural antagonist is an enzyme called thiaminase. When heated, this enzyme is denatured and thus no longer is capable of destroying thiamin. The enzyme has several forms and has been found in fish, shellfish, ferns, betel nuts, and a variety of vegetables. Also found in tea and other plant foods are antithiamin substances that inactivate the vitamin by forming adducts. Tannic acid is one such substance; another is 3,4-dihydroxycinnamic acid (caffeic acid). Some of the flavonoids and some of the dihydroxy derivatives of tyrosine have antithiamin activity.

SOURCES

Thiamin is widely distributed in the food supply. Pork is the richest source, while highly refined foods have virtually no thiamin. Polished rice, fats, oils, refined sugar, unenriched flours are in this group. Many products are made with enriched flour and so provide thiamin to the consumers. Enrichment means that the flour (or other food ingredient) has had thiamin added to it to the level that was there prior to processing. Peas and other legumes are good sources; the amount of thiamin increases with the maturity of the seed. Cereal products contain nutritionally significant amounts of thiamin. Whole grain cereals contain the greater part of thiamin in their outer husks, the part that is removed during milling. Thus, milled grains are enriched with thiamin. Dried brewer's yeast and wheat germ are both rich in thiamin.

ABSORPTION AND METABOLISM

Thiamin is absorbed by a specific active transport mechanism that is energy and Na^+ dependent and carrier mediated. In humans and rats, absorption is most rapid in the proximal small intestine. Thiamin undergoes phosphorylation either in the intestinal lumen or within the intestinal cells. This phosphorylation is closely related to uptake, indicating that the carrier may be the enzyme thiamine pyrophosphokinase. There is, however, some argument about this however. Figure 57 illustrates TPP synthesis.

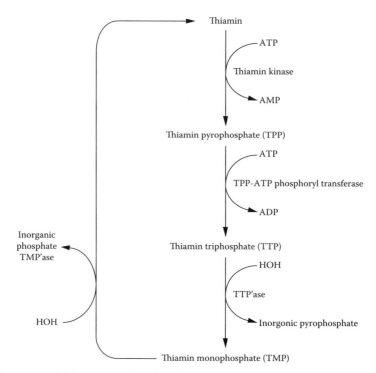

FIGURE 57   Formation of thiamin pyrophosphate through the phosphorylation of thiamin.

While thiamin can accumulate in all cells of the body, there is no single storage site per se. The body does not store the vitamin, and thus a daily supply is needed. Thiamin in excess of need is excreted in the urine. More than 20 metabolites of thiamin have been identified in urine.

FUNCTION

Thiamin is a part of the coenzyme TPP (thiamin with two molecules of phosphate attached to it), also known as cocarboxylase, which is required in the metabolism of carbohydrates. Figure 58 illustrates this function.

The driving force for reactions with thiamin results because of the resonance possible in the thiazolium ring. The thiazolium dipslo ion, known as ylid, will form. Because of the formation of the ylid, the thiazole ring of TPP can serve as a transient carrier of a covalently bound "active" aldehyde group. Mg^{++} is required as a cofactor for these reactions. The metabolism of carbohydrates has three stages at which the absence of thiamin as part of a coenzyme (TPP) leads to a slowing or complete blocking of the reactions.

There are two oxidative decarboxylation reactions of α ketoacids: the formation or degradation of α ketols and the decarboxylation of pyruvic acid to acetyl CoA as it is about to enter the citric acid cycle. This reaction is catalyzed by the pyruvate dehydrogenase complex, an organized assembly of three kinds of enzymes. The mechanism of this action is quite complex. TPP, lipoamide, and FAD serve as catalytic cofactors; NAD and CoA serve as stoichiometric cofactors (Figure 59).

As a consequence of impairment of this reaction in thiamin deficiency, the level of pyruvate will rise. When thiamin is withheld from the diet, the ability of tissues to utilize pyruvate does not decline uniformly, indicating that there are tissue differences in the retention of TPP. Muscle retains more TPP than the brain. This role of thiamin arose from the discovery that

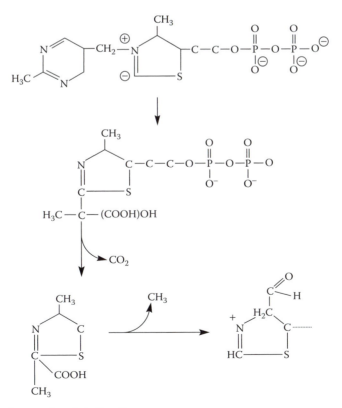

FIGURE 58 Thiamin pyrophosphate function.

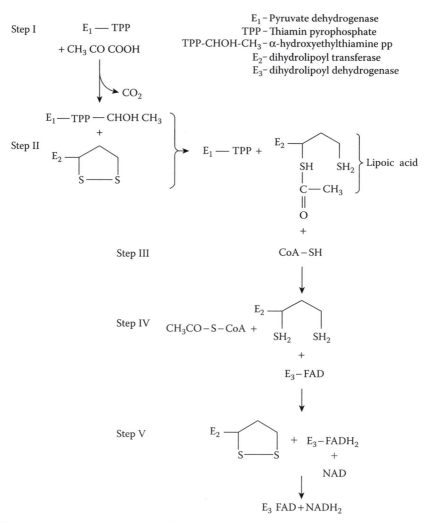

FIGURE 59 Oxidation of pyruvate in the mitochondrial matrix.

thiamin alone promotes nonenzymatic decarboxylation of pyruvate to yield acetaldehyde and CO_2. Studies of this model revealed that the H at carbon 2 of the thiazole ring ionizes to yield a carbanion, which reacts with the carbonyl atom of pyruvate to yield CO_2 and a hydroxyethyl (HE) derivative of the thiazole. The HE may then undergo hydrolysis to yield acetaldehyde or become oxidized to yield an acyl group. Figures 59 and 60 illustrate pyruvate metabolism and show where thiamin plays a role.

Thiamin is also active in the decarboxylation of α-ketoglutaric acid to succinyl CoA in the citric acid cycle. The mechanism of action is similar to that of pyruvate.

Step 1: This step is similar to nonoxidative decarboxylation of pyruvate in alcohol fermentation.
Step 2: The HE group is dehydrogenated, and the resulting acetyl group is transferred to the sulfur atom at C6 of lipoic acid, which constitutes the covalently bound prosthetic group of the second enzyme of the complex lipoate acetyltransferase. The transfer of a pair of H^+ from the HE group of TPP to the disulfide bond of lipoic acid converts the latter to its reduced or dithiol form, dihydrolipoic acid.
Step 3: The acetyl group is enzymatically transferred to the thiol group of CoA. The acetyl CoA so formed leaves the enzyme complex in free form.

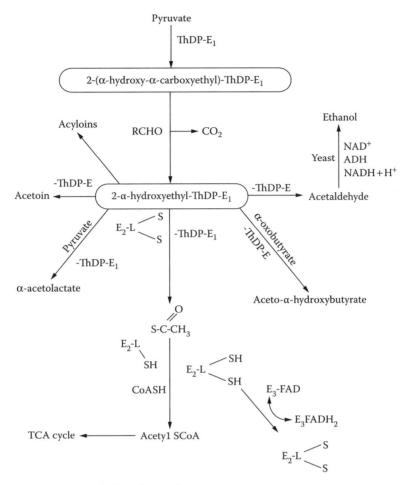

FIGURE 60   Summary of metabolic pathways for pyruvate.

Step 4: The dithiol form of lipoic acid is reoxidized to its disulfide form by transfer of H^+ to the third enzyme of the complex lipoamide dehydrogenase whose reducible prosthetic group is FAD. $FADH_2$, which remains bound to the enzyme, transfers its electron to NAD^+ to form NADH.

E_1 is regulated by PDH kinase and PDH phosphatase. The oxidation of αKG to succinyl CoA is energetically irreversible and is carried out by the αKG DH complex.

$$\alpha KG + NAD^+ + CoA \Leftrightarrow \text{Succinyl CoA} + CO_2 + NADH_2$$
$$\Delta G^1 = 8.0 \text{ kcal mol}^{-1}$$

This reaction is analogous to the oxidation of pyruvate to acetyl CoA and CO_2 and occurs by the same mechanism with TPP, lipoic acid, CoA, FAD, and NAD participating as coenzymes.

The metabolism of ethanol also requires thiamin. The same pyruvate dehydrogenase complex that converts pyruvate to acetyl CoA will also metabolize acetaldehyde (the first product in the metabolism of ethanol) to acetyl CoA. This system probably accounts for only a small part of ethanol degradation.

TPP participates in the transfer of a glycoaldehyde group from D-xylulose to D-ribose-5P to yield D-sedoheptulose-7P and glyceraldehydes-3P, an intermediate of glycolysis. Transketolase contains tightly bound TPP. In this reaction, the glycoaldehyde group (CH_2OH CO) is first transferred from D-xylulose-5P to enzyme-bound TPP to form the αβ dihydroxyethyl derivative of the latter, which is analogous to the α HE derivative formed during the action of PDH. The TPP acts as an intermediate carrier of this glycoaldehyde group, which is transferred to the acceptor molecule D-ribose-5P. This is a reaction in the hexose monophosphate shunt.

From the involvement of vitamin-containing coenzymes in the oxidation of alcohol, it follows that vitamin deficiency could impair the rate of alcohol oxidation and thus increase the retention of alcohol in the blood of malnourished chronic alcoholic subjects. Actually, there is little evidence for this assumption in animals or humans. The rate-limiting step appears to be not the level of vitamin concentration but the amount of alcohol dehydrogenase present.

Large dietary intakes of carbohydrates will require that more thiamin be included in the diet than will small intakes. Ingestion of lipids, on the other hand, is considered thiamin sparing.

DEFICIENCY

The major symptoms of thiamin deficiency are loss of appetite (anorexia), weight loss, convulsions, slowing of the heart rate (bradycardia), and lowering of the body temperature. Loss of muscle tone and lesions of the nervous system may also develop. Because the heart muscle can be weakened, there may be cardiac failure resulting in peripheral edema and ascites in the extremities. The classical pathological condition arising from thiamin deficiency in man is beriberi, formerly quite common in the Orient. Thiamin deficiency can arise not only from poor intake of food but also from its faulty utilization or absorption.

Beriberi is classified into several types: acute, mixed, wet, or dry. The acute, mixed type is characterized by neural and cardiac symptoms producing neuritis and heart failure. In wet beriberi, the edema of heart failure is the most striking sign; digestive disorders and emaciation are additional symptoms. In dry beriberi, loss of functions of the lower extremities or paralysis predominates; it is often called polyneuritis.

Thiamin deficiency is the most common vitamin deficiency seen in chronic alcoholics who prefer alcohol to food. Clinical manifestations of the deficiency vary depending upon the severity of food deprivation. However, in all degrees of deficiency they involve muscle and/or nerve tissue. The most serious form of thiamin deficiency in alcoholics is Wernicke's syndrome. It is characterized by ophthalmoplegia, sixth nerve palsy, nystagmus, ptosis, ataxia, confusion and coma, which may terminate in death. Oftentimes, the confusional state persists after treatment of the acute thiamin deficiency. This is known as Korsakoff's psychosis.

The next most serious level of thiamin deficiency seen in alcoholics is known as alcoholic beriberi. It is seen in those individuals who have a minimal intake of thiamin. It is characterized by symmetrical foot and wrist drop associated with a great deal of muscle tenderness. It may also affect cardiac muscle metabolism and may result in congestive heart failure.

The mildest and most common form of thiamin deficiency is the polyneuropathy affecting only the lower extremities of chronic alcoholics. All forms of thiamin deficiency respond to thiamin treatment unless the pathology is irreversible, a situation not infrequently found with polyneuropathy. The thiamin needs of an individual are influenced by many factors: age, caloric intake, carbohydrate intake, and body weight (see http://www.nap.edu).

TOXICITY

Although thiamin produces a variety of pharmacological effects when administered in large doses, the dose required is thousands of times greater than those required for optimal nutrition. Generally, toxic effects are reported on subcutaneous, intramuscular, intraspinal, or intravenous injections but not oral administration. In rare cases, thiamin has caused reactions resembling anaphylactic shock in humans. However, since these usually develop only in individuals who have been given large intravenous injections, they apparently appear only after a hypersensitivity has developed.

THIAMIN DIPHOSPHATE

Coenyzme form of thiamin, also called thiamin pyrophosphate.

THIAMINASE

An enzyme found in raw fish that destroys thiamin.

THIAZOLIDINEDIONE

A drug that decreases insulin resistance, increases muscle glucose use, decreases gluconeogenesis, increases PPARγ in adipose tissue, and leads to an increase in fatty acid uptake by the adipose tissue.

THIOESTER BOND

An energy-rich bond of the general formula: R-S-C-R-.

THIRST MECHANISM

Control mechanism in which the cells of the anterior hypothalamus of the brain sense a need for water and stimulate drinking behavior.

THREONINE

An essential four-carbon amino acid having a hydroxyl group attached to carbon 3. (See Amino Acids, Table 5.)

THRESHOLD DOSE

The dose required to have a measurable or expected effect.

THROMBOPLASTIN

A substance present in tissues, platelets, and leukocytes that, in the presence of Ca^{++}, brings about the conversion of prothrombin to thrombin and thence the formation of a clot.

THROMBOSIS

Obstruction of a blood vessel by a blood clot.

THROMBUS

A blood clot that obstructs a blood vessel or cavity in the heart.

THYMIC HORMONES

Hormones that play a critical role in the immune system. They include thymosin α, β_2 fraction 5, thymus humoral factor (THG-γ2), and thymopoietin.

THYMIDINE PHOSPHATE (TMP, TDP, TTP)

A nucleotide consisting of thymine (a pyrimidine base) deoxyribose and 1, 2, or 3 phosphate groups.

THYMINE

A pyrimidine base.

THYROCALCITONIN—CALCITONIN

A hormone that regulates blood calcium levels.

THYROIDECTOMY

Removal of the thyroid gland.

THYROIDITIS

Inflammation of thyroid gland.

THYROTOXICOSIS

Hyperactive thyroid gland; excess levels of thyroid hormone also known as Graves' disease. Characterized by elevated oxygen consumption, elevated energy need, increased irritability and nervousness, bulging eyes, and weight loss.

THYROTROPIN

Hormone produced and released by the pars distalis of the anterior pituitary gland that stimulates thyroid gland activity. Also known as TSH.

THYROXINE

See T_4.

TNFα (TUMOR NECROSIS FACTOR α)

A cytokine; levels of this cytokine are high in anorexia nervosa and in obesity. Not all forms of this cytokine have the same effect on all cells.

TOCOPHEROLS

A family of fat-soluble compounds having vitamin E activity.

TOLBUTAMIDE

An hypoglycemic oral agent; a derivative of sulfonylurea that works by stimulating insulin release by the β cells of the pancreas.

TONUS

Tonicity.

TOTAL AREA UNDER CURVE

A means of calculating and comparing the body response to a given stimulus over time as in a glucose tolerance test.

TOTAL HEAT PRODUCTION (HE)

The energy lost from an animal system in a form other than as a combustible compound. Heat production may be measured by either direct or indirect calorimetry. In direct calorimetry, heat production is measured directly by physical methods, whereas indirect calorimetry involves some indirect measure of heat such as the measurement of oxygen uptake and CO_2 production using thermic equivalent of oxygen based on the respiratory quotient (RQ) and theoretical considerations. The commonly accepted equation for indirect computation of heat production from the respiratory exchange is HE = 3.866 (liters oxygen) = 1.200 (liters CO_2) − 1.431 (g urinary nitrogen) − 0.518 (liters methane). Heat production may also be measured as the difference from the determination of total carbon and nitrogen balance or from a comparative slaughter experiment. These methods arrive at total heat production be different calculations and are subject to systematic errors of measurement.

TOTAL IRON-BINDING CAPACITY

The relative saturation of the iron-binding protein transferrin.

TOTAL LUNG CAPACITY

Total amount of gas that the lungs can hold.

TOTAL PARENTERAL NUTRITION (TPN)

Total parenteral nutrition. A method of providing all nutrients needed through a solution infused into a large blood vessel.

TOXEMIA OF PREGNANCY

See Eclampsia and Preeclampsia. A condition associated with pregnancy characterized by hypertension and inadequate renal function.

TOXIC REACTION

A food-intolerance reaction caused by toxic food components. Also known as food poisoning.

TOXICITY

The potential of a chemical to induce an adverse effect in a living organism. Each chemical, and thus also each food component, has its own specific toxicity. In general, information on the toxicity of food components is obtained from studies in experimental animals, in vitro studies, studies in volunteers, or epidemiological studies. The aims of these studies are to determine the type of adverse effect, dose-effect relationships including the no-observed-adverse-effect level, and the mechanism underlying the adverse effect.

TOXICITY OF NUTRIENTS

Some nutrients (fat-soluble vitamins A and D, some minerals) if consumed in excess can elicit undesirable effects. These effects can be life threatening.

TOXINS

Chemicals that elicit symptoms of poisoning. Table 50 lists some of these.

TABLE 50
Some Potentially Poisonous (Toxic) Agents in Food

Poison (Toxin)	Source	Symptoms and Signs	Distribution	Magnitude	Prevention	Treatment	Remarks
Aflatoxins (see Mycotoxins in this table).	Aluminum (Al; also see Minerals.) Food additives, mainly presented in such items as baking powder, pickles, and processed cheeses. Aluminum-containing antacids. Utensils.	Abnormally large intakes of aluminum irritate the digestive tract. Also, unusual conditions have sometimes resulted in the absorption of sufficient aluminum from antacids to cause brain damage. Aluminum may form nonabsorbable complexes with essential trace elements, thereby creating deficiencies of these elements.	Aluminum is widely used throughout the world.	The United States uses more aluminum than any other product except iron and steel. However, known cases of aluminum toxicity are rare.	Based on the evidence presented herein, no preventative measures are recommended.		Aluminum toxicity has been reported in patients receiving renal dialysis.
Arsenic (As)	Consuming foods and beverages contaminated with excessive amounts of arsenic-containing sprays used as insecticides and weed killers. Arsenical insecticides used in vineyards exposing the workers when spraying or by inhaling contaminated dusts and plant debris. Arsenic in the air from three major sources: (1) smelting of metals, (2) burning of coal, and (3) use of arsenical pesticides.	Burning pains in the throat or stomach, cardiac abnormalities, and the odor of garlic on the breath. Other symptoms may be diarrhea and extreme thirst along with a choking sensation. Small doses of arsenic taken into the body over a long period of time may produce hyperkeratosis (irregularities in pigmentation, especially on the trunk), arterial insufficiency, and cancer. There is strong evidence that inorganic arsenic is a skin and lung carcinogen in humans.	Arsenic is widely distributed, but the amount of the element consumed by humans in food and water, or breathed, is very small and not harmful.	Causes of arsenic toxicity in man are infrequent. Two note-worthy episodes occurred in Japan in 1955. One involved tainted powdered milk; the other contaminated soy sauce. The toxic milk caused 12,131 cases of infant poisoning, with 130 deaths. The soy sauce poisoned 220 people.		Induce vomiting, followed by an antidote of egg whites in water or milk. Afterward, give strong coffee or tea, followed by Epsom salts in water or castor oil.	Arsenic is known to partially protect against selenium poisoning. The highest residues of arsenic are generally in the hair and nails. Arsenic in soils may sharply decrease crop growth and yields, but it is not a hazard to people or livestock that eat plants grown in these fields.

Poison (Toxin)	Source	Symptoms and Signs	Distribution	Magnitude	Prevention	Treatment	Remarks
Chromium (Cr)	Food, water, and air contaminated by chromium compounds in industrialized areas.	Inorganic chromium salt reduces the absorption of zinc; hence, zinc deficiency symptoms may become evident in chronic chromium toxicity.	Chromium toxicity is not common.	Chromium toxicity is not very common.	It is unlikely that people will get too much chromium because only minute amounts of the element are present in most foods, the body utilizes chromium poorly, and the toxic dose is about 10,000 times the lowest effective medical dose.		
Copper (Cu)	Diets with excess copper, but low in other minerals that counteract its effects.	Acid foods or beverages (vinegar, carbonated beverages, or citrus juices) that have been in prolonged contact with copper metal may cause acute gastrointestinal disturbances. Acute copper toxicity is characterized by headache, dizziness, metallic taste, excessive salivation, nausea, vomiting, stomachache, diarrhea, and weakness. If the disease is allowed to get worse, there may also be racing of the heart, high blood pressure, jaundice, hemolytic anemia, dark-pigmented urine, kidney disorders, and even death. Chronic copper toxicity may contribute iron-deficiency anemia, mental illness following childbirth (postpartum psychosis), certain types of schizophrenia, and perhaps heart attacks.	Copper toxicity may occur wherever there is excess copper intake, especially when accompanied by low iron, molybdenum, sulfur, zinc, and vitamin C.	The incidence of copper toxicity is extremely rare in man. Its occurrence in significant form is almost always limited to suicide attempted by ingesting large quantities of copper salt or a genetic defect in copper metabolism inherited as an autosomal recessive, known as Wilson's disease.	Avoid foods and beverages that have been in prolonged contact with copper metal.	Administration of copper chelating agents to remove excess copper.	Copper is essential to human life and health, but like all heavy metals, it is also potentially toxic.

(Continued)

TABLE 50 (Continued)
Some Potentially Poisonous (Toxic) Agents in Food

Ergot	Rye, wheat, barley, oats and triticale carry this mycotoxin. Ergot replaces the seed in the heads of cereal grains, in which it appears as a purplish-black, hard, banana-shaped, dense mass from ¼ to ¾ in. (6–9 mm) long.	When a large amount of ergot is consumed in a short period, convulsive ergotism is observed. The symptoms include itching, numbness, severe muscle cramps, sustained spasms and convulsions, and extreme pain. When smaller amounts of ergot are consumed over an extended period, ergotism characterized by gangrene of the fingertips and toes, caused by blood vessel and muscle contraction stopping blood circulation in the extremities. These symptoms include cramps, swelling, inflammation, alternating burning and freezing sensations (St. Anthony's fire), and numbness; eventually the hands and feet may turn black, shrink, and fall off. Ergotism is a cumulative poison, depending on the amount of ergot eaten and the length of time over which it is eaten.	Ergot is found throughout the world, wherever rye, wheat, barley, oats, or triticale are grown.	There is considerable ergot, especially in rye. But, normally, screening grains before processing alleviates ergotism in people.	Consists of an ergot-free diet. Ergot in food and feed grains may be removed by screening the grains before processing. In the United States, wheat and rye containing more than 0.3% ergot are classed as "ergoty." In Canada, government regulations prohibit more than 0.1% ergot in feeds.	An ergot-free diet; good nursing; treatment by a doctor. Six different alkaloids are involved in ergot poisoning. Ergot is used to aid the uterus to contract after childbirth, to prevent loss of blood. Also, another ergot drug (ergotamine) is widely used in the treatment of migraine headaches.

Poison (Toxin)	Source	Symptoms and Signs	Distribution	Magnitude	Prevention	Treatment	Remarks
Fluorine (F) (fluorosis)	Ingesting excessive quantities of fluorine through either the food or water, or a combination of these. Except in certain industrial exposures, the intake of fluoride inhaled from the air is only a small fraction of the total fluoride intake in man. Pesticides containing fluorides, including those used to control insects, weeds, and rodents. Although water is the principal source of fluoride in an average human diet in the United States, fluoride is frequently contained in toothpaste, toothpowder, chewing gums, mouthwashes, vitamin supplements, and mineral supplements.	Acute fluoride poisoning: Abdominal pain, diarrhea, vomiting, excessive salivation, thirst, perspiration, and painful spasms of the limbs. Chronic fluoride poisoning: Abnormal teeth (especially mottled enamel) during the first 8 years of life and brittle bones. Other effects, predicted from animal studies, may include loss of body weight, and altered structure and function of the thyroid gland and kidneys. Water containing 3–10 ppm of fluoride may cause mottling of the teeth. An average daily intake of 20–80 mg of fluoride over a period of 10–20 years will result in crippling fluorosis.	The water in parts of Arkansas, California, South Carolina, and Texas contains excess fluorine. Occasionally, throughout the United States, high-fluorine phosphates are used in mineral mixtures.	Generally speaking, fluorosis is limited to high-fluorine areas. Only a few instances of health effects in man have been attributed to airborne fluoride, and they occurred in persons living in the vicinity of fluoride-emitting industries.	Avoid the use of food and water containing excessive fluorine.	Any damage may be permanent, but people who have not developed severe symptoms may be helped to some extent if the source of excess fluorine is eliminated. Calcium and magnesium may reduce the absorption and utilization of fluoride.	Fluorine is a cumulative poison. The total fluoride in the human body averages 2.57 g. Susceptibility to fluoride toxicity is increased by deficiencies of calcium, vitamin C, and protein. Virtually all foods contain trace amounts of fluoride.

(Continued)

TABLE 50 (Continued)
Some Potentially Poisonous (Toxic) Agents in Food

| Lead (Pb) | Consuming food or medicinal products (including health food products) contaminated with lead. Inhaling the poison as a dust by workers in such industries as painting, lead mining, and refining. Inhaling airborne lead discharged into the air from auto exhaust fumes. Consuming food crops contaminated by lead being deposited on the leaves and other edible portions of the plant by direct fallout. Consuming food or water contaminated by contact with lead pipes or utensils. Old houses in which the interiors were painted with leaded paints prior to 1945, with the chipped wall paint eaten by children. Such miscellaneous sources as illicitly distilled whiskey, improperly lead-glazed earthenware, old battery casings used as fuel, and toys containing lead. | Symptoms develop rapidly in young children, but slowly in mature people. Symptoms of acute lead poisoning include colic, cramps, diarrhea or constipation, leg cramps, and drowsiness. The most severe form of lead poisoning, encountered in infants and in heavy drinkers of illicitly distilled whiskey, is characterized by profound disturbances of the CNS, permanent damage to the brain, damage to the kidneys, and shortened life span of the erythrocytes. Symptoms of chronic lead poisoning include colic, constipation, lead palsy especially in the forearm and fingers, the symptoms of chronic nephritis, and sometimes mental depression, convulsions, and a blue line at the edge of the gums. | Predominantly among children who may eat chips of lead-containing paints, peeled off from painted wood. | The Center for Disease Control, Atlanta, Georgia, estimates that lead poisoning claims the lives of 200 children each year, and 400,000–600,000 children have elevated lead levels in the blood. Lead poisoning has been reduced significantly with the use of lead-free paints. | Avoid inhaling or consuming lead. | Acute lead poisoning: An emetic (induce vomiting), followed by drinking plenty of milk and ½ oz (14 g) of Epsom salts in half a glass of water. Chronic lead poisoning: Remove the source of lead. Sometimes treated by administration of magnesium or lead sulfate solution as a laxative and antidote on the lead in the digestive system, followed by potassium iodide which cleanses the tracts. Currently, treatment of lead poisoning makes use of chemicals that bind the metal in the body and help in its removal. | Lead is a cumulative poison. When incorporated in the soil, nearly all the lead is converted into forms that are not available to plants. Any lead taken up by plant roots tends to stay in the roots, rather than move up to the top of the plant. Lead poisoning can be diagnosed positively by analyzing the blood tissue for lead content; clinical signs of lead poisoning usually are manifested at blood lead concentrations above 80 mg/100 g. |

Poison (Toxin)	Source	Symptoms and Signs	Distribution	Magnitude	Prevention	Treatment	Remarks
Mercury (Hg)	Mercury is discharged into air and water from industrial operations and is used in herbicide and fungicide treatments. Mercury poisoning has occurred where mercury from industrial plants has been discharged into water then accumulated as methylmercury in fish and shellfish. Accidental consumption of seed grains treated with fungicides that contain mercury, used for the control of fungus diseases of oats, wheat, barley, and flax.	The toxic effects of organic and inorganic compounds of mercury are dissimilar. The organic compounds of mercury, such as the various fungicides, affect the central nervous system and are not corrosive. The inorganic compounds of mercury include mainly mercuric chloride, a disinfectant; mercurous chloride (calomel), a cathartic; and elemental mercury. Commonly the toxic symptoms are corrosive gastrointestinal effects, such as vomiting, bloody diarrhea, and necrosis of the alimentary mucosa.	Wherever mercury is produced in industrial operations or used in herbicide or fungicide treatments.	Limited. But about 1200 cases of mercury poisoning identified in Japan in the 1950s were traced to the consumption of fish and shellfish from Japan's Minamata Bay, which was contaminated with methylmercury. Some of the offspring of exposed mothers were born with birth defects, and many victims suffered CNS damage. Still another outbreak of mercury toxicity occurred in Iraq, where more than 6000 people were hospitalized after eating bread made from wheat that had been treated with methylmercury.	Control mercury pollution form industrial operations. Mercury is a cumulative poison. The U.S. Food and Drug Administration prohibits use of mercury-treated grain for food or feed.		Grain crops produced from mercury-treated seed and crops produced on soils treated with mercury herbicides have not been found to contain harmful concentrations of this element.
Polybrominated biphenyls (PBBs), a fire retardant that may cause cancer when taken into the food supply	All of the 1973 Michigan toxicity problem was traced to livestock feed which became contaminated with PBB when the fire retardant was shipped by mistake to a feed manufacturer.	People exposed to PBB in Michigan reported suffering from neurological symptoms such as loss of memory, muscular weakness, coordination problems, headaches, painful swollen joints, acne, abdominal pain, and diarrhea.	In 1973, the accidental contamination of animal feeds exposed many people in Michigan to PBB in dairy products and other foods.	The Michigan incident eventually led to the slaughter and burial of nearly 25,000 cattle, 3,500 hogs, and 1.5 million chickens; and the disposal of about 5 million eggs and tons of milk, butter, cheese, and feed.		Follow the prescribed treatment of a medical doctor.	PBBs are long-term, low-level contaminants, very stable and resistant to decay.

(Continued)

TABLE 50 (Continued)
Some Potentially Poisonous (Toxic) Agents in Food

	Sources of contamination	Clinical effects		Prevention	Treatment	Comments
Polychlorinated biphenyls (PCBs), industrial chemicals; chlorinated hydrocarbons that may cause cancer when taken into the food supply	Sources of contamination to man include contaminated foods, mammals or birds that have fed on contaminated foods of fish, residues on foods that have been wrapped in papers and plastics containing PCBs, milk from cows that have been fed silage from silos coated with PCB-containing paint, eggs from layers fed feeds contaminated with PCBs, and absorption by human beings of PCBs through the lungs, the gastrointestinal tract, and the skin.	The clinical effects of people are an eruption of the skin resembling acne, visual disturbances, jaundice, numbness, and spasms. Newborn infants from mothers who have been poisoned show discoloration of the skin, which regresses after 2–5 months.	PCBs are widespread packaging materials.	Avoid harmfully contaminated food.	People afflicted with PCB should follow the prescribed treatment of their doctor.	Although the production of PCBs was halted in 1977 and the importing of PCBs was banned January 1, 1979, the chemicals had been widely used for 40 years, and they are exceptionally long-lived. PCBs have been widely used in dielectric fluids in capacitors and transformers, hydraulic fluids, and heat transfer fluids. Also, they have more than 50 minor uses, including plasticizers and solvents in adhesives, printing ink, sealants, moisture retardants, paints, and pesticide carriers. PCB will cause cancer in laboratory animals (rats, mice, and rhesus monkeys). It is not known if it will cause cancer in humans. More study is needed to gauge its effects on the ecological food chain and on human health. When fed Coho salmon from Lake Michigan with 10–15 ppm PCB, mink in Wisconsin stopped reproducing or their kits died. In 1977, polar bears at the very top of the Arctic food chain showed PCB levels of up to 8 ppm in their fatty tissue. This indicates that PCBs are spread throughout the atmosphere.

Poison (Toxin)	Source	Symptoms and Signs	Distribution	Magnitude	Prevention	Treatment	Remarks
Salt (NaCl: sodium chloride) poisoning	Consumption of high levels of the salt in food or drinking water.	Salt may be toxic when it is fed to infants or others whose kidneys cannot excrete the excess in the urine, or when the body is adapted to a chronic low-salt diet.	Salt is used all over the world. Hence, the potential for salt poisoning exists everywhere.	Salt poisoning is relatively rare.		Drink large quantities of fresh water.	Even normal salt concentration may be toxic if water intake is low.
Selenium	Consumption of high levels of the element in food or drinking water.	Presence of malnutrition, parasitic infestation, or other factors which make people highly susceptible to selenium toxicity. Abnormalities in the hair, nails, and skin. Children in a high-selenium area of Venezuela showed loss of hair, discolored skin, and chronic digestive disturbances. Normally, people who have consumed large excesses of selenium excrete it as trimethylselenide in the urine and/or as dimethyl selenide on the breath. The latter substance has an odor resembling garlic.	In certain regions of western United States, especially in South Dakota, Montana, Wyoming, Nebraska, Kansas, and perhaps areas in other states in the Great Plains and Rocky Mountains. Also in Canada.	Selenium toxicity in people is relatively rate.		Selenium toxicity may be counteracted by arsenic or copper, but such treatment should be carefully monitored.	Confirmed cases of selenium poisoning in people are rare because only traces are present in most foods, foods generally come from a wide area, and the metabolic processes normally convert excess selenium into harmless substances, which are excreted in the urine or breath.
Tin (Sn)	From acid fruits and vegetables canned in tin cans. The acids in such foods as citrus fruits and tomato products can leach tin from the inside of the can. Then the tin is ingested with the canned food. In the digestive tract tin goes through a methylation process in which nontoxic tin is converted to methylated tin, which is toxic.	Methylated tin is a neurotoxin—a toxin that attacks the CNS; the symptoms are numbness of the fingers and lips followed by a loss of speech and hearing. Eventually, the afflicted person becomes spastic, then coma and death follow.	Tin cans are widely used throughout the world.	The use of tin in advanced industrial societies has increased 14-fold over the last 10 years.	Many tin cans are coated on the inside with enamel or other materials.		Currently, not much is known about the amount of tin in the human diet.

Source: Adapted from Ensminger et al., 1994. *Foods and Nutrition Encyclopedia.* 2nd ed. Boca Raton, FL: CRC Press, pp. 1790–1803.

TRACE ELEMENTS

Minerals needed in trace amounts. (See Minerals.)

TRANS FATTY ACIDS

Fatty acids that assume the chair form rather than the boat form around a double bond. When industrial hydrogenation occurs, as in the manufacture of margarine and shortening, the oils become semisolids or solids, and some of the double bonds are converted into single bonds. However, in the process of hydrogenation, cis fatty acids may be converted to trans fatty acids. The fatty acids in the fats so produced are referred to as industrialized trans fatty acids (ITFAs). Hydrogenation can result in changes in the configuration of some of the fatty acids. These structural changes involve the difference in the placement of the carbon chains and hydrogen atoms on each side of the double bond. In the normal or cis configuration, the carbon chains are on one side of the double bond while the hydrogen atoms are on the other side of the double bond (Figure 2). Under the conditions of hydrogenation, the fatty acid structure changes such that a trans configuration is formed. The hydrogen atoms are on opposite sides of the double bond, and the carbon chains likewise are on opposite sides of the double bond. These fatty acids are called trans fatty acids. In addition to the geometric isomerism that occurs with hydrogenation, there is some change in the shape of the fatty acid. A cis fatty acid is "bent" 120° at the double bond, whereas the trans fatty acid is "straight."

TRANSAMINATION

A process or reaction where the amino group ($-NH_3$) is transferred from one compound to another.

TRANSCRIPTION

The synthesis of mRNA using DNA as a template. (See Protein Synthesis.)

TRANSFER RNA (tRNA)

Small stable RNA molecules that dock onto the mRNA and ribosomes and carry amino acids. Each amino acid has its own specific tRNA. (See Protein Synthesis.)

TRANSFERRIN

Iron-carrying protein in blood.

TRANSGENIC (ANIMAL)

An animal into which a foreign DNA has been inserted into its germ line.

TRANSKETOLASE

An enzyme that catalyzes the transfer of a two-carbon keto group from a keto sugar to an aldehyde sugar.

TRANSLATION

The synthesis of protein using the message for amino acid sequence carried by mRNA. Occurs on the ribosomes.

TRANSLOCASES

Proteins that move smaller molecules through a membrane.

TRAUMA

Injury.

TREE NUT ALLERGY

In several studies, a cross-reactivity has been reported between birch pollen and nuts. This cross-reactivity shows itself in a syndrome that is known as the para-birch syndrome. The complaints of people suffering from this syndrome result from a birch pollen allergy (sneezing, nasal obstruction, and conjunctivitis during the birch pollen season) and also from an allergy to nuts and/or certain fruits. Allergic reactions to these foods mainly cause symptoms such as itching in and around the mouth and pharynx and swelling of the lips. In some cases, however, more severe reactions occur. Related fruits in this context are apple, peach, plum, cherry, and orange. Also, some vegetables such as celery and carrot have been shown to be cross-reactive with the birch allergen. Other known cross-reactivity combinations are grass pollen with carrot, potato, wheat, and celery. A grass pollen–allergic person may become allergic to wheat as well. The exact mechanisms underlying these phenomena are not known.

TREPROSTINIL SODIUM

A drug that is a vasodilator and is used to treat hypertension. Trade name: Remodulin.

TRETINOIN

A synthetic vitamin A derivative used to treat acne. Trade names: Avita, Renova, Retin-A, Retin-A Micro, Stieva-A, Stieva-A Forte.

TRIACYLGLYCEROL (TRIGLYCERIDES)

A lipid consisting of three fatty acids esterified to a glycerol backbone.

TRIAMCINOLONE ACETONIDE

A synthetic glucocorticoid that is used as an anti-inflammatory drug. Trade names: Nasacort, Nasacort AQ.

TRICHINOSIS

A disease caused by a parasite found in pork.

TRICHOTHECENES

The most important mycotoxins produced by the mold *Fusarium*. They can be classified as 12,13-epoxytrichothecenes and macrocyclic resorcyclates (naturally occurring derivatives of b-resorcyclic acid). The production of trichothecenes is shared by the species of *Trichothecium*, *Myrothecium*, *Trichoderma*, and *Cephalosporium*. There are three types of trichothecenes:

(1) monoepoxytrichothecenes (8-deoxymonoepoxytrichothecenes (structure I), including diacetoxy-scirpenol and T-2 toxin; (8-ketomonoepoxytrichothecenes (structure II), including trichothecin and fusarenone; (2) diepoxytrichothecenes (structure III), including crotocin and crotocol; (3) macrocyclic trichothecenes (macrocyclic diesters [structure IV], including the roroidins; and (4) macrocyclic triesters (structure V), including the verrucarins). Most trichothecenes are phytotoxic and zootoxic. The in vitro toxic effects of the trichothecenes include skin necrosis, inflammatory effects, massive hemorrhages, and effects on heart and respiration rates. Furthermore, many of the trichothecenes have been shown to be inhibitors of protein synthesis; the most toxic types inhibiting at the initiation step (e.g., T-2 toxin, diacetoxyscirpenol, many of the verrucarins), the least toxic types at the elongation-termination process (e.g., crotocin, trichothecin, trichodermin). The actual toxicities of some of the trichothecenes were probably demonstrated in the field by both animal and human mycotoxicoses. An example of the latter is alimentary toxic aleukia, a toxic syndrome caused by *Fusarium* spp. This disease was traced to the consumption of grain that was allowed to overwinter in the fields. The grains became invaded by cryophilic molds from which several fungal genera and species were identified. In order to produce toxins, the most important requirement of these molds appeared to be the presence of alternate freezing and thawing cycles. The clinical course of alimentary toxic aleukia occurs in four stages. In the first stage (3–9 days) there is a burning sensation in the mouth and tongue and in the gastrointestinal tract, headache, dizziness, weakness, fatigue. In the latent second stage (2–8 weeks) there is progressive leukopenia, granulopenia, lymphocytosis, anemia, bacterial infections, disturbances in the central and autonomic nervous system, such as weakness, headache, palpitation, asthmatic attacks, icterus, hypotension, dilation of the pupils, soft and labile pulse, diarrhea, or constipation. In the third stage there are petechial hemorrhages in the skin, mucous membranes in the mouth, tongue, gastrointestinal tract and nasal area, necrosis in parts of the buccal cavity, enlargement and edema of the cervical lymph nodes, lesions in the esophagus and epiglottis, and edema in the larynx. In the fourth stage (≥2 months), if death does not intervene, the patient may recover.

TRIMESTER

Three months.

TRIPEPTIDES

Three amino acids joined together via the peptide bonds.

TRISTEARIN

Triacylglyceride having three stearic acids esterified to the glycerol backbone.

TRITIUM (^{3}H+)

Radioactive hydrogen.

TRYPSIN

A proteolytic enzyme that attacks peptide bonds adjacent to arginine or lysine.

TRYPSINOGEN

Precursor of trypsin; trypsin is available after trypsinogen is acted on by enterokinase.

TRYPTOPHAN

An essential amino acid. (see Table 5).

TSH

Thyroid-stimulating hormone. A hormone released by the pituitary that stimulates the thyroid gland to make and release thyroxine.

TUBE FEEDING

See EnteralNutrition.

TULAREMIA

See Rabbit Fever.

2,3,7,8-TETRACHLORODIBENZO-P-DIOXIN (TCDD)

A well-known environmental pollutant formed at high temperatures (as in incinerators) from chlorinated hydrocarbons. It is also a contaminant of the herbicide 2,4,5-trichlorophenoxyacetic acid (2,4,5-T). On acute exposure, it is highly toxic. In experimental animals, it has been shown to induce liver damage, teratogenic effects, immune suppression, enzyme induction, and increased tumor incidence. In man, occupational exposures and industrial accidents involving TCDD have been associated with chloracne, liver damage, and polyneuropathy. The principal sources of TCDD exposure include spraying of crops with 2,4,5-T, ingestion of contaminated feed by livestock, magnification through food chains, and contamination of fruits and vegetables in the proximity of incinerators. The average daily intake of TCDD is set at 10 pg/kg/day.

TXA$_2$

Thromboxane A$_2$. An eicosanoid involved in stimulating platelet aggregation.

TYPES OF ANTINUTRITIVES

TYPE A ANTINUTRITIVES

Substances primarily interfering with the digestion of proteins or the absorption and utilization of amino acids. Also known as antiproteins. People depending on vegetables for their protein supply, as in developing countries, are in danger of impairment by this type of antinutritives. The most important type A antinutritives are protease inhibitors and lectins.

Protease inhibitors, occurring in many plant and animal tissues, are proteins that inhibit proteolytic enzymes by binding to the active sites of the enzymes. Proteolytic enzyme inhibitors were first found in avian eggs around the turn of the century. They were later identified as ovomucoid and ovoinhibitor, both of which inactivate trypsin. Chymotrypsin inhibitors also are found in avian egg whites. Other sources of trypsin and/or chymotrypsin inhibitors are soybeans and other legumes and pulses; vegetables; milk and colostrum; wheat and other cereal grains; guar gum; and white and sweet potatoes. The protease inhibitors of kidney beans, soybeans, and potatoes can additionally inhibit elastase, a pancreatic enzyme acting on elastin, an insoluble protein in meat. Animals given food containing active inhibitors show growth depression. This appears to be due to interference in trypsin and chymotrypsin activities and excessive stimulation of the secretory exocrine pancreatic cells, which become hypertrophic. Valuable proteins may be lost to the feces in this case. In vitro experiments with human proteolytic enzymes have been shown that trypsin inhibitors from bovine colostrum, lima beans, soybeans, kidney beans, and quail ovomucoid were active against human trypsin, whereas trypsin inhibitors originating from bovine and porcine pancreas, potatoes, chicken ovomucoid, and chicken ovoinhibitor were not. The soybean and lima bean trypsin inhibitors are also active against human chymotrypsin. Many protease inhibitors are heat labile, especially with moist heat. Relatively heat-resistant protease inhibitors include the antitryptic factor in milk, the alcohol-precipitable and nondialyzable trypsin inhibitor in alfalfa, the chymotrypsin inhibitor in potatoes, the kidney bean inhibitor, and the trypsin inhibitor in lima beans.

Lectin is the general term for plant proteins that have highly specific binding sites for carbohydrates. They are widely distributed among various sources such as soybeans, peanuts, jack beans, mung beans, lima beans, kidney beans, fava beans, vetch, yellow wax beans, hyacinth beans, lentils, peas, potatoes, bananas, mangoes, and wheat germ. Most plant lectins are glycoproteins, except concanavalin A from jack beans, which is carbohydrate free. The most toxic lectins include ricin in castor bean (oral toxic dose in man: 150–200 mg; intravenous toxic dose: 20 mg) and the lectins of kidney bean and hyacinth bean. The mode of action of lectins may be related to their ability to bind to specific cell receptors in a way comparable to that of antibodies. Because they are able to agglutinate red blood cells, they are also known as hemagglutinins. The binding of bean lectin on rat intestinal mucosal cells has been demonstrated in vitro, and it has been suggested that this action is responsible for the oral toxicity of the lectins. Such bindings may disturb the intestines' absorptive capacity for nutrients and other essential compounds. The lectins, being proteins, can easily be inactivated by moist heat. Germination decreases the hemagglutinating activity in varieties of peas and species of beans.

Type B Antinutritives

Substances interfering with the absorption or metabolic utilization of minerals. Also known as antiminerals. Although they are toxic per se, the amounts present in foods seldom cause acute intoxication under normal food consumption. However, they may harm the organism under suboptimum nutriture. The most important type B antinutritives are phytic acid, oxalates, and glucosinolates.

Phytic acid, or myo-inositol hexaphosphate, is a naturally occurring strong acid that binds to many types of bivalent and trivalent heavy metal ions, forming insoluble salts. Consequently, phytic acid reduces the availability of many minerals and essential trace elements. The degree of insolubility of these salts appear to depend on the nature of the metal, the pH of the solution, and for certain metals, the presence of another metal. Synergism between two metallic ions in the formation of phytate complexes has also been observed. For instance, zinc-calcium phytate precipitates maximally at pH 6, which is also the pH of the duodenum, where mainly calcium and trace metals are absorbed. Phytates are occurring in a wide variety of foods, such as cereals (e.g., wheat, rye, maize, rice, and barley); legumes and vegetables (e.g., bean, soybean, lentil, pea, and vetch); nuts and seeds (e.g., walnut, hazelnut, almond, peanut, and cocoa bean); and spices and flavoring agents (e.g., caraway, coriander, cumin, mustard, and nutmeg). From several experiments in animals and man, it has been observed that phytates exert negative effects on the availability of calcium, iron, magnesium, zinc, and other trace essential elements. These effects may be minimized considerably, if not eliminated, by increased intake of essential minerals. In the case of calcium, intake of cholecalciferol must also be adequate, since the activity of phytates on calcium absorption is enhanced when this vitamin is inadequate or limiting. In many foodstuffs, the phytic acid level can be reduced by phytase, an enzyme occurring in plants, that catalyzes the dephosphorylation of phytic acid.

Oxalic acid is a strong acid that forms water-soluble Na^+ and K^+ salts but less soluble salts with alkaline earth and other bivalent metals. Calcium oxalate is particularly insoluble at neutral or alkaline pH, whereas it readily dissolves in acid medium. Oxalates mainly exert effects on the absorption of calcium. These effects must be considered in terms of the oxalate/calcium ratio (in milliequivalent/milliequivalent): foods having a ratio greater than 1 may have negative effects on calcium availability, whereas foods with a ratio of 1 or below do not. Examples of foodstuffs having a ratio greater than 1 are rhubarb (8.5), spinach (4.3), beet (2.5–5.1), cocoa (2.6), coffee (3.9), tea (1.1), and potato (1.6). Harmful oxalates in food may be removed by soaking in water. Consumption of calcium-rich foods (e.g., dairy products and seafood), as well as augmented cholecalciferol intake, is recommended when large amounts of high-oxalate foods are consumed.

A variety of plants contain a third group of type B antinutritives, the glucosinolates, also known as thioglucosides. Many glucosinolates are goitrogenic. They have a general structure and yield on hydrolysis the active or actual goitrogens, such as thiocyanates, isothiocyanates, cyclic sulfur compounds, and nitriles. Three types of goiter can be identified: (1) cabbage goiter; (2) brassica seed goiter; and (3) legume goiter. Cabbage goiter, also known as struma, is induced by excessive consumption of cabbage. It seems that cabbage goitrogens inhibit iodine uptake by directly affecting the thyroid gland. Cabbage goiter can be treated by iodine supplementation. Brassica seed goiter can result from the consumption of the seeds of brassica plants (e.g., rutabaga, turnip, cabbage, and rape), which contain goitrogens that prevent thyroxine synthesis. This type of goiter can only be treated by administration of the thyroid hormone. Legume goiter is induced by goitrogens in legumes like soybeans and peanuts. It differs from cabbage goiter in that the thyroid gland does not lose its activity for iodine. Inhibition of the intestinal absorption of iodine or the reabsorption of thyroxine has been shown in this case. Legume goiter can be treated by iodine therapy. Glucosinolates, which have been shown to induce goiter, at least in experimental animals, are found in several foods and feedstuffs: broccoli (buds), brussels sprouts (head), cabbage (head), cauliflower (buds), garden cress (leaves), horseradish (roots), kale (leaves), kohlrabi (head), black and white mustard (seed), radish (root), rape (seed), rutabaga (root), and turnips (root and seed). One of the most potent glucosinolates is progoitrin from the seeds of brassica plants and the roots of rutabaga. Hydrolysis of this compound yields 1-cyano-2-hydroxy-3-butene, 1-cyano-2-hydroxy-3,4-butylepisulfide, 2-hydroxy-3,4-butenylisothiocyanate, and (S)-5-vinyl-oxazolidone-2-thione, also known as goitrin. The latter product interferes, together with its R-enantiomer, with the iodination of thyroxine precursors, so that the resulting goiter cannot be treated by iodine therapy.

TYPE C ANTINUTRITIVES

Naturally occurring substances that can decompose vitamins, form unabsorbable complexes with them, or interfere with their digestive or metabolic utilization. Also known as antivitamins. The most important type C antinutritives are ascorbic acid oxidase, antithiamine factors, and antipyridoxine factors.

Ascorbic acid oxidase is a copper-containing enzyme that catalyzes the oxidation of free ascorbic acid to diketogluconic acid, oxalic acid, and other oxidation products. It has been reported to occur in many fruits (e.g., peaches and bananas) and vegetables (e.g., cucumbers, pumpkins, lettuce, cress, cauliflowers, spinach, green beans, green peas, carrots, potatoes, tomatoes, beets, and kohlrabi). The enzyme is active between pH 4 and 7 (optimum pH 5.6–6.0); its optimum temperature is 38°C. The enzyme is released when plant cells are broken. Therefore, if fruits and vegetables are cut, vitamin C content decreases gradually. Ascorbic acid oxidase can be inhibited effectively at pH 2 or by blanching at around 100°C. Ascorbic acid can also be protected against ascorbic acid oxidase by substances of plant origin. Flavonoids, such as the flavonols quercetin and kempferol, present in fruits and vegetables, strongly inhibit the enzyme.

A second group of type C antinutritives are the antithiamine factors, which interact with thiamine. Antithiamine factors can be grouped as thiaminases, catechols, and tannins. Thiaminases, which are enzymes that split thiamine at the methylene linkage, are found in many freshwater and saltwater fish species and in certain species of crab and clam. They contain a nonprotein coenzyme, structurally related to hemin. This enzyme is the actual antithiamine factor. Thiaminases in fish and other sources can be destroyed by cooking. Antithiamine factors of plant origin include catechols and tannins. The most well-known ortho-catechol is found in bracken fern. In fact, there are two types of heat-stable antithiamine factors in this fern, one of which has been identified as caffeic acid, which can also by hydrolyzed from chlorogenic acid (found in green coffee beans) by intestinal bacteria. Other ortho-catechols, such as methylsinapate occurring in mustard seed and rapeseed, also have antithiamine activity. The mechanism of thiamine inactivation by these compounds requires oxygen and is dependent on temperature and pH. The reaction appears to proceed in two phases: (1) a rapid initial phase, which is reversible by the addition of reducing agents (e.g., ascorbic acid), and (2) a slower subsequent phase, which is irreversible. Tannins, occurring in a variety of plants, including tea, similarly possess antithiamine activity. Thiamine is one of the vitamins that is likely to be deficient in the diet. Thus, persistent consumption of antithiamine factors and the possible presence of thiaminase-producing bacteria in the gastrointestinal tract may compromise the already marginal thiamine intake.

A variety of plants and mushrooms contain pyridoxine (a form of vitamin B_6) antagonists. These antipyridoxine factors have been identified as hydrazine derivatives. Linseed contains the water-soluble and heat-labile antipyridoxine factor linatine (g-glutamyl-1-amino-D-proline). Hydrolysis of linatine yields the actual antipyridoxine factor 1-amino-proline. Antipyridoxine factors have also been found in wild mushrooms, the common commercial edible mushroom, and the Japanese mushroom shiitake. Commercial and shiitake mushrooms contain agaritine. Hydrolysis of agaritine by g-glutamyl transferase, which is endogenous to the mushroom, yields the active agent 4-hydroxy-methylphenylhydrazine. Disruption of the cells of the mushroom can accelerate hydrolysis; careful handling of the mushroom and immediate blanching after cleaning and cutting can prevent hydrolysis. The mechanism underlying the antipyridoxine activity is believed to be condensation of the hydrazines with the carbonyl compounds pyridoxal and pyridoxal phosphate (the active form of the vitamin), resulting in the formation of inactive hydrazones.

TYRAMINE

The amine of tyrosine; an amine with vasoactive effects similar to epinephrine. It is found in French cheese, cheddar cheese, yeast, chianti, and canned fish. It can also be produced by microorganisms in the gut. Symptoms of migraine headache and urticaria can occur in sensitive persons.

TYROSINASE

A copper-containing enzyme that catalyzes the conversion of tyrosine to melanin.

TYROSINE

An amino acid that results from the hydroxylation of phenylalanine (see Table 5).

TYROSINOSIS

A rare genetic disorder due to a lack of parahydroxyphenylpyruvic acid oxidase, which catalyzes the conversion of tyrosine to homogentisic acid. Characterized by elevated blood and urine levels of tyrosine, liver damage, mental retardation, and rickets.

U

UBIQUINONE

Coenzyme Q, an electron carrier that is part of the respiratory chain in the mitochondria.

ULCERATIVE COLITIS

A type of inflammatory bowel disease that primarily affects the rectum and colon.

ULTRA TRACE ELEMENTS

Minerals required in extremely small amounts. (See Minerals.)

UMBILICAL CORD

Connection between the developing fetus and the placenta.

UMP, UDP, UTP

Uridine mono-, di- or triphosphate. A high-energy compound essential to glycogen synthesis.

URACIL

Pyrimidine base used in DNA.

UREA

Waste product of amino acid degradation.

UREA CYCLE

A cyclic series of reactions that converts carbamyl phosphate to urea. (See Metabolic Maps, Appendix 2.)

UREMIA

Blood urea levels above 25 mg/dL.

URIC ACID

Crystalline acid, excreted in urine, from purine metabolism.

URIDINE

Uracil with a ribose group attached.

UROLITHIASIS

Urinary tract stone or calculi.

URTICARIA

A vascular reaction of the skin characterized by severe itching and rash.

UTERUS

Womb; vessel that houses the embryo and developing fetus.

V

VACCENIC ACID

A naturally occurring trans fatty acid that has antiatherogenic effects in LDL-receptor–deficient individuals.

VALDECOXIB

A nonsteroidal anti-inflammatory drug that works by inhibiting the COX-2 enzyme. Trade name: Bextra.

VALIDITY (OF A MEASUREMENT)

The concordance between the value of a measurement and the true value. A high reproducibility is a prerequisite for validity but does not automatically imply validity. With regard to the validity of the results of epidemiological studies, a distinction is made between internal and external validity.

VALINE

An essential amino acid (see Table 5).

VALSARTAN

An angiotensin II antagonist that serves as an antihypertensive agent. Trade name: Diovan.

VASOACTIVE COMPOUNDS

Compounds that elicit either vasoconstriction or vasodilation.

VASOCONSTRICTION

Constriction of the vascular tree with the result of an increase in blood pressure.

VASODILATION

Relaxation of the vascular tree with the result of a fall in blood pressure.

VASOPRESSIN

Antidiuretic hormone (ADH) released by the pituitary. Stimulates water reabsorption by the kidney.

VEAL

Meat from an immature bovine.

VECTOR

A plasmid or bacteriophage into which foreign DNA can be introduced for the purposes of cloning.

VEGAN

An individual who subsists on a diet free of meat, milk, egg, cheese, and fish. May be at risk of vitamin B_{12} deficiency.

VEGETABLE ALLERGY

This kind of allergy may be provoked by beans (soy), peas, and peanuts. Peanut allergy is especially well known. Extensive reactions include urticaria, angioedema, nausea, vomiting, rhinitis, and dyspnea. Anaphylactic shock is not uncommon. The peanut allergen is very stable; it is resistant to all kinds of processing. In peanut butter and peanut flour (which is added to quite a few food products), the peanut allergen is still detectable, whereas it is not or seldom present in peanut oil. Similarly, the soy allergen is rarely found in soy oil. Allergy to a particular legume does not invariably imply allergic sensitivity to all members of the legume family.

VEGETARIAN DIET

There are several variants of the vegetarian diet. They include the consumption of all foods except meat but can include fish, eggs, milk, and milk products; the consumption of all foods except meat and fish, but can include eggs, milk, and milk products; and the consumption of fruits and vegetables with the exclusion of all foods of animal origin.

VERY-LOW-CALORIE DIET

Diet containing <1000 calories per day.

VILLI

Fingerlike projections from the small intestinal wall that function in the absorption of nutrients.

VIP

Vasoactive peptide. A neuropeptide originating in the neurons of the gastrointestinal system.

VIRAL HEPATITIS

Inflammation of the liver caused by a viral infection. Five types of viral hepatitis (hepatitis A, B, C, D, and E) have been identified by their unique methods of transmission, onset, and laboratory findings.

VISCERAL PROTEIN

Body protein in components other than muscle tissue such as internal organs and blood.

VITAL CAPACITY

Maximal amount of gas that can be exhaled after a maximal inspiration.

VITAMINS

A group of small organic compounds that cannot be synthesized in the body and, therefore, are considered essential nutrients. They are divided into two groups: (1) fat-soluble vitamins, and (2) water-soluble vitamins. The fat-soluble vitamins include vitamins A, D, E, and K. The water-soluble vitamins include thiamin, riboflavin, niacin, pyridoxine, pantothenic acid, biotin, vitamin B_{12}, choline, and ascorbic acid.

VITAMIN A

Vitamin A is not a single compound. It exists in several forms and is found in a variety of foods such as liver and highly colored vegetables. The International Union of Pure and Applied Chemistry–International Union of Biochemistry (IUPAC–IUB) Commission on Biochemical Nomenclature has proposed the following rules for naming the compounds having vitamin A activity: The parent substance, all-trans vitamin A alcohol, is designated "all-trans retinol." Derivatives of this compound are named accordingly. In Table 51, the major vitamin A compounds are listed.

In foods of animal origin, the vitamin usually occurs as the alcohol (retinol). However, it can also occur as an aldehyde (retinal) or as an acid (retinoic acid). In foods of plant origin, the vitamin is associated with plant pigments and is a member of the carotene family of compounds. These compounds can be converted to vitamin A in the animal body and are known as provitamins. Of the carotenes, β-carotene is the most potent. Figure 61 gives the structure of vitamin A as all-trans retinol.

There are a number of biologically important compounds that have vitamin A activity. All of these compounds have a β-ionene ring to which an isoprenoid chain is attached. This structure is essential if a compound is to have vitamin activity. If any substitutions to the chain or ring occur, then the activity of the compound as vitamin A is reduced. The preparation of a methyl ester or other esters at carbon 15 results in a very stable compound with full vitamin activity. In addition to improving the chemical stability of the compound, these ester forms confer an improved solubility in food oils. These vitamin ester forms are frequently used in food products for vitamin enrichment.

If the side chain is lengthened or shortened, vitamin activity is lost. Activity is also reduced if the unsaturations are converted to saturated bonds or if the side chain is isomerized. Oxidation of the β-ionene ring and/or removal of its methyl groups likewise reduce its vitamin activity. Some of these substituted or isomerized forms are potent therapeutic agents. The provitamin A group consists of members of the carotene family. More than 600 members of the carotenoid family of

---

TABLE 51
Nomenclature of Major Compounds
in the Vitamin A Group

Recommended Name	Synonyms
Retinol	Vitamin A alcohol, axerophthol
Retinal	Vitamin A aldehyde, retinene, retinaldehyde
Retinoic acid	Vitamin A acid
3-Dehydroretinal	Vitamin A_2 (alcohol)
3-Dehydroretinol	Vitamin A_2 aldehyde; retinene
3-Dehydroretinoic acid	Vitamin A_2 acid
Anhydroretinol	Anhydro vitamin A
Retro retinol	Rehydrovitamin A
5,6-Epoxyretinol	5,6-Epoxyvitamin A alcohol
Retinyl palmitate	Vitamin A palmitate

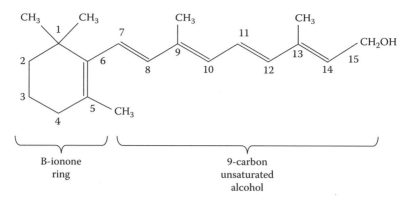

FIGURE 61   Structure of all-trans retinal.

TABLE 52
Carotenoids with Vitamin A Activity[a]

Compound	Relative Potency
β-carotene	100
α-carotene	53
γ-carotene	43
Cryptoxanthin	57
Lycopene	0
Zeaxanthin	0
Xanthophyll	0

[a] Reference compound for subsequent compounds. Note that β-carotene compared to all-trans retinol, is only half as active as all-trans retinol.

pigments exist. However, only 50 or so can be converted (or degraded) into components that have vitamin activity. All these compounds have many conjugated double bonds, and thus each can form a variety of geometric isomers. The vitamin A activity of the provitamin members of the carotene family is variable. Theoretically, β-carotene should provide two molecules of retinol, but it does not because of differences in absorption and inefficient cleavage of the molecule. In general, if consumed in the pure form in an oily solution, the β-carotene molecule will provide about 50% of its quantity as vitamin A. When consumed as part of a food matrix, only one-twelfth of the consumed carotene is available as active vitamin. During its cleavage by the enzyme β-carotenoid 15,15′dioxy-genase, there is some oxidative conversion of the cleavage product to retinal and some oxidation to retinoic acid. This retinoic acid is rapidly excreted in the urine. The carotene content of food varies with the growing conditions and the post harvest storage of the food. Other carotenes are less potent than β-carotene. These compounds are listed in Table 52. Note that some of these compounds, that is, xanthophylls and lycopenes, have no vitamin activity even though they are highly colored and are related chemically to carotene. They may have other biological functions but no vitamin activity.

All-trans retinol is a nearly colorless oil and is soluble in such fat solvents as ether, ethanol, chloroform, and methanol. While fairly stable to the moderate heat needed to cook foods, it is unstable to very high heat, to light, and to oxidation by oxidizing agents. Antioxidants can retard or reduce these vitamin losses.

Retinal, the aldehyde, combines with various amines to form Schiff bases. This reaction is important to the formation of rhodopsin within the visual cycle. All-trans retinal also reacts with both the sulfhydryl and amino groups of cysteine and the amino group of tryptophan to form a five-membered thiazolidine ring. The formation of the thiazolidine ring is enhanced if formaldehyde is present. The resulting compound has a red color, which is bleached upon exposure to light. This reaction, similar to the bleaching of rhodopsin (the visual pigment in the eye) with light exposure, does not utilize the same amino acid that is used in rhodopsin. In the latter, retinal binds to the ε amino group of lysine rather than the amino group of tryptophan or cysteine. Bleaching occurs when the energy transmitted by the light causes a shift in the electrons within the N-retinyl lysine. The same principle is involved in the loss of color with light exposure of N-retinyl cysteine and N-retinyl tryptophan. In nature, vitamin A and carotene are bound to proteins, particularly the lipoproteins. Indeed, the vitamin is stored as an ester in those tissues (notably the liver) that synthesize lipoprotein. Usually retinol is covalently bound to palmitic acid as well as being associated with a protein. The vitamin also complexes with other proteins as part of its mechanism of action at the subcellular level.

One international unit (IU) of vitamin A is defined as the activity of 0.3 μg of all-trans retinol. Because β-carotene must be converted to retinol to be active and because this conversion is not 100% efficient, 1 μg of all-trans β-carotene is equivalent to 0.167 μg of all-trans retinol. For other members of the carotene family, appropriate correction factors must be applied to determine the vitamin A activity in terms of retinol equivalents (REs). In general, however, 1 mg of retinol is roughly equivalent to 6 mg β-carotene and 12 mg of mixed dietary carotenes. The U.S. Institute of Medicine now recommends the use of REs rather than IUs. The use of the term RE allows for the calculation of the vitamin A activity found in a variety of foods, each containing one or more vitamin A compounds. For example, if 100 g of a given food contained 100 mg of α-carotene, which has 53% of the potency of β-carotene, the retinol equivalence would be $100 \times .53 \times 0.167$ or 8.851. Thus, this food would provide 8.851 RE or 29.5 IU of vitamin A (8.851/0.3) per 100 g. Most tables of food composition give the vitamin A content in terms of IU; however, the reader should be aware of how these units are derived and realize that corrections must be made to allow for availability and efficiency of conversion of the provitamin to the active vitamin form, all-trans retinol. Table 53 lists the REs for major A vitamin sources.

Vitamin A and its carotene precursors are present in a variety of foods. Red meat, liver, whole milk, cheese, butter, and fortified margarine are but a few of the foods containing retinol. Carotene-rich foods include the highly colored fruits and vegetables such as squash, carrots, rich green vegetables (peas, beans, etc.), yellow fruits (peaches, apricots), and vegetable oils.

The absorption of the vitamin depends largely on the form ingested, whether food lipids are present, and on the presence and activity of the system responsible for its uptake. It is generally accepted that all-trans retinol is the preferred form for absorption. Retinal and retinoic acid are less well absorbed, although both will disappear from the intestinal contents at a rate commensurate with a rate associated with an active transport system. Absorption requires the presence of food

TABLE 53
REs for Humans[a]

Compound	μg/IU	IU/μg	RE/μg
All-trans retinol	0.300	3.33	1.00
All-trans retinyl acetate	0.344	2.91	–
All-trans retinyl palmitate	0.549	1.82	–
All-trans β-carotene (in a food matrix)	1.800	0.56	0.167[b]
Mixed carotenoids	3.600	0.28	0.083

[a] From Olson, J. A. Vitamin A. In: *Handbook of Vitamins*, 2nd ed., ed. L. J. Machlin, pp. 1–57. New York: Marcel Dekker, Inc.

[b] When pure β-carotene in oily suspension is administered, 2 μg converts to 1 μg of retinol; http://www.nap.edu.

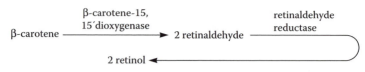

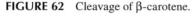

FIGURE 62 Cleavage of β-carotene.

lipid and bile salts and the presence of a transport protein, the retinol-binding protein. Carotenoids are absorbed less efficiently, via diffusion. There is no active carrier for carotene within the luminal cell. The carotenoids are transported by lipoproteins as are the retinyl esters. Carotene is oxidatively cleaved to retinal and to small amounts of longer chain apocarotenoids prior to absorption. The major cleavage products are retinol and retinoic acid (Figure 62).

Both central and eccentric cleavage is possible. The cleavage enzymes are very unstable. They are rapidly inactivated. Two enzymes are involved in the cleavage: The first, β-carotene-15, 15′diox-ygenase, catalyzes the cleavage of the central double bond to yield two molecules of retinaldehyde. The second enzyme, retinaldehyder eductase, catalyzes the reduction of retinaldehyde to retinol. In order for the first enzyme to work, the β-carotene must be solubilized. This means that bile salts and some lipid must be present. Oxygen is also required since this is a dioxygenase type of reaction. The enzyme of the second reaction, retinaldehyder eductase, is also a soluble mucosal cell enzyme. It requires the presence of either NADPH or NADH as donors of REs.

There are two pathways for retinol esterification. In the first, an acyl CoA–independent reaction is used. This involves the formation of a complex between retinol and type II cellular retinol-binding protein (CRBP II). As retinol intake increases there is a corresponding increase in the activity of the enzyme (acyl CoA retinol acyl transferase), which catalyzes the formation of this complex. The CRBP II is found only in the cytosol of the intestinal mucosal cell and, interestingly, its synthesis is influenced by the intake of particular fatty acids. The second pathway is an acyl CoA–dependent pathway whereby retinol is bound to any protein, not just the aforementioned specific CRBP. In both pathways, the retinol is protein bound prior to ester formation.

In food, all-trans retinol is usually esterified to long-chain fatty acids. Palmitic acid is the most common of these fatty acids. The ester is hydrolyzed in the intestine by a specific esterase that is, in some species, activated by the bile salt sodium taurocholate. After the ester has been hydrolyzed, the resulting retinol is actively transported (carrier mediated) into the mucosal cell where it is then reesterified to a long-chain fatty acid (palmitic acid) and incorporated into lymph chylomicrons. The absorption of vitamin A follows the same route as the long-chain fatty acids of the dietary tria-cylglycerides, cholesterol, and cholesterol esters. The chylomicrons are absorbed by the lacteals of the lymphatic system and enter the circulation when the thoracic duct joins the circulatory system at the vena cava. Once in the vascular compartment, the triacylglyceride of the retinol-containing chylomicron is removed, leaving the protein carrier, retinol, and cholesterol. Whereas the triacylg-lycerides are removed from the chylomicrons by the extrahepatic tissues, retinol is removed by the liver. In the liver, hydrolysis and reesterification occur once again as the vitamin enters the hepato-cyte and is stored within the cell associated with droplets of lipid. Retinoic acid is absorbed by the portal system and does not accumulate in the liver. Retinoic acid, because it is not stored, represents only a very small percentage of the body's vitamin A content.

A specific protein is needed for the subsequent transport of retinol from the liver to the peripheral target tissues. This protein is called retinol-binding protein (RBP). RBP is synthesized in the liver. It is a single polypeptide chain (molecular weight: 21,000 Da) and possesses a single binding site for retinol. The mobilization of vitamin A from the liver requires this protein. In plasma, vitamin A circulates bound to the RBP that forms a protein-protein complex with transthyretin, a tetramer that also binds thyroxine in a 1:1 complex. Because this complex contains the vitamin and thyrox-ine, there is an association of thyroid status and vitamin A status. RBP is responsive to nutritional status. In protein-malnourished children it is depressed while in vitamin A–deficient individuals it is elevated. Patients with renal disease have elevated levels of RBP and may be at risk of developing vitamin A toxicity if vitamin A intake is above normal. In the patient with renal disease, the increase in the RBP is probably due to the decreased capacity of the kidney to remove the protein. The kidney is the main catabolic site for RBP. Where protein intakes are low, binding-protein levels are also low, thus explaining the simultaneous observations of symptoms of protein and retinol deficiency in malnourished children. This association is due to the inability of the liver in the protein-malnourished child to synthesize RBP; thus, the child is unable to utilize the hepatic vitamin stores. Once protein is restored to the diet, symptoms of both deficiency syndromes disappear. If dietary retinol (or its precursors) is lacking, serum RBP levels fall while hepatic levels rise. Within minutes after retinol is given to a deficient individual, these changes are reversed: serum levels rise while hepatic levels fall. Compounds that influence the levels of this binding protein influence the mobilization and excretion of retinol. Estrogens increase the level of this protein, whereas cadmium poisoning, because it increases excretion, reduces the level of this protein.

Once the RBP complex arrives at the target tissue, it must then bind to its receptor site on the cell membrane. The retinol is released from the serum RBP and transferred into the cell where it is then bound to intracellular binding proteins. These binding proteins are highly specific for the different vitamin A forms. The CRBP is the cellular RBP, while CRABP is the cellular retinoic acid binding protein. CRLBP is the retinal binding protein and IRBP is the interphotoreceptor or interstitial RBP. The latter is found only in the extracellular space of the retina. CRBP (II) is the RBP found in the mucosal cells of the small intestine. The presence of these binding proteins in different tissues is highly variable. See Table 54 for the features and functions of these binding proteins.

TABLE 54
Retinol Binding Proteins (RBPs)

Acronym	Protein	Molecular Weight (Da)	Location	Function
RBP	Retinol-binding protein	21,000	Plasma	Transports all-trans retinol from intestinal absorption site to target tissues.
CRBP	Cellular retinol-binding protein	14,600	Cells of target tissue	Transports all-trans retinol from plasma membrane to organelles within the cell.
CRBP II	Cellular retinol-binding protein type II	16,000	Absorptive cells of small intestine	Transports all-trans retinol from absorptive sites on plasma membrane of mucosal cells.
CRABP	Cellular retinoic acid–binding protein	14,600	Cells of target tissue	Transports all-trans retinoic acid to the nucleus.
CRALBP	Cellular retinal binding protein	33,000	Specific cells in the eye	Transports 11-cis retinal and 11-cis retinol as part of the visual cycle.
IRBP	Interphotoreceptor or interstitial retinol–binding protein	144,000	Retina	Transports all-trans retinol and 11-cis retinal in the retina extracellular space.
RAR	Nuclear retinoic acid receptor, three main forms (α, β, γ)		All cells α—liver β—brain γ—liver, kidney, lung	Binds retinoic acid and regions of DNA.
RXR	Nuclear retinoic acid receptors, multiple forms			

Vitamin A has several important functions in the body: it plays an essential role in protein synthesis and cell turnover. Some of the earliest reports of retinol deficiency include observations on the changes in epithelial cells of animals fed vitamin A–deficient diets. Normal columnar epithelial cells were replaced by squamous keratinizing epithelium. These changes were reversed when vitamin A was restored to the diet. Epithelial cells, particularly those lining the gastrointestinal tract, have very short half-lives (in the order of 3–7 days) and as such are replaced frequently. Thus, in vitamin A deficiency, changes in these cells, as well as other cells having a rapid turnover time, indicates that the vitamin functions at the level of protein synthesis and cellular differentiation. Protein catabolism, in general, increases in vitamin A–deficient rats as does the activity of the urea cycle enzymes. Table 55 lists a number of cellular proteins regulated by retinoic acid. Vitamin A (as retinoic acid) plays an essential role in gene expression. Retinol is converted to retinoic acid, which regulates cell function by binding to nuclear and mitochondrial retinoic acid receptors that in turn bind to DNA. Two distinct families of receptors have been identified; both of these families, called RAR and RXR, have multiple forms, and both are structurally similar to the receptor that binds the steroid and thyroid hormones. These receptors function as ligand-activated transcription factors (see Table 54) that regulate mRNA transcription. In some instances these factors stimulate transcription, and in other instances they suppress the process. There is also an interaction of vitamin A with other vitamins. For example, the synthesis of the calcium-binding protein calbindin is usually regulated by vitamin D. This protein, found in the intestinal mucosal cells and the kidney, is also found in the brain. In the brain its synthesis is regulated by retinoic acid rather than vitamin D.

TABLE 55
Retinoic Acid Responsive Proteins

I. Proteins that have their synthesis increased due to RA-receptor effect on the transcription of their mRNA

Growth hormone	Neuronal cell
Transforming growth factor β2	Calcium-binding protein
Transglutaminase	Calbindin DZ8K
Phosphoenolpyruvate carboxykinase	Ornithine decarboxylase
Gsα	Osteocalcin
Alcohol dehydrogenase	
t plasminogen activator	
Glycerophosphate dehydrogenase	

II. Retinoic acid proteins that function in mRNA transcription

1,25-$(OH)_2D_3$ receptors
Retinoic acid receptors β
c-Fos[a]
Progesterone receptors[a]
Zif 268 transcription factor
AP-2 transcription factor
MSH receptors
Interleukin-6 receptors[a]
Interleukin-2 receptors
EGF receptors (corneal endothelium)
EGF receptors (corneal epithelium)[a]
Peroxisomal proliferator–activated receptors

[a] The activity of these proteins are suppressed when the RA-receptor is bound to them.

In vitamin A–deficient brain cells, additions of retinoic acids increased the mRNA for calbindin synthesis. Additions of vitamin D were without effect. The retinoic acid receptors contain zinc finger protein sequence motifs, which mediate its binding to DNA. The carboxyl terminal end of the receptor functions in this ligand binding. Retinoic acid binding to nuclear receptors sets in motion a sequence of events that culminate in a change in transcription of the cis-linked gene. That is, proteins are synthesized and these proteins bind to regions of the promoter adjacent to the start site of the DNA that is to be transcribed. Such binding either activates or suppresses transcription and, as a result, there are corresponding increases or decreases in the mRNA coding for specific proteins, which in turn lead to changes in cell function. Table 56 lists a number of enzymes that have been reported to be affected by the deficient state. In each of these instances, it could be assumed that the reason for the change in activity could be explained by the effect of vitamin A on the synthesis of these enzymes. Where there is an increase, it is likely that transcription and hence synthesis is usually suppressed (or kept within normal bounds) when vitamin A intake is adequate.

There is another aspect of vitamin A nutriture that is of importance when the function of this vitamin is considered. This concerns the structure and function of the nuclear retinoic acid-binding protein, the RA receptor. Should this receptor not be synthesized, as can occur in the absence of retinoic acid, the whole cascade of events dependent on the binding of the RA-receptor complex will not occur. Further, should the receptor itself be aberrant in amino acid sequence, both its capacity to bind RA and its affinity for specific regions of the DNA will be affected.

REPRODUCTION AND GROWTH

The role of vitamin A in the growth process is related to its function in RNA synthesis as described earlier. Epithelial cells of the mouth and gastrointestinal system are affected, particularly those cells that secrete lubricating and digestive fluids in the mouth, stomach, and intestinal tract. The lack of lubrication due to atrophy of these important cells affects food intake and results in poor growth. The vitamin has a role in reproduction that is related to its role in RNA and protein synthesis. Several of the enzymes listed in Table 56 are involved in the synthesis of reproduction hormones. Of the other enzymes listed, three (ATPase, arginase, and xanthine oxidase) relate primarily to energy or protein wastage, as would be expected in a deficient animal, and which are increased in the

TABLE 56
Enzymes That Are Affected by Vitamin A Deficiency

Enzyme	Reaction	Effect
ATPase	ATP $\leftrightarrow$ ADP + Pi	Increase
Arginase	L-arginine $\rightarrow$ ornithine + urea	Increase
Xanthine oxidase	Hypoxanthine $\rightarrow\rightarrow$ uric acid	Increase
Alanine amino transferase	L-alanine α-ketoglutarate $\rightarrow$ pyruvate + L-glutamate	No change
Aspartate amino transferase	L-aspartate + αketoglutarate $\rightarrow$ oxaloacetate + L-glutamate	No change
Vitamin A palmitate hydrolase	Vitamin A palmitate $\rightarrow$ vitamin A + palmitic acid	No change
Vitamin A ester synthetase	Vitamin A + fatty acid $\rightarrow$ ester	No change
$\Delta^{5,3}$ β-hydroxysteroid dehydrogenase	Removal of H progesterone, glucocorticoid, estrogen, testosterone	Decrease
11β-steroid hydroxylase	Synthesis of steroid hormones	Decrease
ATP sulfurylase sulfotransferase	ATP + SO_4 $\rightarrow$ adenyl sulfate + PPi^{-3} Transfers sulfuryl groups to −O and −N of suitable groups	Decrease
	Synthesis of mucopolysaccharides	Decrease
L-γ-gulonolactone oxidase	L-gulonolactone $\rightarrow$ L-ascorbic acid	Decrease
p-hydroxyphenol pyruvate oxidase	p-hydroxyphenyl pyruvate $\rightarrow$ homogentisic acid	Decrease

deficient animal. The levels of transferase and the enzymes of retinol metabolism are unchanged, while those of the enzymes for the synthesis of mucopolysaccharides are decreased. Observations of increases in the phospholipid content of a variety of cellular and subcellular membranes in vitamin A–deficient rats suggest that enzymes of lipid metabolism are also affected. Cholesterol absorption is increased in the deficient rat, and this increase may in turn affect phospholipid synthesis and membrane phospholipid content since mammalian plasma membranes consist largely of cholesterol and phospholipids. The secondary characteristics of vitamin A deficiency again are probably related to the role of the vitamin in protein synthesis as described earlier. The primary characteristics of decreased dark adaptation, poor growth, reduced reproductive capacity, xerophthalmia, kerotomalacia, and anemia are all related. Vitamin A deficiency in developing mammals affects the central nervous system. Features of neurodegenerative disorders have been reported to occur in severely malnourished deficient animals.

VISION

Of the various functions vitamin A serves, its role in the maintenance of dark adaptation was the first to be fully described on a molecular basis. When animals are deprived of vitamin A, the amount of rhodopsin in the retina declines. This is followed by decreases in the amount of the protein opsin. Rhodopsin is present in the rod cells of the retina of most animals. All-trans retinol is transported and transferred into the cell, and then converted to all-trans retinal. All-trans retinal is isomerized to the active vitamin 11-cis retinal, which combines with opsin to form rhodopsin. Rhodopsin is an asymmetric protein with a molecular weight of about 38,000 Da. It has both a hydrophilic and a hydrophobic region with a folded length of about 70Å. It spans the membrane of the retina via seven helical segments that cross back and forth and comprises about 60% of the membrane protein. The light-sensitive portion of the molecule resides in its hydrophobic region. When rhodopsin is exposed to light it changes its shape. The primary photochemical event is the very rapid isomerization of 11-cis retinal to a highly strained trans form, bathorhodopsin. Note that the alcohol (retinol) and the aldehyde (retinal) are interchangeable with respect to the maintenance of the visual function.

Retinoic acid is ineffective primarily because there are no enzymes in the eye to convert the retinoic acid to the active 11-cis retinal needed for the formation of rhodopsin. The 11-cis retinol is also involved in the formation of iodopsin in the cones, and the photochemical isomerization of the 11-cis isomer triggers the visual process. In the rhodopsin breakdown process, an electrical potential arises and generates an electrical impulse that is transmitted via the optic nerve to the brain.

Because the vitamin is stored in the liver, it is possible to develop a toxic condition when high levels of the vitamin are consumed. In humans, hypervitaminosis A is characterized by increased intracranial pressure resulting in headaches, blurring vision, vomiting, lack of muscular coordination, abnormal liver function, and pain in the weight-bearing bones and joints. In young children, a bulging fontanel has been observed. Because of the limitation in the conversion of carotenes to retinol, vitamin A intoxication is less likely with large intakes of carotene; however, reports of yellowing of the skin of persons consuming large amounts of carrot juice have appeared. This yellowing is likely due to the deposition of carotene in subcutaneous fat.

There is no treatment except for the discontinuance of vitamin A consumption for the hypervitaminosis state. Elevated tissue levels fall only slowly after intake has stopped as the body has a tendency to conserve its vitamin store. Intakes of retinol that are higher than normal but not overtly toxic may have adverse consequences. Data from population studies have suggested that intakes in excess of the RDI for retinol may reduce bone mineralization and contribute to the development of osteoporosis. The relative risk of hip fracture, for example, appears to increase relative to the excess of retinol consumed but not with the increase in carotenoid consumption. The Institute of Medicine has recommended an upper limit for retinal intake based on life stage. For infants, the upper limit is 600 μg/day; for children, 600–900 μg/day; for adolescents, 1700–3000 μg/day; and for pregnant and lactating women, 2800–3000 μg/day. These upper limits are two to three times the recommended intake levels for these life stage groups.

VITAMIN B$_1$

See Thiamine.

VITAMIN B$_2$

See Riboflavin.

VITAMIN B$_3$

See Niacin.

VITAMIN B$_6$

See Pyridoxine.

VITAMIN B$_{12}$

Vitamin B$_{12}$ is a very complex structure, as shown in Figure 63. The term B$_{12}$ is the generic descriptor for all corrinoids, or those compounds having a corrin ring. Cyanocobalamin is the trivial designation for this compound. In order to have vitamin activity, it must contain a cobalt-centered corrin ring. There are a number of structural analogs that have vitamin activity. The ring consists of four reduced pyrrole rings linked by three methylene bridges and one direct bond. The cobalt atom is in the 3$^+$ state and can form up to six coordinate bonds. It is tightly bound to the four pyrrole N atoms and can also bond a nucleotide and a small ligand below and above the ring, respectively.

Vitamin B$_{12}$ is moderately soluble in water (12.5 mg/mL). It is insoluble in fat solvents. It is a heat-stable red crystal but will decompose at temperatures above 210°C. The crystal will melt at temperatures above 300°C. It is unstable to ultraviolet light, acid conditions, and in the presence of metals such as iron and copper. Organ meats are good sources of B$_{12}$. It is synthesized in the gastrointestinal system by the resident flora.

The process of absorption begins in the stomach where preformed B$_{12}$ is bound to a carrier protein called intrinsic factor. As B$_{12}$ is made by the gut flora, it too is bound to a carrier protein. Whether this carrier is identical to that available in the stomach is not known. Actually, there are four structurally distinct B$_{12}$ carrier proteins. Intrinsic factor is one of these and another, called R binder, is found in the proximal part of the alimentary tract. The R binder is degraded by the pancreatic peptidases and proteases, while the intrinsic factor–B$_{12}$ complex proceeds intact to the distal portion of the ileum where in the presence of calcium and neutral pH the complex binds to a receptor (called IF) on the surface of the luminal epithelial cell. Subsequent to binding of the complex to IF, the vitamin appears in the portal blood bound to a fourth transcobalamin II (TCII). The blood contains an additional R-type protein called transcobalamin I (TCI), which assists in the transport of the vitamin to its target cells. Although absorption occurs mainly in the distal ileum, it also occurs in the large intestine. This takes advantage of the fact that B$_{12}$ is synthesized by the intestinal flora in this part of the intestinal tract. The mechanism of absorption by the ileum is likely an active one mediated by the intrinsic factor; however, the details of this mechanism are unknown except for the need for the carriers as described earlier. Similarly, the transport of B$_{12}$ through the enteral cell likely involves these carriers and probably involves divalent ions. Calcium is needed for the attachment of the intrinsic factor–B$_{12}$ complex to its cognate receptor on the enteral cell plasma

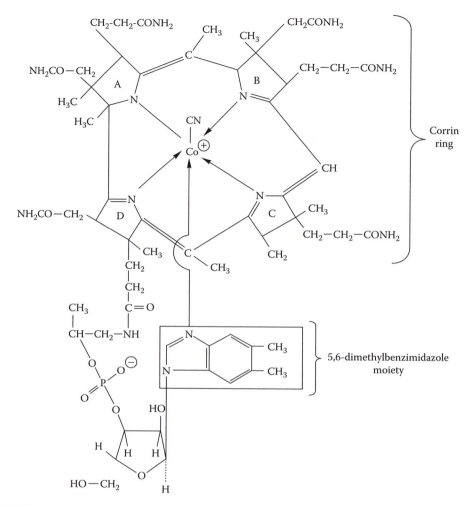

FIGURE 63 Structure of vitamin B$_{12}$.

membrane. It is likely that other factors are also involved; persons with a variety of diseases such as pancreatitis, tropical sprue, fluoroacetate poisoning, and pancreatic insufficiency do not absorb B$_{12}$ efficiently and often show signs of pernicious anemia until provided with oral B$_{12}$ supplements or injected with B$_{12}$. Absorption by the large intestine likely occurs via passive diffusion.

Once absorbed, B$_{12}$ is transported in the blood bound to one of three transport proteins: TCI, TCII, or TCIII. Small amounts are stored (as methylcobalamin) in the liver, kidney, heart, spleen, and brain. Thus, if an individual lacks intrinsic factor due perhaps to a genetic disease or surgical loss of the stomach (gastrectomy), or, as described earlier, has one of the diseases that affect B$_{12}$ absorption, an injection of B$_{12}$ can be given once a month and this will correct the problem of inadequate supply. As people age, there is a decline in B$_{12}$ status.

B$_{12}$ is a cobalt-containing coenzyme for two types of reactions. In the first type of reaction, it participates in methyl group transfer as in the methylation of homocysteine to reform methionine. This reaction also requires folacin as N-5-methyltetrahydrofolate. Not only is methionine regenerated in this reaction but so too is tetrahydrofolate. This reaction is essential to hemoglobin synthesis. In the second type of reaction, 5′-adenosylcobalamin is required for the action of methyl malonyl mutase, which converts methylmalonyl-CoA to succinyl CoA. This is the final step in the oxidation of odd-numbered fatty acids.

Vitamin B$_{12}$ participates as a coenzyme in reactions that utilize 5′-deoxyadenosine linked covalently to the cobalt atom (adenosylcobalamin). It also participates as a coenzyme in reactions that utilize the attachment of a methyl group to the central cobalt atom (methylcobalamin). The conversion of cobalamin to methylcobalamin is catalyzed by the enzyme B$_{12}$ coenzyme synthetase. It catalyzes the reduction of the molecule, then catalyzes the reaction with deoxyadenosyl mostly derived from ATP. In addition to ATP, this reaction needs a diol or a dithiol group and a reduced flavin or a reduced ferredoxin as the biological alkylating agent. The enzymes requiring B$_{12}$ as a coenzyme are listed in Table 57. One of the characteristics of the B$_{12}$-deficient state is an anemia characterized by few mature red cells. Immature nucleated cells (megaloblasts) can be found but not the mature ones. Among the other enzymes listed in Table 57 is methylmalonyl CoA mutase, which participates in propionate metabolism. Propionate metabolism, although a minor pathway in monogastric animals, is of some importance in neural tissue. Loss of this metabolic activity may explain the peripheral neural coat loss that characterizes long-term B$_{12}$ deficiency.

Methylmalonic aciduria characterizes the B$_{12}$-deficient individual. Studies with rats made B$_{12}$ deficient show an increase in odd-numbered fatty acids in the neural and hepatic lipids and low hepatic methylmalonyl CoA mutase activity. Replacement of B$_{12}$ in the diet corrects both these responses. The effect of B$_{12}$ on mutase activity is such that it is likely that the vitamin not only serves as the coenzyme in the reaction but also serves a role in the synthesis of that enzyme. Several reports of B$_{12}$ activity vis-á-vis protein synthesis have appeared in the literature in addition to the one concerning the synthesis of the mutase. Whether this relates to the role of B$_{12}$ in DNA and RNA synthesis, that is, the synthesis of pyrimidines and purines, or whether a B$_{12}$–protein complex acts as a cis- or transacting factor in the pathway for the expression of the specific genes for these enzymes is unknown.

The deficiency state has as its main characteristic pernicious anemia. While inadequate B$_{12}$ intake can result in this anemia, this is a rather unusual nutritional state because most foods of animal origin contain B$_{12}$ and so little B$_{12}$ is needed. A more common cause of pernicious anemia is a genetically determined deficiency of intrinsic factor. This trait is inherited as an autosomal dominant trait and occurs in about 1 in 1000. It can be treated with monthly B$_{12}$ injections (~60–100 µg/dose). In the absence of this trait, the people most at risk for pernicious anemia are those who abstain from eating foods of animal origin. In addition to these are those people who have had one of the illnesses described earlier that impair absorption. Humans that have had a gastrectomy, some disease of the gastric mucosa, or some disease resulting in malabsorption are in this category.

Following the development of pernicious anemia, which is reversible, is the irreversible loss of peripheral sensation. This is due to the degenerative changes in these nerves including demyelination

---

TABLE 57
Enzymes Requiring B$_{12}$ as a Coenzyme

N^5-methyltetrahydrofolate homocysteine methyltransferase

Acetate synthetase

Glutamate mutase

Methylmalonyl-CoA mutase

α-Methyleneglutarate mutase

Dioldehydrase a

Dioldehydrase b

Glycerol dehydratase

Ethanolamine ammonia-lyase

L-β-lysine mutase

D-α-lysine mutase

Ornithine mutase

L-β-leucine aminomutase

---

or loss of the lipid protective coat that surrounds the nerve tracts. Once the myelin is lost the nerve dies. Neural loss begins in the feet and hands and progresses upward to the major nerve trunks such that a progressive neuropathy can be followed. Because both folate and B_{12} are interactively involved in DNA and RNA synthesis, it used to be difficult to segregate one deficiency anemia from the other. However, given the presence of methylmalonic aciduria and differential analysis of the red cell one can determine the cause of the anemia. In addition to deficient intakes of folacin and B_{12}, deficient intakes of iron, copper, and zinc can also explain anemia. (See Anemia.)

Daily requirements for B_{12} are very small (see http://www.nal.edu). The normal turnover rate is about 2.5 µg/day; thus the recommendation for adults is close to this turnover rate or 2 µg/day. The need for B_{12} is also related to the intake of ascorbic acid, thiamin, carnitine, and fermentable fiber. Each of these nutrients affects the production of propionate, and in their absence or relative deficiency propionate production is increased, which in turn drives up the need for B_{12}. As already mentioned, the needs for B_{12} and folate are related.

VITAMIN C

See Ascorbic Acid.

VITAMIN D

Like vitamin A, vitamin D is not a single compound. The D vitamins listed in Table 58 are a family of 9,10 secosteroids, which differ only in the structures of their side chains. There is no D_1 because when the vitamins were originally isolated and identified, the compound identified as D_1 turned out to be a mixture of the other D vitamins rather than a separate entity.

Since the other D vitamins were already described and named, the D_1 designation was deleted from the list. All the D vitamers are related structurally to the four-ring compounds cyclopentanoperhydrophenanthrenes from which they were derived by a photochemical reaction. The chief structural prerequisite of compounds serving as D provitamins is the sterol structure, which has an opened B ring that contains a $D_{5,6}$ conjugated double bond. No vitamin activity is possessed by the compound until the B ring is opened. This occurs as a result of exposure to ultraviolet light. In addition, vitamin activity is dependent on the presence of a hydroxyl group at carbon 3 and upon the presence of conjugated double bonds at the 10–19, 5–6, and 7–8 positions. If the location of these double bonds is shifted, vitamin activity is substantially reduced. A side chain of a length at least equivalent to that of cholesterol is also a prerequisite for vitamin activity. If the side chain is replaced by a hydroxyl group, for example, the vitamin activity is lost. The potency of the various D vitamins is determined by the side chain. D_5, for example, with its branched 10-carbon side chain, is much less active with respect to the calcification of bone. Of the compounds shown in Figure 64, the most common form is that of D_2, ergocalciferol,

TABLE 58
D Vitamers

Precursor	D vitamer
Ergosterol	D_2 (ergocalciferol)
7-Dehydrocholesterol	D_3 (cholecalciferol)
22,23-Dihydroergosterol	D_4
7-Dehyrositosterol	D_5
7-Dehydrostigmasterol	D_6
7-Dehydrocompesterol	D_7

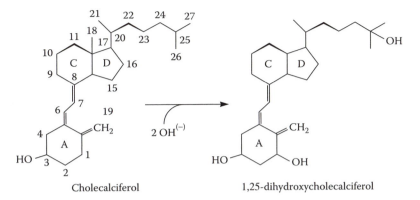

Cholecalciferol   1,25-dihydroxycholecalciferol

FIGURE 64 Chemical structure of vitamin D.

so called because its parent compound is ergosterol. Ergosterol can readily be prepared from plant materials and, thus, serves as a commercially important source of the vitamin. Vitamin D_3, cholecalciferol, is the most important member of the D family because it is the only form that can be generated in vivo. Cholesterol, from which cholecalciferol takes its name, serves as the precursor of this vitamin. The 7-dehydrocholesterol at the skin's surface is acted upon by ultraviolet light and is converted to vitamin D_3. In the absence of sunshine (or in the presence of sunblockers), this conversion does not take place.

The comparative potency of the D vitamers depends on several factors, such as the species consuming the vitamer and the particular function assessed. With respect to species specificity, in mammalian species both the D_2 and D_3 are equivalent and both would be given a value of 100 if rickets prevention were used as the functional criteria. However, should these two vitamers be compared in chicks as preventers of rickets, D_2 would be given a value of perhaps 10 while D_3 would be given 100. In this instance, it is clear that species differ in their use of these two vitamers. A related sterol, dihydroachysterol, which is a product of irradiated ergosterol, would have only 5%–10% of the activity of ergocalciferol. In contrast, the activated forms of D_3 (25-hydroxy and 1,25-dihydroxycholecalciferol) are far more potent (2–5 times and 5–10 times, respectively) than their parent vitamer D_3. The synthetic analog of D_3, 1α-hydroxycholecalciferol, likewise has 5–10 times the potency of cholecalciferol.

Active vitamin D is given in IU. One IU uses cholecalciferol, D_3, as the reference standard where 1 g of a cottonseed oil solution of D_3 contains 10 mg of the vitamin or 400 USP units. Thus, 1.0 IU of vitamin is 0.025 μg, which is equivalent to 65.0 pmol. The recommendation is that all of the various forms of the vitamin be stated in relation to their equivalent molar unit of the parent vitamin D_3. The current recommended intake for infants and children, adolescents, adults, and pregnant and lactating women is 200 IU/day (5 μg/day). For adults over the age of 51 the recommendation is for twice that amount or 400 IU/day (10 μg/day). After the age of 70 the intake recommendation is further increased to 600 IU/day (15 μg/day). This further increase in recommended intake with age is based on the observations that there is an age-related decrease in the activity of the conversion of previtamin D to 25-hydroxy vitamin D in the skin.

Dietary vitamin D is passively absorbed with food fats and is dependent on the presence of bile salts and a vitamin D transport protein. Any disease that results in an impairment of fat absorption likewise results in an impairment of vitamin D absorption. Absorption of the vitamin is a passive process that is influenced by the composition of the gut contents. Vitamin D is absorbed with long-chain fatty acids and is present in the chylomicrons of the lymphatic system. Absorption takes place primarily in the jejunum and ileum. This has a protective effect on vitamin D stores since the bile, released into the duodenum, is the chief excretory pathway of the vitamin; reabsorption in times of vitamin need can protect the body from undue loss. However, in times of vitamin excess this reabsorptive mechanism may be a detriment rather than a benefit. The vitamin is absorbed in either the hydroxylated or the unhydroxylated form.

Because the body can completely synthesize dehydrocholesterol and ergosterol, convert it to D_2 or D_3, and then hydroxylate it to form the active form, an argument against its essentiality as a nutrient can be developed. In point of fact, because the active form is synthesized in the kidney and from there distributed by the blood to all parts of the body, this active form meets the definition of a hormone and the kidney, its site of synthesis, meets the definition of an endocrine organ. Thus, whether vitamin D is a nutrient or a hormone is dependent on the degree of exposure to ultraviolet light. Lacking exposure, vitamin D must be provided in the diet and thus is an essential nutrient.

Once absorbed, vitamin D is transported in a nonesterified form bound to a specific vitamin D–binding protein (DBP). This protein (DBP) is nearly identical to the $\alpha2$ globulins and albumins with respect to its electrophoretic mobility. All of the forms of vitamin D (25-hydroxy D_3, 24,25-dihydroxy D_3, and 1,25-dihydroxy D_3) are carried by this protein, which is a globulin with a molecular weight of 58,000 Da. Its binding affinity varies with the vitamin form. The DNA sequence analysis of DBP shows homology with a fetoprotein and serum albumin. DBP also has a high affinity for actin but the physiological significance for this cross-reactivity is unknown.

METABOLISM

Once absorbed or synthesized at the body surface, vitamin D is transported via DBP to the liver. It is hydroxylated here via the enzyme vitamin D hydroxylase at carbon 25 to form 25-hydroxycholecalciferol. Figure 65 illustrates the pathway from cholesterolto 1,25-dihydroxycholecalciferol.

With the first hydroxylation a number of products are formed, but the most important of these is 25-hydroxycholecalciferol. The biological function of each of these metabolites is not known completely. As mentioned earlier, the hydroxylation occurs in the liver and is catalyzed by a cytochrome P-450–dependent mixed-function monooxygenase. This enzyme has been found in both mitochondrial and microsomal compartments. It is a two-component system that involves flavoprotein and a cytochrome P-450 and is regulated by the concentration of ionized calcium in serum. The hydroxylation reaction can be inhibited if D_3 analogs having modified side chains are infused into the animal fed a rachitic diet and a D_3 supplement.

The 25-hydroxy D_3 is then bound to DBP and transported from the liver to the kidney where a second hydroxyl group is added at carbon 1. This hydroxylation occurs in the kidney proximal tubule mitochondria catalyzed by the enzyme 25-OH-D_3-1α-hydroxylase. This enzyme has been characterized as a three-component enzyme involving cytochrome P-450, an iron sulfur protein (ferredoxin), and ferredoxin reductase. The reductant is $NADPH_2$. Considerable evidence has shown that 1,25-dihydroxycholecalciferol is the active principle that stimulates bone mineralization, intestinal calcium uptake, and calcium mobilization. Because this product is so active in the regulation of calcium homeostasis its synthesis must be closely regulated. Indeed, product feedback regulation not only on the activity of this enzyme but also at the level of its transcription has been shown. In both instances the level of 1,25-dihydroxycholecalciferol negatively affects 1α-hydroxylase activity and suppresses mRNA transcription of the hydroxylase gene product. In addition, control of the hydroxylase enzyme is also exerted by the parathyroid hormone (PTH). When plasma calcium levels fall PTH is released, and this hormone stimulates 1α-hydroxylase activity while decreasing the activity of 25-hydroxylase. In turn, PTH release is downregulated by rising levels of 1,25-dihydroxycholecalciferol and its analog, 24,25-dihydroxycholecalciferol. Insulin, growth hormone, estrogen, and prolactin are additional hormones that stimulate the activity of 1α-hydroxylase. The mechanisms that explain these stimulatory effects are less well known and are probably related to their effects on bone mineralization as well as on other calcium-using processes. Instead of 1,25-dihydroxy D_4, 24,25-dihydroxy D_3 may be formed and may serve to enhance bone mineralization and embryonic development and suppress PTH release. 24,25-Dihydroxy D_3 arises by hydroxylation of 25-hydroxy D_3. When 25-OH D_3

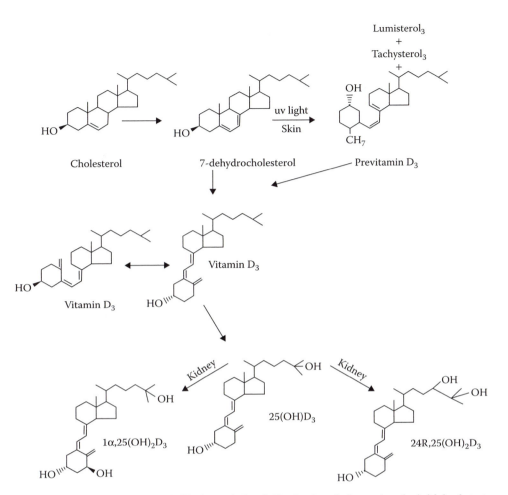

FIGURE 65 Synthesis of active 1,25-dihydroxycholecalciferol using cholesterol as the initial substrate.

1α-hydroxylase activity is suppressed, 24,25-hydroxylation is stimulated. This hydroxylase is substrate inducible through the mechanism of increased enzyme protein synthesis and has been found in kidney, intestine, and cartilage. The 24,25-dihydroxy D_3 may represent a "spillover" metabolite of D_3. That is, a metabolite is formed when excess 25-hydroxy D_3 is present in the body. Other D_3 metabolites such as 25-hydroxy D_3 26,23-lactose also can be regarded as spillover metabolites since measurable quantities are observed under conditions of excess intake. While 24,25-dihydroxy D_3 does function in the bone mineralization process, it is not as active in this respect as is 1,25-dihydroxy D_3.

The question of whether a hydroxyl group at carbon 25 is a requirement for vitamin activity has been posed since several D_3 metabolites, as per Table 58, lack this structural element. Studies utilizing fluro-substituted D_3 showed conclusively that while maximal activity is shown by the 1,25-dihydroxy D_3, activity can also be shown by compounds lacking this structure. In part, the structural requisite for vitamin activity may relate to the role the 25-hydroxy substituents play in determining themolecular shape of the compound. This shape must conform to the receptor shape of the cellular membranes in order for the D_3 to be utilized. Specific intracellular receptors for 1,25-dihydroxy D_3 have been found in parathyroid, pancreatic, pituitary, and placental tissues. All these tissues have been shown to require D_3 for the regulation of their function. For example, in D_3 deficiency pancreatic release of insulin is impaired. Insulin release is a calcium-dependent process.

When discussing vitamin D metabolism, it is important to recognize that 7-hydroxycholesterol irradiated by ultraviolet light becomes a cholecalciferolthat is transported to liver, converted to

25-hydroxycholecalciferol, transported to the kidney, and converted to 1,25-dihydroxycholecalciferol, which is in fact the active principle. This compound is then distributed throughout the body, exerting its effect on a variety of tissues. Because the body can indeed synthesize the active compound and because this synthesis takes place in an organ distal to the tissues upon which it acts, this compound is more truly a hormone rather than an essential nutrient. Of course, if irradiation does not or cannot occur sufficiently to effect the conversion of 7-hydroxycholesterol, as happens in aged individuals, then cholecalciferol must be provided in the diet and then, by definition, becomes a required nutrient. As seen in Figure 66, several pathways exist for the degradation of the active 1,25-dihydroxycholecalciferol. These include oxidative removal of the side chain, additional hydroxylation at carbon 24, the formation of a lactone (1,25 OH_2D_2-26,23 lactone), and additional hydroxylation at carbon 26. While 25-hydroxy cholecalciferol can accumulate in the heart, lungs, kidneys, and liver, 1,25-dihydroxycholecalciferol does not accumulate. The active form is not stored appreciably but is found in almost every cell and tissue type.

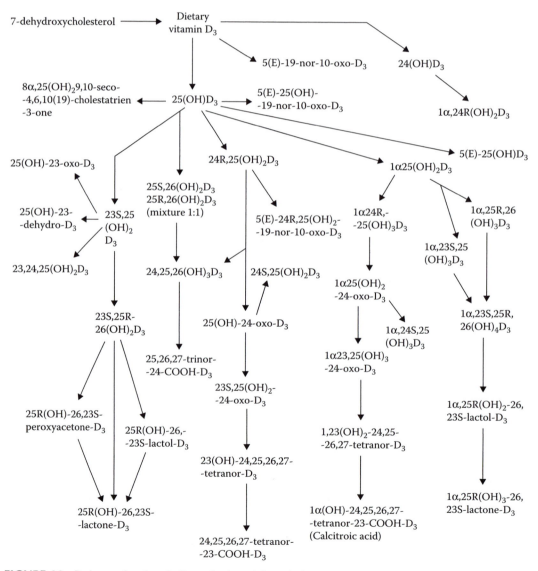

FIGURE 66   Pathways for vitamin D synthesis and degradation.

FUNCTION

Until the recognition of the central role of the calcium ion in cellular metabolic regulation, it was thought that vitamin D's only function was to facilitate the deposition of calcium and phosphorus in bone. This concept developed when it was recognized that the bowed legs of rickets were due to inadequate mineralization in the absence of adequate vitamin D intake or exposure to sunlight.

Studies of in vivo calcium absorption by the intestine revealed that D-deficient rats absorb less calcium than D-sufficient rats and that rats fed very high levels (10,000 IU/day) absorbed more calcium than did normally fed rats. These observations of the vitamin effects on calcium uptake led to work designed to determine the mechanism of this effect. It was soon discovered that vitamin D ($1,25$-dihydroxy D_3) served to stimulate the synthesis of a specific protein in the gut cells that was responsible for calcium uptake. This protein, called the calcium-binding protein (calbindin) was isolated from the intestine and later from brain, bone, kidney, uterus, parotid gland, parathyroid glands, and skin. Several different calcium-binding proteins have been found, but not all of these binding proteins are vitamin D dependent. That is, once formed, their activity with respect to calcium binding was unaffected by vitamin deficiency. Most, however, are dependent on vitamin D for their synthesis. Thus, these calcium-binding proteins are molecular expressions of the hormonal action of the vitamin.

As animals age, their levels of calcium-binding protein fall. Yet, when calcium intake levels fall, the synthesis and activity of the binding proteins rise. This mechanism explains how individuals can adapt to low-calcium diets. Interestingly, calcium deprivation stimulates the conversion of cholecalciferol to 25-hydroxycholecalciferol in the liver and to 1,25-dihydroxycholecalciferol in the kidney. Aging, however, seems to affect this regulatory mechanism. As humans age, they are less able to absorb calcium and may develop osteoporosis, a condition analogous to rickets in children and characterized by demineralization of the bone. In osteoporotic patients, intestinal absorption of calcium is decreased, but when $1,25$-dihydroxy D_3 is administered, calcium absorption is increased. It would appear, therefore, that one of the consequences of aging is an impaired conversion of 25-hydroxy D_3 to $1,25$-dihydroxy D_3, and since less of the latter is available less calcium-binding protein is synthesized. Measures of calcium-binding protein in aging rats, using an immunoassay technique, have shown that this is indeed the case.

Vitamin D also increases intestinal absorption of calcium by mechanisms apart from the synthesis of calcium-binding protein. It does this as part of its general tropic effect as a steroid on a variety of cellular reactions. Vitamin D affects membrane permeability to calcium at the brush border, perhaps through a change in the lipid (fatty acid) component of the membrane. It stimulates the $Ca^{++}Mg^{++}$ ATPase on the membrane of the cell wall, increases the conversion of ATP to cAMP, and increases the activity of the alkaline phosphatase enzyme. All these effects in the intestinal cell are independent of the vitamin's effect on calcium-binding protein synthesis.

In addition to its role in calcium absorption, vitamin D serves to induce the uptake of phosphate and magnesium by the brush border of the intestine. The effect on phosphate uptake is independent of its effect on calcium absorption and is due to an effect of the vitamin on the synthesis of a sodium-dependent membrane carrier for phosphate. The effect of vitamin D on magnesium absorption is incidental to its effect on calcium absorption since the calcium-binding protein has a weak affinity for magnesium. Thus, if synthesis of the calcium-binding protein results in an increase in calcium uptake, it also results in a significant increase in magnesium uptake.

REGULATION OF SERUM CALCIUM LEVELS

Serum calcium levels are closely regulated in the body so as to maintain optimal muscle contractility and cellular function. Several hormones are involved in this regulation: $1,25$-dihydroxy D_3, produced by the kidney; PTH released by the parathyroid gland; and thyrocalcitonin released by the thyroid C cells. Each has a specific function with respect to serum calcium levels and the functions of all three are interdependent. Vitamin D_3 increases blood calcium by increasing intestinal calcium uptake and decreases blood calcium by increasing calcium deposition in the bone. In the relative absence of vitamin D, PTH increases serum calcium levels by increasing the activity of the kidney 1α-25-hydroxylase with the result of increasing blood levels of 1,25-dihydroxy D_3 and through enhancing bone mineral mobilization and phosphate diuresis. PTH in the presence of vitamin D has the reverse action on bone. When both hormones (parathormone and 1,25 D_3) are present, bone mineralization is stimulated. Even though PTH stimulates the production of 1,25-dihydroxy D_3, D_3 does not stimulate PTH release. Thyrocalcitonin serves to lower blood calcium levels through stimulating bone calcium uptake, and its effect is independent of PTH yet dependent on the availability of calcium from the intestine. If serum calcium levels are elevated through a calcium infusion, thyrocalcitonin will be released and will stimulate bone calcium uptake even in animals lacking both PTH and D_3.

MODE OF ACTION AT THE GENOMIC LEVEL

The process of vitamin D (1,25 dihydroxycholecalciferol)-receptor binding to specific DNA sequences follows the classic model for steroid hormone action. Like vitamin A, vitamin D binds to a receptor protein in the nucleus. The receptor protein then acquires an affinity for specific DNA sequences located upstream from the promoter sequence of the target gene. These specific DNA sequences are called response elements and consist of a structure in which two zinc atoms are coordinated in two fingerlike domains. The N-terminal finger confers specificity to the binding while the second finger stabilizes the complex. When bound, transcription of the cognate protein mRNA is activated. Several response elements have been identified with each being specific for a specific gene product. The response elements have in common imperfect direct repeats of six-base pair half elements separated by a three-base pair spacer. Affinity of the nuclear receptor protein for vitamin D is modified by phosphorylation. Two sites of phosphorylation have been found both on serines. One site located in the DNA-binding region at serine 51 between two zinc finger DNA-binding motifs appears to reduce DNA binding when phosphorylated by proteinkinase C (or a related enzyme). The second site is located in the N-terminal region of the hormone-binding region at Ser 208. It has the opposite effect. When phosphorylated, probably by casein kinase II or a related enzyme, transcription is activated.

The vitamin-protein receptor complex that binds to the DNA consists of three distinct elements: 1,25-dihydroxycholecalciferol (the hormone ligand), the vitamin receptor, and one of the retinoid X receptors. Here is an instance where, once again, a vitamin D–vitamin A interaction can occur. It has been reported that 9-cis retinoic acid can attenuate transcriptional activation by the vitamin D–receptor binding to the vitamin D responsive element. Perhaps 9-cis retinoic acid has this effect because when it binds to the retinoid X receptor it blocks or partially occludes the binding site of the vitamin D–protein for DNA. Figure 67 illustrates the mode of vitamin D action at the genomic level. To date, the nuclear vitamin D receptor has been found in 34 different cell types and it is quite likely that it is a universal nuclear component.

Probably this is because every cell has a need to move calcium into or out of its various compartments as part of its metabolic control systems. Thus, calcium-binding proteins whose synthesis is vitamin D dependent are needed. Among the proteins thus far identified are osteocalcin, vitamin D–binding protein, osteoportin, 24-hydroxylase γ^3 interferon, calbindin, prepro PTH, calcitonin type II collagen, fibronectin, bone matrix GLA protein, interleukin-2 and interleukin-G, transcription factors (GM-CSF, c-myc, c-fos, c-fms), vitamin D receptors, calbindin D_{28x} and $_{9x}$, and prolactin. The transcription of the genes for each of these proteins are affected or regulated by vitamin D.

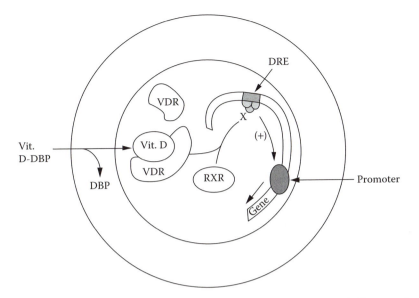

FIGURE 67   Schematic representation showing vitamin D bound to vitamin D–binding protein (DBP).

VITAMIN D DEFICIENCY

As discussed earlier, bone deformities are the hallmarks of the vitamin D–deficient child while porous, brittle bones are indications of the deficiency in the adult. The 1,25-dihydroxy D_3 must be provided to the anephric patient, since these patients cannot synthesize this hormone. Until the realization that the kidney served as the endocrine organ for 1,25-dihydroxy D_3 synthesis, renal disease was almost always accompanied by disturbed calcium balance and osteoporosis. Low vitamin D levels have recently been shown to be associated with decreased immune function. Persons with chronic inflammatory diseases such as obesity have been found to have subnormal levels of circulating vitamin. These reports have stimulated the discussion of appropriate intake recommendations. See http://www.nap.edu for the latest recommendations for vitamin D intake.

HYPERVITAMINOSIS D

Since the vitamin is fat soluble it, like vitamin A, can be stored. The storage capacity of the liver for the D precursor is much less than its capacity for A, and toxic conditions can develop if large amounts of D (in excess of need and storage capacity) are consumed over extended periods of time. Excessive amounts of vitamin D are not available from natural sources. Those individuals given supplements are those at risk for vitamin toxicity. This is a concern in the treatment of patients with hypoparathyroidism, vitamin D–resistant rickets, renal osteodystrophy, osteoporosis, psoriasis, and some cancers and of those who take vitamin supplements for nonmedical reasons. Because vitamin D's main function is to facilitate calcium uptake from the intestine and tissue calcium deposition, excess vitamin D in the toxic range will result in excess calcification not only of bone but of soft tissues as well. Symptoms of intoxication include hypercalcemia, hypercalciuria, anorexia, nausea, vomiting, thirst, polyuria, muscular weakness, joint pain, diffuse demineralization of bones, and disorientation. If the supplements are not stopped immediately upon recognition of the problem, death can occur. Renal stones and calcification of the heart, major vessels, muscles, and other tissues have been shown in experimental animals as well as in humans. Seelighas described a series of patients who were unusually sensitive to vitamin D either in utero or in infancy. These patients had multiple abnormalities in soft tissues and bones and were mentally retarded. Whether excess vitamin D intake provokes mild, moderate, or severe abnormalities is related not only to the individual's genetic background but also to his or her calcium, magnesium, and phosphorus intake. If any of these are consumed in excess of the others, vitamin D intoxication becomes more apparent. If caught early, these effects of intoxication can be reversed.

VITAMIN E

The most active naturally occurring form of vitamin E is d-α-tocopherol. Other tocopherols having varying degrees of vitamin activity have been isolated. Figure 68 shows the molecular structures of α-tocopherol and α-tocotrienol. Figure 69 shows the other tocopherols and tocotrienols and their relationship to α-tocopherol.

To have vitamin activity, the compound must have the double-ring structure (chromane nucleus) as shown in Figures 68 and 69 and must also have a side chain attached at carbon 2 and methyl groups attached at carbons 5, 7, or 8. β-Tocopherols have methyl groups attached at all three positions and represent the most active vitamin compounds. γ-Tocopherols have methyl groups attached to carbons 5 and 8; γ-tocopherols have methyl groups attached at carbons 7 and 8, and δ-tocopherols have only one methyl group attached at carbon 8. If the side chain attached to carbon 2 is saturated then the compound is a member of the tocol family of compounds; if unsaturated, it belongs to the trienol family. All forms have a hydroxyl group at carbon 6 and a methyl group at carbon 2. Other forms, ε, ζ, and η, have their methyl groups at carbons 5, 5 and 7, and 7, respectively. Naturally occurring vitamin E is in the D form whereas synthetic vitamin E preparations are mixtures of the D and L forms. Both tocols and trienols occur as a variety of isomers.

The IU of vitamin E activity uses the activity of 1 mg of dl-α-tocopherol acetate (all-rac) in the rat fetal absorption assay as its reference standard. Even though d-α-tocopherol is 36% more active than the dl form, the latter was selected as the reference substance because it is more readily available as a standard of comparison.

The tocopherols are slightly viscous oils that are stable to heat and the action of alkalis. They are slowly oxidized by atmospheric oxygen and rapidly oxidized by iron or silver salts. The addition of acetate or succinate to the molecule adds stability toward oxidation. The tocopherols are insoluble in water but soluble in the usual fat solvents. Ultraviolet light destroys its vitamin activity.

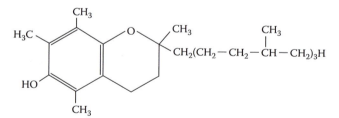

α-tocopherol (5, 7, 8-trimethyl tocol)

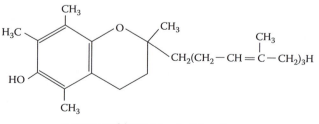

α-tocotrienol (5,7,8-trimethyltrienol)

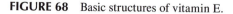

FIGURE 68 Basic structures of vitamin E.

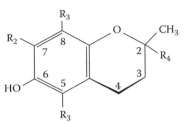

$R_1R_2R_3 = CH_3$ or H

$R_4 = CH_2(CH_2CH_2\overset{CH_3}{CH}CH_2)_3H$ (Tocols)

or $CH_2(CH_2CH = \overset{CH_3}{C}CH_2)_3H$ (Tocotrienols)

α-Tocol or Tocotrienol have $R_1R_2R_3 = CH_3$

β-Tocol or Tocotrienol have $R_1R_3 - CH_3$, $R = H$

γ-Tocol or Tocotrienol have $R_2R_3 = CH_3$, $R_1 = H$

δ-Tocol or Tocotrienol have $R_3 = CH_3$, $R_1R_2 = H$

ϵ-Tocol or Tocotrienol have $R_1 = CH_3$ $R_2R_3 = H$

ζ-Tocol or Tocotrienol have $R_1, R_2 = CH_3$ $R_3 = H$

η-Tocol or Tocotrienol have $R_2 = C+_3$, $R_1R_3 = H$

FIGURE 69   Structures of naturally occurring compounds having vitamin E activity.

The tocopherols have been isolated from a number of foods. Almost all are from the plant kingdom with wheat germ oil being the richest source. European wheat germ oil contains mostly β-tocopherols while American wheat germ oil contains mostly α-tocopherols. Corn oil contains α-tocopherols and soybean oil δ-tocopherols. Olive and peanut oil are poor sources of the vitamin. Some animal products such as egg yolk, liver, and milk contain tocopherols; but, in general, foods of animal origin are relatively poor sources of the vitamin. Vegetable oils vary from 100 µg/g (olive oil) to nearly 1200 µg/g (wheat germ oil).

Because of its lipophilicity, vitamin E, like the other fat-soluble vitamins, is passively absorbed via the formation of chylomicrons and subsequent uptake by the lymphatic system. The tocopherols are transported as part of the lipoprotein complex. Absorption is relatively poor. In humans, studies of labeled tocopherol absorption have shown that less than half of the labeled material appears in the lymph and up to 50% of the ingested vitamin may appear in the feces. Efficiency of absorption is enhanced by the presence of food fat in the intestine. Within this macronutrient class, efficiency of absorption is enhanced by saturated fat and decreased by the presence of polyunsaturated fatty acids. The use of water-miscible preparations enhances absorption efficiency particularly in those individuals whose fat absorption is impaired, that is, persons with cystic fibrosis or biliary disease. The commercially prepared tocopherol acetate or palmitate loses the acetate or palmitate through the action of a bile-dependent mucosal cell esterase prior to absorption. The pancreatic lipases, bile acids, and mucosal cell esterases are all important components of the digestion and absorption of vitamin E from food sources. The same processes required for the digestion and absorption of food fat apply here for the tocopherols.

In addition, there are gender differences in absorption efficiency: females are more efficient than males. Unlike the food fats (cholesterol and acylglycerides), hydrolysis is not followed by reesterification in the absorption process. To date, a specific tocopherol transport protein has not been identified or described. It appears that the tocopherols are bound to all of the lipid-carrying proteins in the blood and lymph. An excellent antioxidant, vitamin E serves this function very well as it is transported (from enterocyte to target tissue) with those lipids that could be peroxidized and thus require protection. Some cardiovascular researchers have suggested that one important function of vitamin E is to prevent the peroxidation of lipids in the blood, which would in turn suppress possible endothelial damage to the vascular tree and thus suppress some of the early events in plaque formation. Whether this hypothesis about the role of vitamin E in preventing such degenerative disease is true remains to be proven.

Although no specific transport protein has been found for the tocopherols in blood and lymph, there appears to be such a protein within the cells. A 30-kDa α-tocopherol-binding protein has been found in the hepatic cytosol and another 14.2-kDa one in the heart and liver that specifically binds to α-tocopherol and transfers it from liposomes to mitochondria. Having the vitamin in these two organelles protects them from free radical damage. One of the targets of free radicals is the genetic material DNA while the other is the membrane phospholipid. In either instance, damage to these vital components could be devastating. The smaller of the two binding proteins is similar in size to the intracellular fatty acid–binding protein (FABP). This protein also binds some of the eicosanoids but not α-tocopherol. The other tocopherols (β, γ, etc.) are not bound to the tocopherol-binding proteins to the same extent as α-tocopherol, nor are these isomers retained as well. Tocopherols are found in all of the cells in the body with adrenal cells, pituitary cells, platelets, and testicular cells having the most per cell. Adipose tissue, muscle, and liver serve as reservoirs, and these tissues will become depleted should intake levels be inadequate to meet the need. The rate of depletion with dietary inadequacy varies considerably. Since its main function is as one of several antioxidants, other nutrients that also serve in this capacity can affect vitamin depletion. The intake of β-carotene and ascorbic acid and also the level of polyunsaturated fatty acid intake can markedly affect the rate of use of α-tocopherol as an antioxidant. Increased intakes of β-carotene and ascorbic acid protect against α-tocopherol depletion whereas increased intakes of polyunsaturated fatty acids drive up the need for antioxidants. A further consideration is the intake of selenium. This mineral is an integral part of the glutathione peroxidase system that suppresses free radical production. In selenium-deficient animals, the need for α-tocopherol is increased and vice versa. The α-tocopherol-deficient animal has a greater need for selenium. In addition, α-tocopherol protects against iron toxicity in another instance of a mineral-vitamin interaction. In this instance, high levels of iron drive up the potential for free radical formation, and this can be overcome with increases in vitamin E intake.

Upon entry into the cell very little degradation occurs. Usually less than 1% of the ingested vitamin (or its metabolite) appears in the urine. Compounds called Simon's metabolites appear in the urine. These are glucuronates of the parent compound. The major excretory route is via the intestine. The excretory pathway is shown in Figure 70. As mentioned, the main function of vitamin E is as an antioxidant. This function is shared by β-carotene, ascorbic acid, the selenium-dependent glutathione peroxidase, and the copper-manganese- and magnesium-dependent super-oxide dismutase.

Glutathione peroxidase has been found in cells other than red blood cells. It is present in adipose tissue, liver, muscle, and glandular tissue, and its activity is complementary to that of catalase, another enzyme that uses peroxide as a substrate. Together these enzymes and vitamin E protect the integrity of the membranes by preventing the degradation, through oxidation, of the membrane lipids. This function of vitamin E is seen more clearly in animals fed high levels of polyunsaturated fatty acids. As the intake of these acids increase, they are increasingly incorporated into the membrane lipids, which in turn become more vulnerable to oxidation. Unless protected against oxidation, the functionality of the membranes will be impaired, and if uncorrected the cell will die. Disturbances in the transport of materials across membranes have been shown in liver with respect to cation flux. Liver slices from E-deficient animals lost the ability to regulate sodium-potassium exchange and calcium flux. Investigators have shown a decline in mitochondrial respiration in vitamin E–deficient rats. Such a decline probably represents a decline in the flux of adenosine diphosphate (ADP) or calcium into the mitochondria to stimulate oxygen uptake by the respiratory chain. Such a decline would permit more oxygen to remain in the cytosol to serve in the oxidation of lipids. In addition to peroxidative damage to the membrane, there is also damage to the DNA

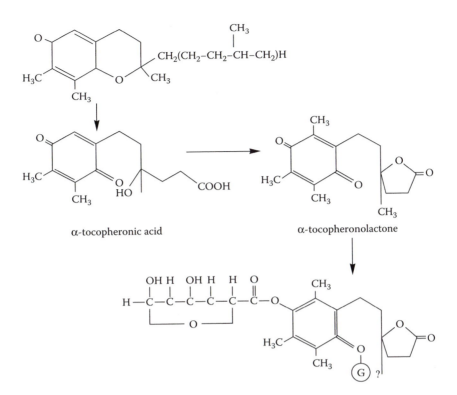

FIGURE 70   Excretory pathway for the tocopherols.

with the possible result of aberrant gene products. Thus, a whole cascade of responses to vitamin E insufficiency can be envisioned. Interestingly, in diseases manifested by an increased hemolysis of the red cells and a decreased ability of the hemoglobin to carry oxygen, red cell vitamin E levels are low. This has been shown in patients with sickle cell anemia and in patients with cystic fibrosis. In patients with sickle cell anemia, the low vitamin E level in the erythrocytes is accompanied by an increased level of glutathione peroxidase activity. It has been suggested that the increase in enzyme activity was compensatory to the decrease in vitamin E content.

Vitamin E and zinc have been found to have interacting effects in the protection of skin lipids. In zinc-deficient chicks, supplementation with vitamin E decreased the severity of the zinc-deficiency state, suggesting that zinc also may have antioxidant properties or that there may be an interacting effect of zinc with the vitamin.

In addition to the aforementioned main function of vitamin E, there are other roles for this substance. One involves prostaglandin synthesis. Thromboxane (TXA_2), a platelet-aggregating factor, is synthesized from arachidonic acid (20:4) via a free radical–mediated reaction. This synthesis is greater in a deficient animal than in an adequately nourished one. Vitamin E enhances prostacyclin formation and inhibits the lipooxygenase and phospholipase reactions. This effect is secondary to the vitamin's role as an antioxidant. As mentioned, phospholipase A_2 is stimulated by lipid peroxides. Other secondary functions also are related to its antioxidant function. Oxidant damage to DNA in bone marrow could explain red blood cell deformation as well as the fragility (due to membrane damage) of these cells. In turn, this would explain why enhanced red cell fragility is a characteristic of the deficient state.

Steroid hormone synthesis as well as spermatogenesis, both processes that are impaired in the deficient animal, could be explained by the damaging effects of free radicals on DNA, which are corrected by the provision of this antioxidant vitamin.

Even though vitamin E is a fat-soluble vitamin like A and D, there is little evidence that high intakes will result in toxicity in humans. Excess is excreted in feces; however, vitamin E toxicity has been produced in chickens. It is characterized by growth failure, poor bone calcification, depressed hematocrit, and increased clotting times. These symptoms suggest that the excess vitamin E interferes with the absorption and/or use of other fat-soluble vitamins since these symptoms are those of the vitamin A-, D-, and K-deficiency states. This suggests that advocates of megadoses of vitamin E as treatment for heart disease, muscular dystrophy, and infertility (among other ailments) may unwittingly advocate the development of additional problems associated with an imbalance in fat-soluble vitamin intake due to these large vitamin E intakes.

One of the first deficiency symptoms recorded for the tocopherols was infertility, followed by the discovery that the white muscle disease or a peculiar muscle dystrophy could be reversed if vitamin E was provided. Later, it was recognized that selenium also played a role in the muscle symptoms.

VITAMIN K

A large number of compounds, all related to a 2-methyl-1,4 napthaquinone, possess vitamin K activity (Figure 71). Compounds isolated from plants have a phytyl radical at position 3 and are members of the K_1 family of compounds. Phylloquinone (2-methyl-3-phytyl-1,4 napthaquinone (II)) is the most important member of this family. The K vitamins are identified by their family and by the length of the side chain attached at position 3. The shorthand designation uses the letter K with a subscript to indicate family and a superscript to indicate the side chain length. Thus, K_2^{20} indicates a member of the family of compounds isolated from animal sources having a 20-carbon side chain. The character of the side chain determines whether a compound is a member of the K_1 or K_2 family. K_1 compounds have a saturated side chain whereas K_2 compounds have an unsaturated side chain. Chain lengths of the K_1 and K_2 vitamins can vary from 5 to 35 carbons.

A third family of compounds is the K_3 family. These compounds lack the side chain at carbon 3. Menadione is the parent compound name and it is a solid crystalline material (a salt), menadione

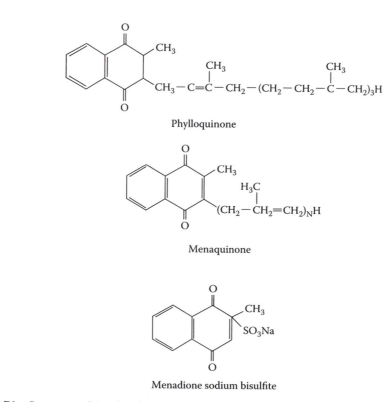

Phylloquinone

Menaquinone

Menadione sodium bisulfite

FIGURE 71   Structures of the vitamin K_1 (phylloquinone), K_2 (menaquinone), and K_3 (menadione).

sodium bisulfite. Other salts are also available. These salts are water soluble and thus have great use in diet formulations or mixed animal feeds. Menadiol sodium diphosphate is clinically useful. The use of this compound must be very carefully monitored as overdoses can result in hyperbilirubinemia and jaundice. When consumed as a dietary ingredient the quinone structure is converted by the intestinal flora to a member of the K_2 family.

There are several structural requirements for vitamin activity: There must be a methyl group at carbon 2 and a side chain at carbon 3. The benzene ring must be unsubstituted. The chain length can vary; however, optimal activity is observed in compounds having a 20-carbon side chain. K_1 and K_2 compounds with similar chains have similar vitamin activities. The vitamin can exist in either the cis or the trans configuration. All trans phylloquinone is the naturally occurring form whereas synthetic phylloquinone is a mixture of the cis and trans forms.

The various compounds with vitamin activity are not equivalent with respect to potency as a vitamin. The most potent compound of the phylloquinone series is the one with a 20-membered side chain. Compounds having fewer or greater numbers of carbons are less active. The most potent compound in the menaquinone series is the one with a 25-membered unsaturated side chain.

Phylloquinone (K_1^{20}) is a yellow viscous oil. The physical state of menaquinone (K_2^{20}) depends on its side chain length. If the side chain is 5 or 10 carbons long, it is an oil; if longer, it is a solid. Menadione (K_3) is a solid. All three families of compounds are soluble in fat solvents. Menadione can be made water soluble by converting it to a sodium salt. All the vitamin K compounds are stable to air and moisture but unstable to ultraviolet light. They are also stable in acid solutions but are destroyed by alkali and reducing agents. These compounds possess distinctive absorption spectra because of the presence of napthaquinone.

All of the natural forms of the K vitamins can be stored in the liver. Menadione is not stored as such but is stored as its conversion product, menaquinone. Menadione metabolism by the liver occurs at the expense of the redox state. When menadione is metabolized by Ca^{++}-loaded mitochondria, there is a rapid oxidation and loss of pyridine nucleotides and a decrease in the ATP level. The effects of menadione on Ca^{++} homeostasis are probably initiated by NAD(P)H: (quinone-acceptor) oxido reductase. Large amounts of menadione have been shown to alter the surface structure and reduce the thiol content of the liver cell. Because of these changes, menadione is cytotoxic in large quantities.

Vitamin K's most important function is in the blood-clotting process. It serves to bind calcium, thus promoting clot formation. Its actions can be inhibited by dicumarol, a substance first isolated from spoiled clover. It is marketed as coumarin. Another use is as a rodenticide, marketed as warfarin.

ABSORPTION

The mechanism by which the K vitamins are absorbed and the rate at which this occurs is species dependent. Species such as the chicken, which have a rapid gut passage time, absorb the vitamin more rapidly than do species such as the rat, which have a long gut passage time. The absorption of K_1 and K_2 analogs is generally thought to occur via an active, energy-dependent transport process, whereas K_3 (menadione) analogs are absorbed by passive diffusion. The absorption of K_1 and K_2 requires a protein carrier, and again species differ in the saturability of the carrier. In rats, the carrier is saturated at far lower vitamin concentrations than occurs in chickens. In contrast to the absorption of phylloquinone and the menaquinones, menadione appears to be absorbed primarily in the large intestine where the gut bacteria convert it to a form with a side chain. Without the side chain the absorption of K_3 is a passive process.

Absorption of the K vitamins is dependent on the presence of lipid, which stimulates the release of bile and pancreatic lipases. As lipids are absorbed into the lymphatic system, so too are the K vitamers. If there is any impairment in the lipid absorption process, less vitamin K will be absorbed. For example, patients with biliary obstruction have been shown to absorb substantially less vitamin K than normal subjects.

METABOLISM AND FUNCTION

Vitamin K serves as an essential cosubstrate in the posttranslational oxidative carboxylation of glutamic acid residues in a small group of specific proteins, most of which are proteins involved in blood coagulation. These proteins are the blood-clotting factors II, VII, IX, and X; a calcium-binding bone protein, osteocalcin, and plasma proteins C and S. Posttranslational oxidative carboxylation of proteins at selected glutamic acid residues occurs as a cyclic process. As the vitamin serves as a cosubstrate, it is metabolized by the hepatic microsomes. Its metabolism is dependent on adequate intakes of niacin and riboflavin that are components of the redox systems important in the transfer of reducing equivalent (REs). Vitamin K is reduced to the hydroquinone (vitamin KH_2) with NADH as the coenzyme (NADH is a niacin-containing coenzyme). There are two pathways for vitamin K reduction: (1) the reduction pathway—warfarin sensitive—irreversible by coumarin, and (2) DT diaphorase and microsomal dehydrogenase. This pathway is important to counteract coumarin toxicity. Upon reduction, it is then oxidized to form an epoxide. The epoxide is converted back to the quinone form by an epoxide reductase. This enzyme is a two-component cytosolic enzyme that catalyzes the reduction of the vitamin K epoxide using dithiothreitol as either a primary or secondary source of REs. Warfarin, an antivitamin, interferes with both the reduction of vitamin K to the hydroquinone and the conversion of the epoxide back to the original compound. Warfarin is bound to a protein (likely the epoxidase and the reductase). When fed to deficient rats, the epoxide has an activity similar to that of the vitamin in inducing protein carboxylation and prothrombin synthesis. This similarity is probably due to the conversion of the epoxide to the hydroquinone. The epoxidation reaction is coupled to the carboxylation of the glutamic acid residues protruding from peptides having clusters of this amino acid.

Aspartyl residues can also be carboxylated. The epoxidation reaction can be coupled to the oxidation of other peptides as well; however, only those having the clusters of glutamic acid will be oxidatively carboxylated. Unless the proteins are carboxylated they are unable to bind calcium. For example, the precursor of prothrombin, acarboxyprothrombin, has within the first 33 amino acids at the amino terminal end 10 tightly clustered glutamic acid residues and binds less than 1 mol of calcium per mole of protein. When carboxylated to prothrombin, the glutamic acid residues are converted to a carboxyglutamic acid residue, and now each mole of the protein can bind 10–12 moles of calcium. The carboxylated glutamic acid-rich region serves an important function in clot formation. Prior to activation by the protease factor Xa, both the prothrombin and the protease are absorbed onto the phospholipids of the damaged cells by way of calcium bridges. Without carboxylation, these bridges will not form and the adherence or absorption of the prothrombin to the phospholipids of the injured cell walls does not take place. The phospholipids are not only important to the binding of prothrombin to the injured cell wall but are also important determinants of carboxylase activity. Phosphatidyl choline has been found to be an essential component of the carboxylase enzyme system. When depleted of phospholipid, the enzyme loses activity; when repleted, its activity is restored.

Proteins other than those involved in the coagulation process have also been shown to be vitamin K dependent. Carboxylated proteins have been found in bone matrix. Up to 20% of the noncollagenous proteins (or 1%–2% of the total bone protein) is a carboxylated protein called osteocalcin. Another is called bone gla protein (BGP). Osteocalcin is synthesized in bone tissue. Bone microsomes are responsible for the posttranslational vitamin K–dependent oxidative carboxylation reaction. The synthesis of osteocalcin is highest during rapid growth periods and coincides with detectable bone mineralization. The osteocalcin appears prior to mineralization and, like the blood coagulation proteins, shows a remarkable avidity for calcium. It will also bind (in order of preference after calcium) magnesium, strontium, barium, and lanthanide. In addition to its ability to bind divalent ions, osteocalcin also binds strongly to hydroxyapatite, the major calcium phosphate salt of the bone. Whether osteocalcin has a direct role in bone mineralization has not been conclusively shown; however, studies of embryonic chicks treated with warfarin showed a decrease in both osteocalcin and mineralization. Warfarin-treated animals in contrast do not show this same effect;

osteocalcin levels are low but bone mineralization is normal. Because the overwhelming effects of vitamin K deficiency induced either through diet or warfarin treatment results in lethal bleeding, this secondary effect on bone mineralization is difficult to study except in systems utilizing embryonic tissues. Evidence of warfarin injury has been reported in humans. Mothers consuming warfarin during pregnancy have given birth to infants having defective bone development such as stippled epiphyses, "saddle" nose, punctate calcifications, and frontal bossing.

BGP is a 49-residue, vitamin K–dependent protein involved in the regulation of bone calcium homeostasis rather than bone formation. It is secreted by osteosarcoma cells having an osteoblastic phenotype and appears in calcifying tissues 1–2 weeks after mineral deposition, and at the approximate time that the maturation of bone mineral to hydroxyapatite is thought to occur. The synthesis and secretion of BGP from osteosarcoma cells are regulated by vitamin D. The 9-cis retinoic acid reduces 1α-25-dihydroxycholecalciferol-induced renal calcification by altering vitamin K–dependent γ-carboxylation of matrix γ-carboxyglutamic acid protein. The renal cortex also contains a microsomal vitamin K–dependent oxidative carboxylation system. Its function is to produce a carboxy glutamic acid–rich protein, which serves to bind calcium. It is located in the renal tubule and may function in the conservation of calcium. There is also a matrix gla protein that has an inhibitory role in the calcification of the arterial tree. In vitamin K–supplemented men and women, there is a reduced rate of arterial calcification due to the inhibitory action of matrix gla protein on this process. In addition to its function as described earlier, vitamin K serves a role in the inhibition of the carcinogenic properties of benzopyrene. Menadione inhibits aryl hydrocarbon hydroxylase, thus reducing the levels of carcinogenic and mutagenic metabolites in the cell with resultant reduction in tumor formation.

DEFICIENCY

Due to the fact that intestinal synthesis of vitamin K usually provides sufficient amounts of the vitamin to the body, primary vitamin K deficiency is rare. However, secondary deficiency states can develop as a result of biliary disease, which results in an impaired absorption of the vitamin. Deficiency can also occur as a result of long-term broad-spectrum antibiotic therapy, which may kill the vitamin K–synthesizing intestinal flora, or as a result of anticoagulant therapy using coumadin, which, as described earlier, interferes with the metabolism and function of the vitamin. The primary characteristic of the deficiency state is a delayed or prolonged clotting time. Deficient individuals may have numerous bruises indicative of subcutaneous hemorrhaging in response to injury. Newborn infants, because they do not yet have established their vitamin K–synthesizing intestinal flora, have delayed coagulation times.

VLDL

Very-low-density lipoprotein. A lipid-protein complex involved in the transport of lipids from the liver and gut to storage sites.

VOLATILE FATTY ACIDS

Short-chain (carbons fewer than eight) fatty acids that volatilize at room temperature.

VON GIERKE'S DISEASE

A rare genetic disorder characterized by excess glycogen stores in liver and muscles due to a mutation in the gene for the enzyme glucose-6-phosphatase. Also called type I glycogen storage disease.

W

WARFARIN SODIUM

A coumarin derivative that is used as an anticoagulant. Warfarin is also the active ingredient in rat poison. Trade names: Coumadin, Panwarfin, Sofarin, Warfilone.

WATER BALANCE

The water intake is equal to the water loss. For a description of the control of water balance, see ACE Inhibitors.

WATER INTOXICATION

Excess water intake.

WATER MISCIBLE

Substance or liquid that mixes freely with water.

WATER OF METABOLISM

Water produced in the course of a metabolic reaction, such as the splitting of a peptide bond.

WERNICKE-KORSAKOFF SYNDROME

Condition resulting from severe deficiency of thiamine marked by loss of memory and personality changes. Alcoholism usually precedes this development.

WESTERN BLOT

A method for transferring proteins to a nitrocellulose filter on which the proteins can be detected using specific antibodies.

WHEAT ALLERGY

A condition where the individual is intolerant to wheat products in the diet. Wheat contains water, starch, lipids, and the proteins albumin, globulins, and gluten. Gluten consists of gliadin and glutenine. The various proteins in wheat can cause different symptoms. One example is the so-called baker's asthma in bakers allergic to wheat albumin. This reaction occurs when wheat dust is inhaled. In food allergy, globulins and glutenine are the most important allergens. Allergic reactions can occur following the ingestion of wheat. In celiac disease, an allergy to gliadin plays an important role in the pathogenesis. After exposure to gluten, infiltration of eosinophils and neutrophils, along with edema and an increase in vascular permeability of the mucosa of the small intestine, can be observed. If the allergic reaction is chronic, the infiltration consists mainly of lymphocytes and plasma cells. Furthermore, flattening of the mucosal surface is found. The disorder manifests itself typically 6–12 months after introduction of gluten into the diet. It is characterized initially by intermittent symptoms such as abdominal pain, irritability, and diarrhea. If not treated, anemia, various deficiencies, and growth failure may occur as a result of malabsorption. Improvement is seen about 2 weeks after elimination of gluten from the diet. In addition to the immunological reaction to gluten, a direct toxic effect may also play a role in causing the disease.

WHEAT GERM

The fatty portion of the wheat grain; rich source of vitamin E.

WHEY

Proteins in milk that separate out when milk is coagulated with renin. These are the proteins that comprise cheese.

WHOLE GRAIN CEREALS

Cereals that contain all parts of the grain from which it is made.

WILSON'S DISEASE

Abnormal accumulation of copper in tissues due to an impaired incorporation of copper into ceruloplasmin and decreased biliary excretion of copper. The disease is a rare genetic disease where there is a mutation in the P-type ATPase cation transporter.

WOLFRAM SYNDROME

A rare genetic disease that starts with type 1 diabetes followed by optic atrophy and severe neurodegeneration; prevalence: 1:1,000,000.

X

XANTHINE

Nitrogenous extract formed during the metabolism of nucleoproteins. Three methylated xanthines include caffeine, theophylline, and theobromine.

XEROPHTHALMIA

Vitamin A deficiency; one of the leading causes of blindness in the world.

Z

ZEARALENONE

A mycotoxin produced by *Fusarium tricinctum*, *Fusarium gibbosum*, *Fusarium roseum*, and three subspecies of the latter, *Fusarium roseum culmorum*, *Fusarium roseum equiseti*, and *Fusarium roseum graminearum*. In animals, it has been shown to possess oestrogenic and anabolic properties. The production of zearalenone by *Fusarium roseum* required alternating high (24°C–27°C) and low (12°C–14°C) temperatures. The lower temperature is necessary for the induction of the biosynthetic enzyme for zearalenone, whereas the higher temperature is important in the proceeding of the biosynthesis. Food types involved in the contamination of zearalenone include maize, wheat, flour, and milk.

ZELLWEGER SYNDROME

A rare fatal genetic disease. Victims of this disorder do not make bile acids or plasmalogens, nor are they able to shorten the very long fatty acids. These biochemical deficiencies are seemingly unrelated to the structural abnormalities observed in liver, kidney, muscle, and brain.

ZINC

A cofactor of a variety of enzymes mediating metabolic pathways, such as alcohol dehydrogenation, lactic dehydrogenation, superoxide dismutation, and alkaline phosphorylation. It occurs especially in meat, (whole) grains, and legumes. The DRI varies from 8 to 12 mg/day, depending on the age, while the zinc intake is about 10 mg/day. See http://www.nap.edu for age and gender recommendations. Zinc deficiency affects DNA damage, oxidative stress, antioxidant defenses, and DNA repair. Acute toxicity, including gastrointestinal irritation and vomiting, has been observed following the ingestion of 2 g or more of zinc in the form of sulfate.

ZYMOGEN

An inactive enzyme.

Appendix 1
General Guidelines for Food Selection to Optimize Health

Before one can provide general statements about food choice we must recognize that these choices are not only due to the recognition of the need for food to avoid starvation but also due to a variety of nonfood, nonhealth considerations. Among these are food availability, ethnic identity, economic status, education, occupation, gender, age, physiological status, religious beliefs, and individual factors of likes, dislikes, tolerances, and intolerances. Advertising of specific food products, peer pressure, and the availability of restaurants and takeout food producers also influence food acceptance and food choice. Having acknowledged the above, there are some general guidelines that, if followed, will result in a healthy diet. In the United States, the Department of Agriculture has developed a food guide called the Food Guide Pyramid. This consists of six groups of foods arranged in order of the number of servings per day as follows:

Food	Servings
Bread, cereal, rice, pasta	6–11 servings/day
Fruits	2–4 servings/day
Vegetables (including potatoes)	3–5 servings/day
Meat, poultry, fish, dry beans, nuts, eggs	2–3 servings/day
Milk, yogurt, cheese	2–3 servings/day
Fats, oils, sweets	Use sparingly

What does this food guide mean? A serving can be defined in varying amounts. Is a serving of meat 4 or 8 oz? One can use this guide to translate desired energy intakes into a real diet:

Energy Intake (kcal)	1600	2200	2800
Bread	6	9	11
Vegetable	3	4	5
Fruits	2	3	4
Meats	2	2	3
Milk	2	2	3

Note: A serving of bread = 1 slice bread or 1/2 cup pasta, rice, cereal
A serving of vegetable = 1/2 cup cooked vegetable, 1 cup raw
A serving of fruit = 1/2 cup
A serving of meat = 2–3 oz
A serving of milk = 8 fluid oz or cheese equivalent (1.5 oz)

RESTRICTED ENERGY DIETS

Weight loss will be achieved if energy intake is exceeded by energy expenditure. Energy expenditure = basal energy need (see Table 14) + activity increment (see Table 2). Energy restriction plus an increase in energy expenditure (increase in physical activity) is better than energy restriction alone. An increase in activity builds muscle, which in general uses more energy than does fat tissue.

To reduce energy intake, avoid as much as possible fat and sugar. Substitute reduced-fat products for regular products; substitute artificially sweetened products for products containing sucrose or fructose; select lean meat; substitute chicken (without skin), turkey, or fish for well-marbled meat; avoid fried foods; substitute broiling, boiling, or steaming cooking methods for deep fat frying methods or grilling methods for food preparation; substitute raw unprocessed fruits and vegetables for cooked or prepared fruits and vegetables; and substitute skim milk for whole milk. Making these substitutions to the 1600 kcal diet described above will result in a 20%–30% reduction in energy intake. If the energy intake is less than 1200 kcal, the individual may not be well nourished with respect to micronutrients. A supplement may be needed under these conditions. See Table 37 to assess nutritional status.

LOW-INCOME DIETS

Diets for people under economic stress are difficult to prescribe because of local factors that influence food cost. However, using the Food Guide Pyramid, some general suggestions can be made:

1. Avoid prepared or processed foods. If a kitchen is available, it is generally less expensive to make a given dish than to buy it already prepared.
2. Substitute eggs, cheese, chicken, peanut butter, dried beans, and peas for beef, veal, and pork.
3. Avoid snack foods; they are high-cost items with little nutritional value.
4. Use fresh fruits and vegetables in season when their cost is lowest.
5. If good storage is possible, buy large volumes of foods that store well, that is, potatoes, root vegetables, apples, and oranges in season. These items need cool, well-ventilated storage and will last several months.

DIETS FOR THE ELDERLY

Food choices for the elderly are not much different from those for younger adults, provided these elders have good teeth (or well-fitting dentures) and are not constrained by degenerative disease or economic and social factors. The elderly may have more fixed ideas about food choice and may also need to reduce their energy intake, yet they may need larger amounts of essential micronutrients. They may also use more prescription drugs, and these can affect appetite as well as nutrient use. Malnutrition in the elderly can result if one ignores these factors.

DIETS FOR INFANTS AND CHILDREN

Again, the Food Guide Pyramid can be used as a general guide. Infants usually consume milk as their main source of nutrients. Solid foods are gradually introduced such that by the age of two, a variety of foods is consumed. Because young children are far more sensitive to flavors and textures than adults, the foods offered to children should be monitored with these factors in mind. Highly seasoned items may be rejected as well as items that are tough, gritty, or roughly textured. Children may develop food "jags," which means that they wish to eat only certain food items over many days. These behaviors change with time.

Appendix 2
Metabolic Maps

The many pathways in metabolism have been studied extensively for more than 50 years. The details of their regulation can be found in most comprehensive biochemistry texts. The entire metabolic map with all its details for both plants and animals has been published by the Boehringer Manheim Company* and can be obtained from them at a low cost. The maps in this appendix are quite general and lack the detail found in the Boehringer Mannheim maps. They are provided to the reader only as a general guide to intermediary metabolism as it relates to nutrition.

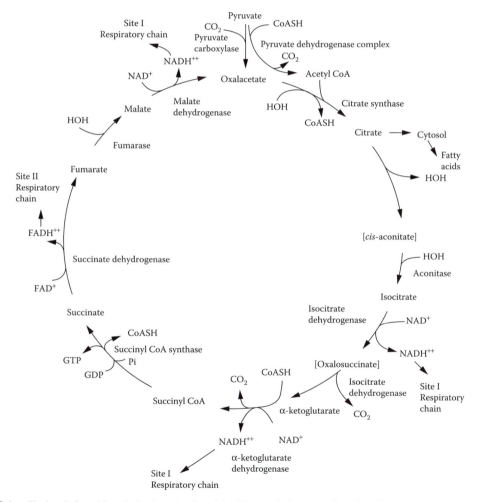

MAP 1   Krebs citric acid cycle in the mitochondria. This cycle is also called the tricarboxylate cycle (TCA).

---

* Boehringer Mannheim, PO Box 31, 01 20, D-6800 Manheim, Germany.

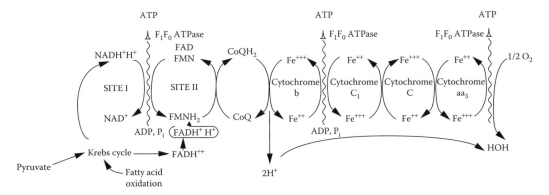

MAP 2   The respiratory chain showing the points where sufficient energy has been generated to support the synthesis of one molecule of ATP from ADP and P_i. Each of the segments generates a proton gradient. This energy is captured by the F_0 portion of the ATPase and transmitted to the F_1 portion of the ATPase. If uncouplers are present, the proton gradient is dissipated and all of the energy is released as heat.

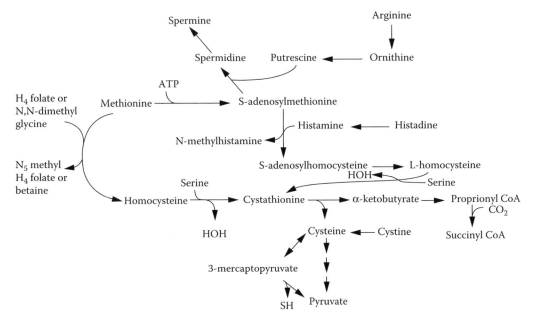

MAP 3   Conservation of SH groups via methionine-cysteine interconversion. Spermine, putrescine, and spermidine are polyamines that are important in cell and tissue growth.

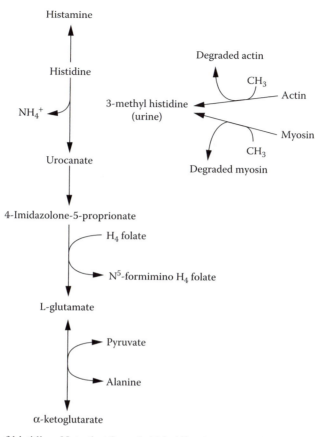

MAP 4   Catabolism of histidine. Note that 3-methyl histidine is not part of the pathway. This metabolite is formed in the muscle when the contractile proteins actin and myosin are methylated.

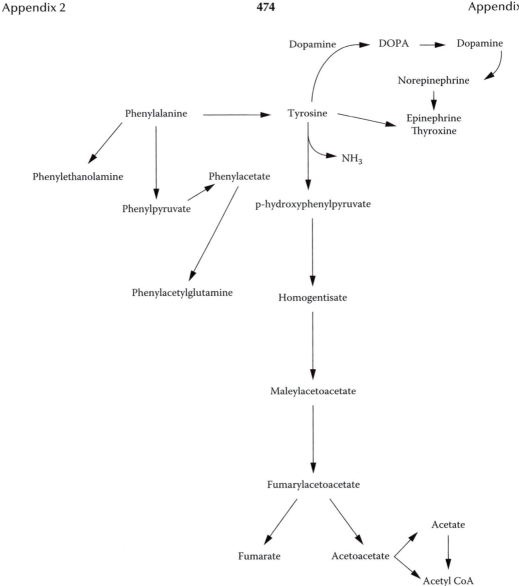

MAP 5 Phenylalanine and tyrosine catabolism. This pathway has a number of mutations resulting in a variety of genetic diseases.

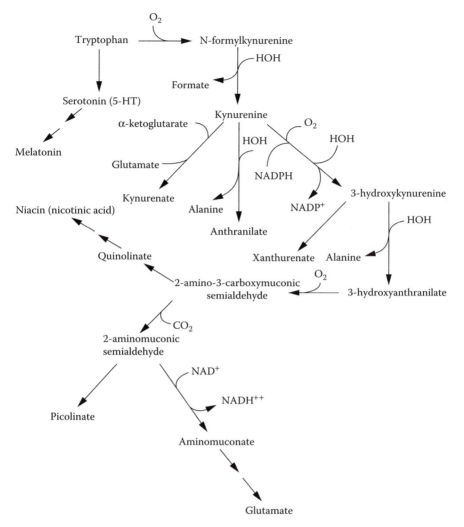

MAP 6 Catabolism of tryptophan showing conversion to the vitamin niacin. This conversion is not very efficient. Tryptophan catabolism also results in picolinate, which is believed by some to play a role in trace mineral conservation.

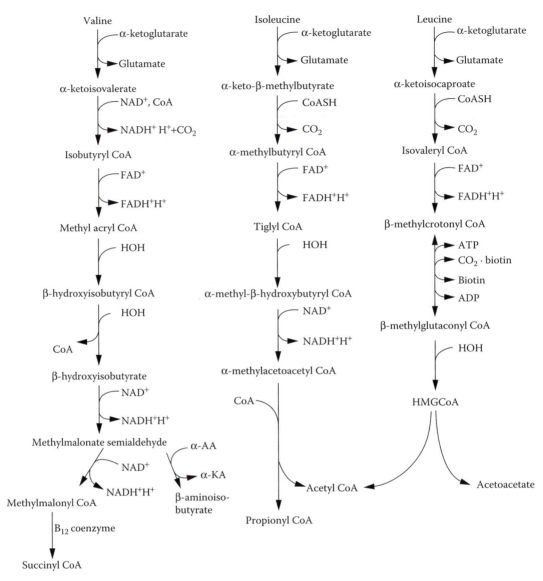

MAP 7   Catabolism of branched-chain amino acids showing their use in the production of metabolites that are either lipid precursors or metabolites that can be oxidized via the Krebs cycle.

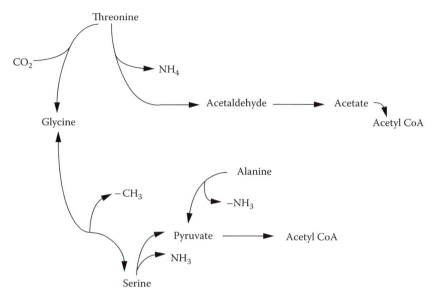

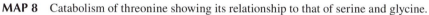

MAP 8   Catabolism of threonine showing its relationship to that of serine and glycine.

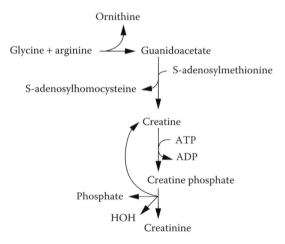

MAP 9   Formation of creatine phosphate.

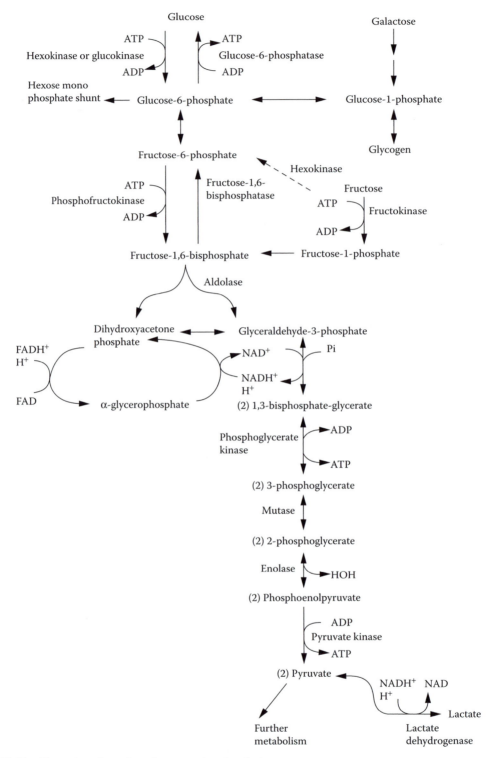

MAP 10 The series of reactions that comprise glycolysis.

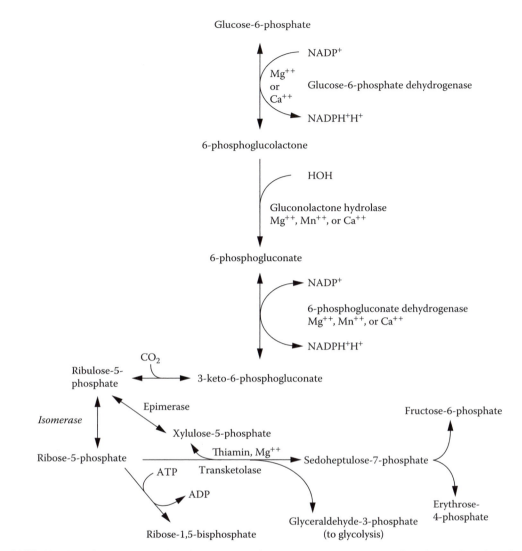

Glucose-6-phosphate

NADP⁺

Mg⁺⁺
or   Glucose-6-phosphate dehydrogenase
Ca⁺⁺

NADPH⁺H⁺

6-phosphoglucolactone

HOH

Gluconolactone hydrolase
Mg⁺⁺, Mn⁺⁺, or Ca⁺⁺

6-phosphogluconate

NADP⁺

6-phosphogluconate dehydrogenase
Mg⁺⁺, Mn⁺⁺, or Ca⁺⁺

NADPH⁺H⁺

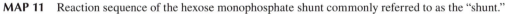

MAP 11   Reaction sequence of the hexose monophosphate shunt commonly referred to as the "shunt."

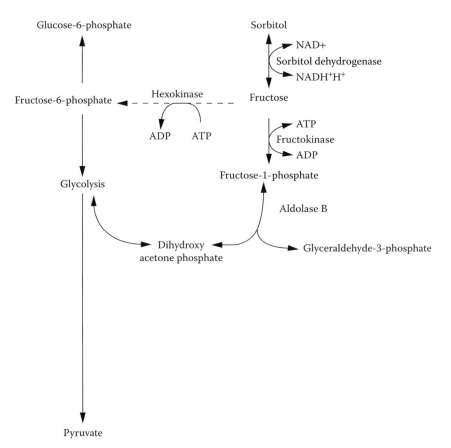

MAP 12   Metabolism of fructose.

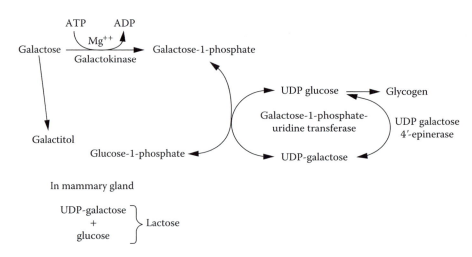

MAP 13   Conversion of galactose to glucose.

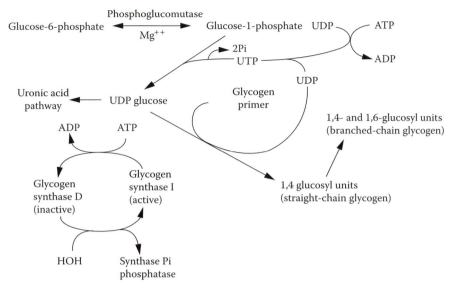

MAP 14   Glycogen synthesis (glycogenesis).

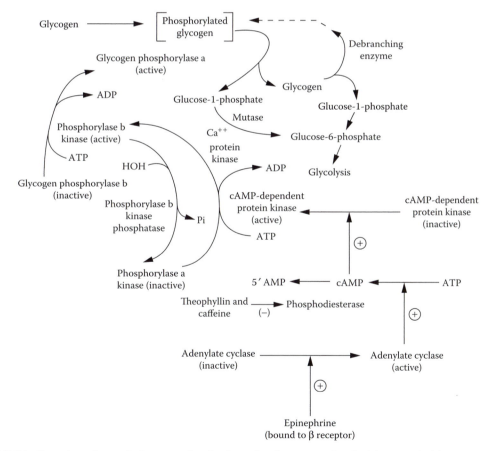

MAP 15   Stepwise release of glucose molecules from the glycogen molecule (glycogenolysis).

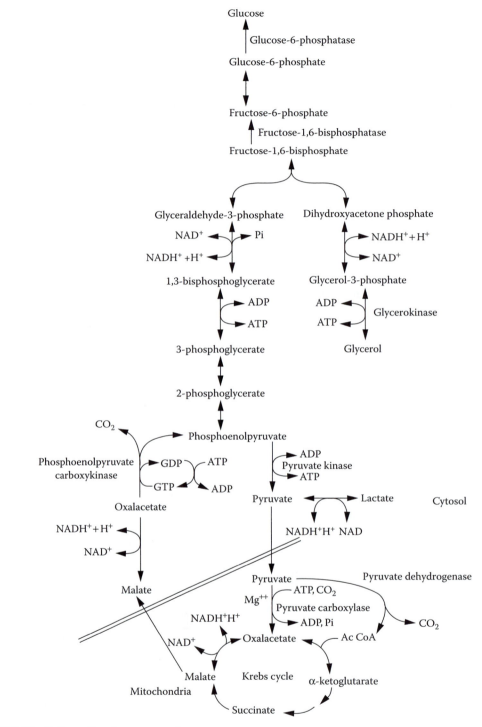

MAP 16   Pathway for gluconeogenesis.

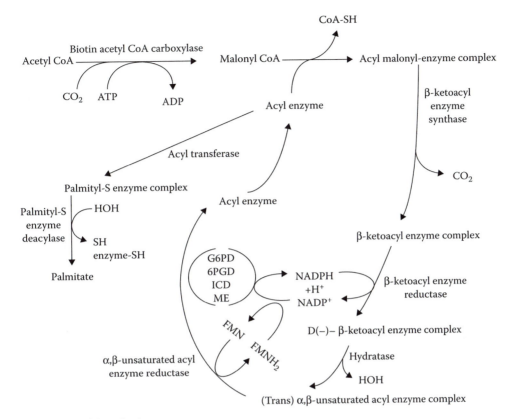

MAP 17   Fatty acid synthesis.

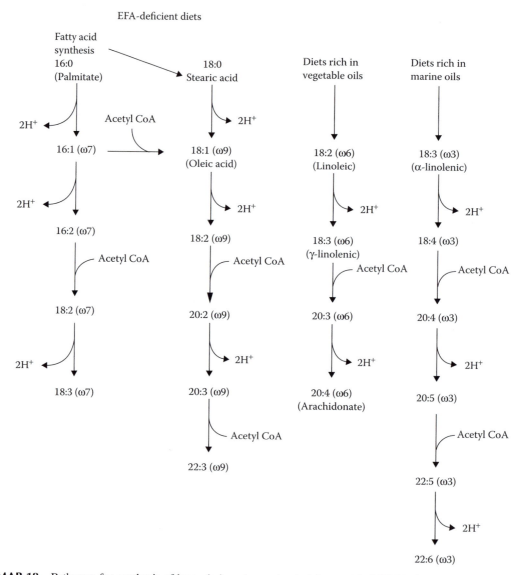

MAP 18   Pathways for synthesis of long-chain polyunsaturated fatty acids (PUFA) through elongation and desaturation. Not all of these reactions occur in all species. The ω symbol is the same as the n symbol. Thus, 18:2 ω 6, linoleic acid, could also be written 18:2n6. Mammals cannot convert oleic acid to linoleic or linolenic acid; felines cannot convert oleic acid to linoleic and then to arachidonic acid.

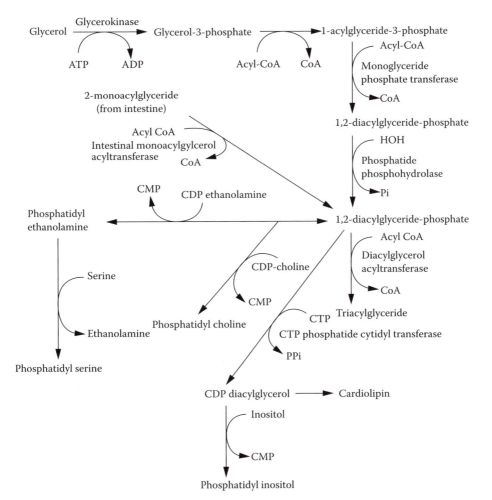

MAP 19   Pathways for synthesis of triacylglycerides and phospholipids.

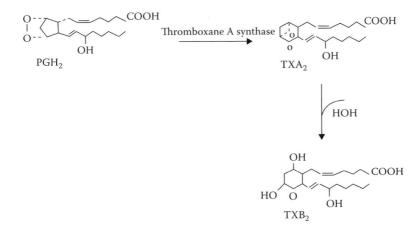

MAP 20   Reaction sequence that produces thromboxane A_2 (TXA_2) and thromboxane B_2 (TXB_2).

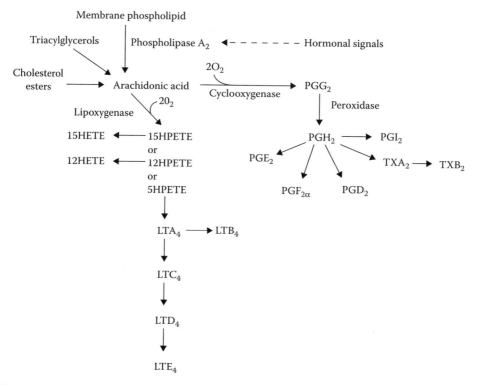

MAP 21   Eicosanoid synthesis from arachidonic acid.

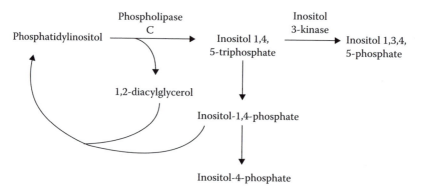

MAP 22   Phosphatidylinositol (PIP) cycle.

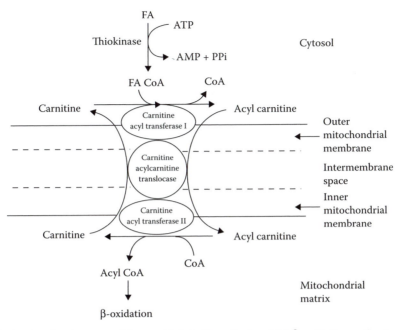

MAP 23   Mechanism for the entry of fatty acids into the mitochondrial β-oxidation pathway.

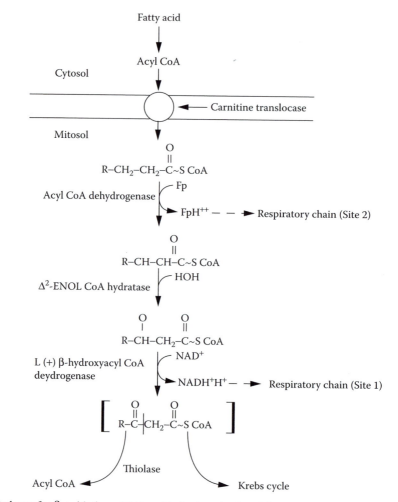

MAP 24 Pathway for β-oxidation of fatty acids in the mitochondria.

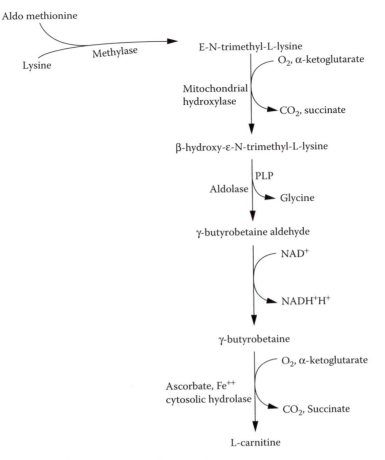

MAP 25 Synthesis of carnitine from lysine and methionine.

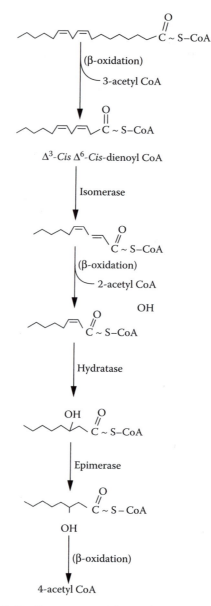

MAP 26   Modification of β-oxidation for unsaturated fatty acid.

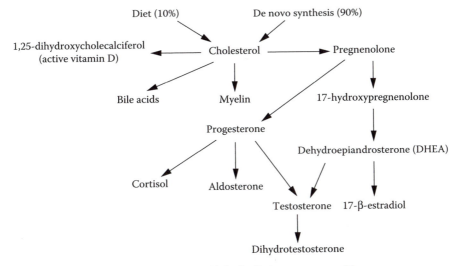

MAP 27   Overview of cholesterol conversion to biologically important steroids.

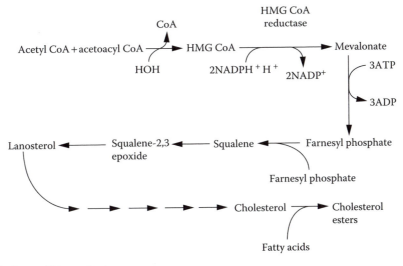

MAP 28   Cholesterol biosynthesis.

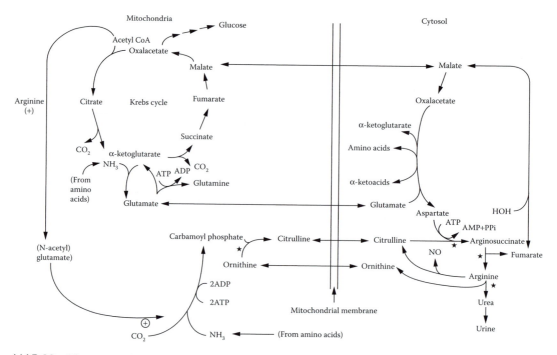

MAP 29 The urea cycle. Locations of mutations in the urea cycle enzymes are indicated with a ⋆. Persons with these mutations have very short lives with evidence of mental retardation, seizures, coma, and early death due to the toxic effects of ammonia accumulation.